Facilitating Resilience and Recovery
Following Trauma

Facilitating Resilience and Recovery Following Trauma

Edited by

LORI A. ZOELLNER
NORAH C. FEENY

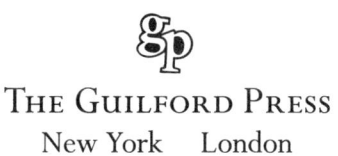

THE GUILFORD PRESS
New York   London

© 2014 The Guilford Press
A Division of Guilford Publications, Inc.
72 Spring Street, New York, NY 10012
www.guilford.com

Printed in the United States of America

This book is printed on acid-free paper.

Last digit is print number: 9 8 7 6 5 4 3 2 1

The authors have checked with sources believed to be reliable in their
efforts to provide information that is complete and generally in accord
with the standards of practice that are accepted at the time of publication.
However, in view of the possibility of human error or changes in
behavioral, mental health, or medical sciences, neither the authors, nor
the editors and publisher, nor any other party who has been involved in
the preparation or publication of this work warrants that the information
contained herein is in every respect accurate or complete, and they are
not responsible for any errors or omissions or the results obtained from
the use of such information. Readers are encouraged to confirm the
information contained in this book with other sources.

Library of Congress Cataloging-in-Publication Data

Facilitating resilience and recovery following trauma / edited by Lori A. Zoellner,
Norah C. Feeny.
    pages cm
  Includes bibliographical references and index.
  ISBN 978-1-4625-1350-5 (hardcover)
  1. Resilience (Personality trait). 2. Adjustment (Psychology). 3. Psychic trauma.
I. Zoellner, Lori A. II. Feeny, Norah C.
  BF698.35.R47F33 2014
  155.2′4—dc23
                                                                    2013032862

For those coming together to end trauma
and its consequences

About the Editors

Lori A. Zoellner, PhD, is Professor in the Department of Psychology and Director of the Center for Anxiety and Traumatic Stress at the University of Washington. Her research and clinical experience focus on the prevention and treatment of chronic posttraumatic stress disorder (PTSD), with particular expertise in the area of information processing. Dr. Zoellner has published extensively on PTSD and on its cognitive-behavioral treatment, and has given many workshops for practitioners on the prevention and treatment of chronic PTSD.

Norah C. Feeny, PhD, is Professor in the Department of Psychological Sciences and Director of the PTSD Treatment and Research Program at Case Western Reserve University. Her clinical and research interests and over 100 publications focus on the delivery and evaluation of cognitive-behavioral treatments for PTSD, treatment preferences, and treatment processes.

Contributors

Karen Appleyard Carmody, PhD, LCSW, is a Licensed Psychologist and Assistant Professor at the Center for Child and Family Health in the Department of Psychiatry and Behavioral Sciences at Duke University Medical Center. She received the 2012 Early Career Award from the American Psychological Association's (APA) Section on Child Maltreatment, as well as the 2005 Martin S. Wallach Outstanding Clinical Intern Award from the University of North Carolina at Chapel Hill's School of Medicine. Dr. Appleyard Carmody's research focuses on the correlates and consequences of attachment and parenting, developmental processes and risk and protective factors underlying resilience following early adversity, and implementation science and empirically based interventions relating to trauma and attachment. Her publications address these topics, with the goal of advancing interventions with high-risk children.

Gordon J. G. Asmundson, PhD, is a Registered Doctoral Psychologist, Full Professor in the Department of Psychology, and Director of the Anxiety and Illness Behaviours Lab at the University of Regina. He holds several editorial posts, including Editor-in-Chief of *Cognitive Behaviour Therapy*, and serves on the editorial boards for nine other journals. In addition to numerous prestigious awards received over the course of his career, in 2009 Dr. Asmundson received the highest accolade available to scientists and scholars in Canada: induction as a Fellow of the Royal Society of Canada. His research and clinical interests are in assessment and basic mechanisms of fear, the anxiety disorders, and chronic pain, and the association of these with each other, maladaptive coping, and disability. Dr. Asmundson has published over 300 peer-reviewed journal articles and book chapters as well as six books.

J. Gayle Beck, PhD, is the Lillian and Morrie Moss Chair of Excellence in the Department of Psychology at the University of Memphis. She is Editor of *Clinical Psychology: Science and Practice* in addition to serving on other editorial boards. Dr. Beck is a Past President of the Society of Clinical Psychology (Division 12) of the APA and the Association for Behavioral and Cognitive Therapies (ABCT). A Fellow of APA and the American Psychological Society, she has contributed extensively to the literature on psychopathology of posttraumatic stress disorder (PTSD) and related health and mental health disorders following interpersonal and noninterpersonal traumas, as well as the treatment literature on these disorders. Most recently, Dr. Beck coedited the *Oxford Handbook of Traumatic Stress Disorders*.

Ernestine C. Briggs, PhD, is Assistant Professor in the Department of Psychiatry and Behavioral Sciences at Duke University School of Medicine. She is also the Director of the Trauma Treatment and Research Program at the Center for Child and Family Health and Director of the Data and Evaluation Program at the National Center for Child Traumatic Stress. Her research interests include minority mental health, resiliency, implementation research, health disparities, family violence, and child traumatic stress.

Richard A. Bryant, PhD, is Scientia Professor and Australian Research Council Laureate Fellow at the University of New South Wales and Director of the Traumatic Stress Clinic in Sydney. He served on the DSM-5 committee for traumatic stress diagnoses and serves on the comparable committee for ICD-11. Dr. Bryant has won the Robert Laufer Award from the International Society for Traumatic Stress Studies, the Founders Medal from the Australian Society for Psychiatric Research, and the Scientific Achievement Award from the Australian Psychological Society for his research in traumatic stress. His research has addressed assessment and diagnosis issues, biological and cognitive processes, and psychological treatment, with particular emphasis on early identification and treatment of people after trauma. Dr. Bryant has published over 350 articles on the topics of diagnosis, treatment, and mechanisms of posttraumatic stress.

Joshua D. Clapp, PhD, is Assistant Professor in the Department of Psychology at the University of Wyoming. His primary research interests include trauma-related affective processes, the impact of emotional dysregulation on interpersonal functioning, and the conceptualization and measurement of trauma-related psychopathology. Dr. Clapp has published papers on a range of topics, including trauma-related emotional functioning, factors contributing to the mutual maintenance of PTSD and chronic pain, behavioral consequences of driving-related anxiety, and the treatment of PTSD within specialized populations.

Joop T. V. M. de Jong, MD, PhD, is Professor of Cultural and International Psychiatry at the VU University Amsterdam and the University of Amsterdam,

Adjunct Professor of Psychiatry at Boston University School of Medicine, and Visiting Professor at Rhodes University, South Africa. Dr. de Jong worked for years in Africa as a public health expert, a psychiatrist, and a psychotherapist. He was the founder and director of the Transcultural Psychosocial Organization, a nongovernmental organization that developed psychosocial and mental health programs in armed conflict and natural disaster areas in more than 20 countries in Africa, Asia, Europe, and Latin America. Over the past decades Dr. de Jong worked part time with immigrants and refugees in The Netherlands. He has (co)authored over 250 chapters and papers in the field of cultural psychiatry and psychotherapy, epidemiology, public mental health, and medical anthropology.

Rianne de Kleine, MSc, is a psychologist and researcher at the Overwaal Center for Anxiety Disorders, Pro Persona. She is a PhD student at the Behavioural Science Institute in the Department of Experimental Psychopathology and Treatment at Radboud University Nijmegen and is affiliated with the Nijmegen Center for Anxiety Research and Expertise. Ms. de Kleine's research focuses on the treatment of PTSD, especially cognitive enhancement of exposure treatments. In addition, she studies the role of dissociation, especially freezing and tonic immobility, in relation to threat-related psychopathology and treatment response. Ms. de Kleine is interested in the treatment of conversion disorder and was involved in the development of cognitive-behavioral treatment programs for that disorder. She has published in *Biological Psychiatry* and the *European Journal of Psychotraumatology.*

John A. Fairbank, PhD, is Professor of Medical Psychology in the Department of Psychiatry and Behavioral Sciences at Duke University Medical Center and Director of the VA Mid-Atlantic Mental Illness Research, Education and Clinical Center, located at the VA Medical Center, Durham, North Carolina. He serves as Co-Principal Investigator for the Millennium Cohort Family Study sponsored by the U.S. Department of Defense and is Co-Director of the National Center for Child Traumatic Stress, sponsored by the Substance Abuse and Mental Health Services Administration. Dr. Fairbank's research and clinical interests have focused on understanding the nature, assessment, and treatment of trauma.

Frank J. Farach, PhD, is a Postdoctoral Fellow in the Department of Psychology at the University of Washington. In 2008, he received a Dissertation Grant Award from the Society for a Science of Clinical Psychology. Dr. Farach's current research examines the roles of fear learning and attention as potential biomarkers of response to psychotherapy and pharmacotherapy in PTSD.

Norah C. Feeny, PhD. *See* "About the Editors."

Mathew G. Fetzner, MA, is a PhD student in Clinical Psychology at the University of Regina, working under the supervision of Gordon J. G. Asmundson. He was awarded the prestigious Vanier Canada Graduate Scholarship to fund his dissertation research examining the anxiolytic effects of aerobic exercise for PTSD. Mr. Fetzner's research interests include precipitating and perpetuating factors for PTSD among military and peace officer populations.

Edna B. Foa, PhD, is a Professor of Clinical Psychology in Psychiatry at the University of Pennsylvania and Director of the Center for the Treatment and Study of Anxiety. She was chair of the DSM-IV subcommittees for obsessive–compulsive disorder (OCD) and PTSD. Dr. Foa has published several books and over 300 articles and book chapters and has lectured extensively around the world. Her work has been recognized with numerous awards and honors, including the Lifetime Achievement Award from the International Society for Traumatic Stress Studies, the Lifetime Achievement Award from the ABCT, and the Outstanding Career Achievement Award from the International OCD Foundation. Dr. Foa has devoted her academic career to the study of psychopathology and the treatment of anxiety disorders, primarily OCD and PTSD, and is one of the world's leading experts in these areas.

Lydia Gómez-Pérez, PhD, is a Postdoctoral Fellow in the Anxiety and Illness Behaviours Lab in the Department of Psychology at the University of Regina. Her research interests include the study of the basic mechanisms of chronic pain as well as the association of this pervasive condition with anxiety disorders, stress, and trauma exposure.

Johanna K. P. Greeson, PhD, MSS, MLSP, is Assistant Professor in the School of Social Policy and Practice at the University of Pennsylvania. Her research interests include the transition to adulthood among youth who age out of foster care, natural mentoring and other supportive relationships for vulnerable youth, child traumatic stress, applied community-based intervention research and translation of research to practice, and neurobiological mechanisms of resiliency-focused interventions.

Muriel Hagenaars, PhD, is Assistant Professor at the Behavioural Science Institute in the Department of Experimental Psychopathology and Treatment at Radboud University Nijmegen and is affiliated with the Nijmegen Center for Anxiety Research and Expertise. She is also a licensed psychotherapist and is associated with the Jelgersma Center for Personality Disorders. Dr. Hagenaars's current research focuses on human freezing responses and their role in the development of threat-related psychopathology such as PTSD. She is also interested in the formation of trauma memories and factors that contribute to the development of intrusive memories. Dr. Hagenaars has published in the *Journal of Behavior Therapy and Experimental Psychiatry*, the *Journal of Affective Disorders*, and the *Journal of Experimental Psychology: General*.

Stevan E. Hobfoll, PhD, is Professor and Chair of the Department of Behavioral Sciences at Rush University Medical Center. The author and editor of numerous books, journal articles, and book chapters, he has been a frequent workshop leader on stress and has received funding for his research on stress and health. Dr. Hobfoll has also been involved with the problem of stress in Israel. He received special commendation for his research on the psychology of women and for his AIDS prevention programs with ethnic-minority populations, and was cited by the *Encyclopedia Britannica* for his contribution to knowledge and understanding for his volume *The Ecology of Stress*. Dr. Hobfoll was cochair of the APA Commission on Stress and War during Operation Desert Storm, helping plan for the prevention of prolonged distress among military personnel and their families.

Jason Jacobs-Lentz, BA, worked for several years as a research technician at Stanford University School of Medicine/Veterans Administration Palo Alto, California, prior to beginning doctoral studies in the Clinical Psychology program at the University of Memphis. His current research interests include the use of transdisciplinary methods to investigate how social processes such as stigma contribute to the development and maintenance of PTSD and substance use disorders.

Judiann McNiff Jones, MS, is a doctoral candidate in the Clinical Psychology program at the University of Memphis, where she works as a Graduate Assistant for an ongoing study examining the psychological consequences of domestic violence. She is a member of both the APA and the ABCT, and holds the position of Treasurer of the ABCT Posttraumatic Stress Disorder and Trauma Special Interest Group. Ms. Jones's research interests include interpersonal trauma and the psychological aftereffects of experiencing a lifetime history of abuse. She is also interested in how trauma exposure affects cognitive processing.

Janie J. Jun, MS, is a graduate student in Clinical Psychology at the Center for Anxiety and Traumatic Stress at the University of Washington. Her research interests focus on understanding the processes of change in treatment for PTSD. Specifically, Ms. Jun is interested in seeing how cognitive and emotional processing is associated with symptom change in psychotherapy for PTSD and its effects on treatment outcome.

Brett T. Litz, PhD, is a clinical psychologist and Professor in the Departments of Psychiatry and Psychology at Boston University. He is also Director of the Mental Health Core of the Massachusetts Veterans Epidemiological Research and Information Center at the VA Boston Healthcare System. Dr. Litz is the principal investigator on numerous research projects funded by the U.S. Department of Defense and the National Institute of Mental Health. His research focuses on military trauma and early intervention for trauma and traumatic loss.

Elizabeth H. Marks, MS, is a doctoral Clinical Psychology graduate student at the Center for Anxiety and Traumatic Stress at the University of Washington.

She is primarily interested in memory processes in individuals with PTSD. More specifically, Ms. Marks's research focuses on elements of memory reconsolidation and their role in fear extinction. She has coauthored articles on post-trauma cognitions in PTSD and information processing in PTSD. She has also coauthored several articles on social anxiety disorder.

Carmen P. McLean, PhD, is Assistant Professor of Clinical Psychology in Psychiatry at the Center for the Treatment and Study of Anxiety (CTSA) at the University of Pennsylvania Perelman School of Medicine. She completed a postdoctoral fellowship at the National Center for PTSD at the Boston VA. Dr. McLean now serves as the Web Editor for the Association for Behavioral and Cognitive Therapies and as the Coordinator of Research Activities at the CTSA. Her research interests include gender effects in anxiety disorders, treatment augmentation, and novel treatment delivery methods.

William P. Nash, MD, is a retired Navy psychiatrist and principal author of current Navy and Marine Corps combat and operational stress control doctrine. He currently serves as a consultant in military and veteran psychological health promotion to the U.S. Departments of Defense and Veterans Affairs, and holds an appointment as Assistant Clinical Professor of Psychiatry at the University of California, San Diego. Dr. Nash's research focuses on prevention and treatment of war-zone PTSD in service members, veterans, and their families.

Angela Nickerson, PhD, is a Lecturer in the School of Psychology at the University of New South Wales and Director of the Refugee Trauma and Recovery Program in Sydney, Australia. Her research interests include the examination of mechanisms underlying posttraumatic psychological distress in refugee and postconflict populations, better understanding posttraumatic stress and grief responses, and developing treatment interventions for psychological disorders in refugees. Dr. Nickerson is the recipient of the 2012 National Medical Health and Research Council Early Career Clinical Research Fellowship, and previously held the American Australian Association Sir Keith Murdoch Postdoctoral Fellowship. She has published numerous peer-reviewed journal articles and book chapters in the areas of refugee mental health and psychological responses to trauma.

Shira A. Olsen, PhD, is a research clinician at a private treatment center in Seattle, Washington. She is a member of the APA and the ABCT. Dr. Olsen was awarded the David Caul Graduate Research Grant from the International Society for the Study of Trauma and Dissociation to support her research on dissociation and trauma. Her current research interests include cognitive factors in the development and maintenance of psychopathology, and the dissemination of empirically supported treatments for PTSD and comorbid disorders.

Larry D. Pruitt, PhD, is a Postdoctoral Fellow at the Center for Anxiety and Traumatic Stress at the University of Washington. His research interests include the role of emotion regulation in the pathogenesis of chronic anxiety as well as the optimization and dissemination of empirically supported behavioral interventions.

Nina K. Rytwinski, PhD, is a licensed psychologist in Ohio and a Research Associate in the Department of Psychological Sciences at Case Western Reserve University. Her research, which has been published in international journals, has largely explored the factors that contribute to the onset and maintenance of mood and anxiety disorders.

Denise M. Sloan, PhD, is Associate Director of the Behavioral Science Division at the National Center for PTSD. She is also Professor of Psychiatry at the Boston University School of Medicine. Her research expertise is in psychosocial treatments for PTSD and emotion in psychopathology. She has received funding for her work from several organizations, including the National Institute of Mental Health and the Department of Veterans Affairs. Dr. Sloan is a member of several editorial boards, including *Behavior Therapy*, *Behaviour Research and Therapy*, the *Journal of Abnormal Psychology*, and *Psychosomatic Medicine*.

Hillary L. Smith, BS, is the Research Coordinator for the Center for Anxiety and Traumatic Stress at the University of Washington. Her recent research investigates the role of self-compassion and the efficacy of an expressive writing paradigm in the course of emotional recovery following divorce. Ms. Smith's current research investigates the role and course of anger in the treatment of PTSD. She has published on emotion recovery following relationship termination in *Psychological Science*.

Maria M. Steenkamp, PhD, is a Postdoctoral Clinical Research Fellow at the Massachusetts Veterans Epidemiological Research and Information Center at the VA Boston Healthcare System. Her research focuses on prevention and treatment of military-related PTSD.

Agnes van Minnen, PhD, is a licensed clinical psychologist and Professor at the Behavioural Science Institute in the Department of Experimental Psychopathology and Treatment at Radboud University Nijmegen. She is also affiliated with the Nijmegen Center for Anxiety Research and Expertise and works at the Overwaal Center for Anxiety Disorders, Pro Persona. Dr. van Minnen is associate editor of the *European Journal of Psychotraumatology*. She is coeditor of the *Dutch CBT Standard Books of Treatment Manuals* for adults with psychiatric disorders. Dr. van Minnen's research focus is on treatment of PTSD, especially in comorbid populations. She is also interested in anxiety regulation problems, as seen in dissociation disorders and conversion disorder.

Dr. van Minnen has published in the *Archives of General Psychiatry*, *Biological Psychiatry*, and *Behaviour Research and Therapy*.

Blair E. Wisco, PhD, is Assistant Professor in the Department of Psychology at the University of North Carolina at Greensboro. Her research interests include information-processing biases and emotion regulation processes in depression and PTSD, with a focus on self-relevant cognition. Dr. Wisco has published in journals including *Behaviour Research and Therapy*, *Perspectives on Psychological Science*, *Clinical Psychology Review*, and *Cognition and Emotion*.

Briana A. Woods, PhD, is Assistant Professor in the Department of Community and Behavioral Health at the University of Iowa College of Public Health. Her research interests include African American adolescent health, co-occurring traumatic stress and health risk behaviors, community-based participatory research, health disparities, and implementation research.

Lori A. Zoellner, PhD. *See* "About the Editors."

Preface

The evening news reports after yet another mass trauma: "Counselors are on the scene."

A concerned friend of a rape survivor sadly notes, "She is going to be in therapy for years."

A trauma specialist tells an audience of counselors: "PTSD rarely goes away on its own."

A combat veteran proclaims, "I'm always going to have PTSD. There is no treatment. You just have to learn to live with it."

What do we make of these statements? Are they correct? The perceived need for therapy after horrific events is almost commonplace in our media. The number of therapists willing to provide therapy to help trauma survivors is at an all-time high. PTSD (posttraumatic stress disorder) is no longer an abbreviation known only to experts, but is used widely by the general public.

Yet, for thousands of years, the world has experienced horrific events in the form of earthquakes, tsunamis, war, torture, rape, and so forth. Similarly, for thousands of years, relatives, friends, neighbors, and even strangers have been coming together to help those who are physically and psychologically wounded from these traumatic events. Before recent times, how did we as a people ever get by without psychiatrists, psychologists, social workers, or even formal diagnostic labels seeking to quantify patho- logical reactions to traumatic events and treat them? In fact, the world hasn't changed that much, and principles promoting resilience and under- lying recovery known informally over the years are just as sound now as they were thousands of years ago. What may be different is that over years, the field of traumatic stress has continued to identify principles underlying informal processes and develop more formal therapeutic processes that facilitate resilience and promote recovery following some of life's worst, most traumatic events. Trauma is ubiquitous and, as stated above, there are a lot of beliefs about reactions following trauma circulating among trauma survivors, their friends and family, the media, politicians, public policy and public health experts, medical professionals, clergy, counselors, social workers, psychologists, and psychiatrists. If you are such a professional, or are in training to become one, your work will likely bring you alongside trauma survivors in their greatest time of need. This book is for you.

In this book we choose not to pathologize reactions following trauma exposure and focus on promoting resilience and recovery. We specifically concentrate on principles underlying resilience and recovery rather than therapeutic camps or specific treatment protocols (though both are mentioned). Most importantly, we choose to focus on modifiable risk and resilience factors. Some factors, particularly individual differences prior to trauma exposure and traumatic event characteristics, cannot be changed. However, other factors that are often present after trauma exposure—such as how someone discloses to others about the trauma, what is remembered in regard to the trauma memory, beliefs about one's self and the world, avoidance of trauma reminders, physical pain, dissociation, and the nature of social support—are potentially modifiable through either formal or informal interventions. These modifiable risk factors can be mobilized to facilitate resilience or promote recovery.

We have pulled together some of the world's experts in the field of traumatic stress and asked them to provide real-world clinical examples, summarize the existing research in an accessible manner, highlight emerging and underlying principles of resilience and recovery, and identify clear clinical recommendations for fostering resilience and recovery. In doing this, we have focused on issues of timing, paying attention to both immediately after (acute intervention) and months or years after (chronic intervention) trauma exposure, working with specific populations (e.g., children, military, cultural), and, as mentioned above, special modifiable risk and resilience topics.

We hope readers find this book both cutting-edge in its scholarly review of the research and practically useful in facilitating resilience and recovery for both mass trauma and individual trauma survivors. Our goal is to advance the understanding of principles underlying resilience and recovery and to place these principles in the hands of people who can use them to help mitigate the psychological consequences of trauma exposure.

Contents

PART III. FACILITATING NATURAL
AND THERAPEUTIC RECOVERY:
MODIFIABLE RISK AND RESILIENCE FACTORS

PART IV. INTEGRATION
AND FUTURE DIRECTIONS

Part I

PRINCIPLES UNDERLYING NATURAL AND THERAPEUTIC RECOVERY

Chapter 1

Conceptualizing Risk and Resilience Following Trauma Exposure

Lori A. Zoellner *and* Norah C. Feeny

Mora's sister had cancer for the last 3 years. Periodically throughout the battle, Mora had taken care of her sister's two young children. Mora's own marriage was still intact, but shaky; however, her sister's husband had had an affair and left her during her illness. In the months before Mora's sister's death, Mora had become deeply depressed. She stopped going into town to go to church, stopped attending her spin class, no longer spoke with her friends, and only went out of the house to attend to her sister, get groceries, or shuttle her kids to various activities. After her sister died, Mora's depression only grew worse, and her husband started to worry about whether she would commit suicide. Mora said that her faith and her kids kept her from killing herself, though she saved an old bottle of sleeping pills just in case and thought often about taking the whole bottle and being reunited with her sister.

One day Mora was driving her sister's station wagon. As she was making a left turn off of a country highway, a van tried to pass her on the left-hand side of the road. The van crashed into the side of Mora's car, sending it into a large utility pole. She hardly knew what had happened. She felt the impact and may have even temporarily blacked out. When she regained her senses, her first thought was for her kids in the back seat, but she couldn't move. The windshield had shattered and there was glass and blood everywhere. She screamed for her kids,

3

telling them to get out of the car. The kids responded, saying they were okay, but they weren't going to leave her. Fearing the car catching on fire, she again screamed for them to go. By that time, another car pulled over, and the man in the car came over and helped the children out. Still another man came up and tried to get Mora out of the car but couldn't. As she sat there, she couldn't feel anything and was terrified that the car was going to catch on fire. She kept thinking to herself, "I'm going to die. I'm going to die." The man held her hand, told her that they had called 911, and the fire department should be there shortly. Mora didn't know how much time had passed, feeling at times disconnected from what was going on around her, but the man never left and kept on talking to her. The fire department eventually came and cut her out of the vehicle. At the hospital, she was treated for facial lacerations; rib, femur, and pelvic fractures; and a hemothorax. Her son, who was also on the struck side of the vehicle, had multiple facial and arm lacerations but sustained no serious injuries. Her daughter, who was in the rear, nonstruck side of the vehicle, was shaken up but also sustained no serious injuries.

In the days after the crash, Mora was in the hospital. Her friends from church, her spinning class, and her kids' friends' parents all came to visit and chipped in together to help with food and taking care of the kids. The driver of the van had left the scene of the accident, and the investigation was still ongoing. She couldn't get over the fact that the driver of the other vehicle had left her and her family after the crash. She wondered if he or she had been drunk. Most of all she felt grateful that she was alive and her kids were okay. She also cherished each day she had been given. However, whenever she thought about what happened, a wave of fear would come over her. She would wake up at night, having dreamed that the crash was happening again; she had a hard time watching anything with car accidents on TV; and she did not like riding in cars. However, as soon as she was able, she started going to church, reaching out to her friends, and began physical rehabilitation. Although her marriage was still having difficulties, she was committed to improving it. Her earlier depression dissipated, and she threw out the bottle of pills. Similarly, over the next few months, her fears around having another car accident also started to disappear. Although she thought about the crash on occasion, she started to drive as soon as she was medically cleared.[1]

Contrary to popular belief, resilience is the norm following trauma exposure (e.g., natural disaster, rape, car accident, combat). Indeed, this is

---

[1] This case represents a mixture of various clients whom we have seen in our clinical work. Any resemblance to a specific individual is purely coincidental.

one of the remarkable findings emerging from the study of psychological reactions to traumatic events. These events do have profound impacts on people's lives, but, for the majority of trauma survivors, long-term psychiatric problems and impaired psychosocial functioning are unlikely. In fact, some trauma survivors like Mora actually experience improved psychological and social functioning. By all accounts, Mora was at risk for developing long-term psychological consequences: being a woman, having a previous psychiatric history, having a sense of life threat and dissociation during the event, being severely injured, and having ongoing life stress after the event (e.g., ongoing physical rehabilitation, ongoing crime investigation, marriage problems).

How then do we understand varying trajectories following trauma exposure, and how do we promote psychological health and functioning after such events? In this book, we focus on two things: (1) understanding the nature of resilience, natural recovery, and therapeutic recovery; and (2) understanding common and unique principles underlying these processes of resilience and recovery, particularly focusing on principles that are modifiable either by trauma survivors themselves, others, and the community surrounding trauma survivors, or by professionals or paraprofessionals providing active interventions or treatment. It is through our understanding of these processes of resilience and recovery that we will be better able to promote psychological health and functioning in the aftermath of trauma exposure.

RESILIENCE, NATURAL RECOVERY, AND THERAPEUTIC RECOVERY FOLLOWING TRAUMA EXPOSURE

Resilience

When we see or hear the word *resilience*, we all assume we know what it means. *Is Mora resilient?* If resilience means little or no immediate reaction to the traumatic event, then Mora is decidedly not resilient. If resilience means the absence of initial psychological reactions or functional impairment after a traumatic event, then Mora is also not resilient. However, if resilience means the absence of long-term psychopathology or impairment after a traumatic event, then Mora is resilient. Similarly, if resilience means an ability to cope with and adapt to adversity, then Mora is also resilient. And, if resilience means the ability to move beyond pretrauma levels of functioning to improved levels of functioning, then Mora is indeed resilient. Defining this term we all assume we know is actually complicated.

The *Oxford English* and *Merriam–Webster* dictionaries provide similar definitions for the term. In fact, both dictionaries give two definitions. In the *Oxford English Dictionary*, resilience is defined as (1) the ability of a substance or object to spring back into shape; elasticity; and (2) the capacity to recover quickly from difficulties; toughness. In the *Merriam–Webster Dictionary*, resilience is defined as (1) the capability of a strained body to recover its size and shape after deformation caused especially by compressive stress; and (2) an ability to recover from or adjust easily to misfortune or change. In neither definition does resilience reflect a lack of reaction or impairment. Rather, resilience reflects rebounding, with the words *quickly* and *easily* being used as modifiers. Furthermore, in no definition does resilience imply anything more than recovery or a return to a previous state.

These points are critical when additional terms such as *psychological resilience* or *posttraumatic growth* are used to describe processes after trauma exposure. Probably the most commonly used definition of psychological resilience comes from Bonanno (2004, p. 20), reflecting "the ability of adults in otherwise normal circumstance who are exposed to an isolated and potentially highly disruptive event, such as the death of a close relation or a violent or life-threatening situation, to maintain relatively stable, healthy levels of psychological and physical functioning." For Bonanno, resilience and recovery are not the same thing. Recovery implies a moderate-to-severe initial reaction followed by a return to psychological health and functioning; resilience implies little or no initial reaction and no real change in psychological health or functioning. As noted by Litz (2004), Bonanno also intimates a degree of equivalence between bereavement and trauma. It is relatively easy to agree with Bonanno's definition of resilience after relatively common events such as the death of a loved one from a chronic illness or old age. However, the vast majority of individuals following an acute, personally life-threatening trauma of a given magnitude (e.g., torture, rape) have initial profound reactions, which, as will be discussed below, are expected and normal. By Bonanno's definition, the presence of a temporary, normative reaction to a personally life-threatening event would make the person not resilient. Posttraumatic growth, in contrast, refers to a shift toward more optimal functioning as a result of a traumatic event (e.g., Calhoun & Tedeschi, 2006; Linley & Joseph, 2004). This shift typically refers not just to recovering previous functioning but ending up with *more* adaptive functioning and a change in the way an individual views his or her place in the world. The term *posttraumatic growth*, then, refers to positive changes in functioning and personal meaning for the individual (e.g., Janoff-Bulman, 2004).

Clearly, some of the confusion in the traumatic stress field comes from the overlap and imprecise usage of these terms. In this overlap, psychopathology (e.g., depression, posttraumatic stress disorder [PTSD], anxiety), functioning (e.g., work, social, and family functioning), and belief systems (e.g., about the world, self, others) are not always distinguished. And in the real world, they do not always covary with one another. Further precision in construct definition and longitudinal studies in our field will undoubtedly help in understanding resilience, recovery, and growth processes after traumatic events.

Is Mora resilient? We would say "yes." Mora experienced a relatively "quick" (e.g., within a few months) and "easy" (e.g., no formal intervention) recovery (e.g., psychopathology, functioning) and likely also experienced posttraumatic growth (e.g., improved functioning, more adaptive personal beliefs). Our definition of resilience allows for an initial profound reaction to a traumatic stressor. A lack of a reaction to a personally life-threatening event (e.g., rape, torture) would not be normative and could even indicate an abnormal reaction. For us, resilience also includes a pattern of recovery to prior functioning that occurs naturally in the initial months following trauma exposure. So, one can experience disruptive, trauma-related difficulties that resolve relatively quickly and still be resilient.

Natural Recovery

Prospective studies consistently document a natural recovery process that occurs for the majority of trauma-exposed individuals regardless of the type of traumatic events. Notably, immediately after trauma exposure, many individuals show symptoms consistent with PTSD, anxiety, and depression and related functional impairment. However, within the first 3 months, in particular, and through the first year after trauma exposure, for the majority of individuals, these symptoms decrease without formal psychological or psychiatric treatment (e.g., Kessler, Sonnega, Bromet, Hughes, & Nelson, 1995; Riggs, Rothbaum, & Foa, 1995; Rothbaum, Foa, Riggs, Murdock, & Walsh, 1992). Based on these data, the likelihood of recovery is the strongest in the first 3 months and continues through 1 year; however, after 3 months, the slope of recovery flattens considerably, suggesting that if an individual has not recovered during this initial period, the likelihood of natural recovery decreases substantially. Approximately one-third of trauma-exposed individuals do not recover with time (Kessler et al., 1995).

Two large meta-analyses have examined factors underlying natural recovery (e.g., Brewin, Andrews, & Valentine, 2000; Ozer, Best, Lipsey, & Weise, 2003). Although these meta-analyses are dated, they pooled data from thousands of trauma-exposed individuals and explored a variety of predictors of PTSD. Across both studies, pretrauma factors (i.e., prior trauma, prior adjustment, history of psychopathology, family history of psychopathology, female gender, lower socioeconomic status, lack of education, low intelligence, child abuse, and adverse childhood) carried only a small amount of the variance in predicting who developed PTSD. This is in stark contrast with common clinical lore, which suggests that these factors are primarily responsible for who will and will not develop long-term psychopathology after trauma exposure. Most notably, trauma-related factors (i.e., trauma severity, perceived life threat, peritraumatic emotions, and peritraumatic dissociation) and posttrauma factors (i.e., perceived support, lack of social support, life stress) carried more of the variance of who will develop long-term psychopathology. Since these meta-analyses, the role of peritraumatic dissociation has been questioned (e.g., Marshall & Schell, 2002). New studies have highlighted the role of hyperarousal after trauma exposure (e.g., Solomon, Horesh, & Ein-Dor, 2009) and have replicated the importance of event and postevent factors such as trauma severity, per-ceived lack of support, and ongoing stressful life events (e.g., Smid, van der Velden, Gersons, & Kleber, 2012). Clearly, no single factor consistently predicts the development of chronic psychopathology and impaired func-tioning after trauma exposure with a high degree of accuracy. As suggested by Brewin and colleagues (2000), the impact of pretrauma factors on later PTSD is likely mediated by responses to the trauma or pretrauma factors that interact with responses to the trauma to increase the risk of PTSD. This is consistent with an earlier resilience–recovery model put forth by King, King, Fairbank, Keane, and Adams (1998) highlighting the media-tional role of postevent hardiness (e.g., sense of control, commitment, and change as challenge), postevent structural and functional social support, and additional negative life events posttrauma. Taken together, there are a number of postevent factors that may reduce the likelihood of PTSD, anxiety, depression, and impaired functioning that occur in the immediate aftermath or months after the trauma that are *potentially modifiable and may have the ability to enhance natural recovery.*

Therapeutic Recovery

For those who do not naturally recover and suffer trauma-related prob-lems (e.g., PTSD, depression, anxiety) months and years after such an event, specific psychotherapies (e.g., cognitive-behavioral therapy) and pharmacotherapies (e.g., selective serotonin reuptake inhibitors [SSRIs]) have been found to reduce psychological difficulties and improve overall quality of life, while other therapies such as general support and relax-ation do not produce clinically meaningful changes (e.g., Institute of Medi-cine, 2007; National Institute for Health and Clinical Excellence, 2005; U.S. Department of Defense and Department of Veterans Affairs, 2003). Clearly, though, individuals differ in their likelihood to respond to ther-apeutic interventions. However, predictors of therapeutic outcome for chronic PTSD have been relatively elusive. Bradley, Greene, Russ, Rusta, and Westen (2005), in their meta-analysis of psychotherapy approaches for PTSD, found that trauma type, specifically combat trauma, showed lower effect sizes than heterogeneous or assault samples; however, this study did not examine other patient-related moderators. This latter finding also has not been replicated, where in another meta-analysis for prolonged exposure, a type of cognitive-behavioral therapy, factors such as time since the trauma, therapeutic dosage, or type of trauma did not reliably alter the observed effects (Powers, Halpern, Ferenschak, Gillihan, & Foa, 2010). Taken together, seemingly disparate therapeutic approaches such as various cognitive and behavioral therapies and SSRIs are able to meaningfully reduce trauma-related psychopathology and improve functioning for many. The similar efficacy of these different approaches may point to both unique and shared principles underlying therapeutic recovery.

SHIFTING FOCUS TO UNDERLYING PRINCIPLES

Comorbidity and Heterogeneity

For well over 20 years, our field has recognized that we suffer from twin challenges (e.g., Clark, Watson, & Reynolds, 1995): comorbidity between disorders and heterogeneity within disorders. Reactions following trauma exposure and resultant psychopathology such as PTSD, depression, substance abuse, and anxiety are no exception. For example, PTSD shares diagnostic symptoms with major depressive disorder (MDD), including anhedonia, difficulty sleeping, irritability, and difficulty concentrating. Not surprisingly, epidemiological data shows that between 48 and 55% of people with PTSD have comorbid MDD (e.g., Elhai, Grubaugh, Kashdan, & Frueh, 2008; Kessler et al., 1995). PTSD and MDD are significantly associated with one another (.50), showing a similar degree of association to other anxiety disorders with MDD (.42–.60; Kessler, Chiu, Demler, & Walters, 2005). Indeed, some have suggested that PTSD and co-occurring PTSD and MDD after trauma exposure may be the same construct and that their separation may be arbitrary (e.g., O'Donnell, Creamer, & Pattison, 2004). Although depressive disorders are the most common comorbidity with PTSD, substance disorders and anxiety disorders are also commonly seen with PTSD (Kessler et al., 1995), highlighting that comorbidity in PTSD, like many other disorders, is normative.

Besides substantial comorbidity, there is also significant heterogeneity within PTSD. The diagnosis of PTSD in the fourth edition of the *Diagnostic and Statistical Manual of Mental Disorders* (DSM-IV), indeed, has been criticized for being too heterogeneous (Rosen & Frueh, 2007). The PTSD diagnosis uses polythetic criteria (e.g., 1 of 5, 2 of 7), which allows for considerable variability. Specifically, using this polythetic criterion, there are 79,794 possible ways to have the diagnosis of PTSD. With MDD, which is also often criticized for being too heterogeneous, there are only 126 minimal and 256 possible combinations (Miller, 2010). Notably, with the increase in number of PTSD symptoms in the fifth edition (DSM-5) resulting in even more possible combinations, this problem of observed heterogeneity within PTSD will only increase. Accordingly, the variability of symptom combinations of who will qualify for a diagnosis of PTSD will increase; and both clinicians and researchers will need to pay better attention to the varying *processes* driving various observed symptom presentations.

Emerging Scientific Advances

Given these patterns of high levels of observed comorbidities and within-diagnosis heterogeneity, both clinicians and researchers are recognizing the need to better understand common principles underlying the presence and reduction of psychopathology. Two emerging scientific developments provide the backdrop for our focus on principles underlying resilience and recovery following trauma exposure and, although not explicitly stated up to now, our focus on broader outcomes beyond PTSD as the sole psychiatric response following trauma exposure. These specific scientific advancements are the development of research-domain criteria aimed at identifying transdiagnostic constructs and a growing emphasis on empirically supported principles underlying therapeutic recovery. Although these scientific shifts are not the explicit focus of this book, they underlie the core thinking behind our focus on broad principles of recovery/resilience and merit a brief discussion to highlight our scientific foundation.

The National Institute of Mental Health has started the development of research domain criteria, called RDoC (see Insel et al., 2010). RDoC seeks to define basic transdiagnostic constructs across multiple units of analysis from genes to neural circuits to behaviors in order to rapidly develop an integrative understanding of psychopathology and improve treatment development. This shift to a dimensional system that is agnostic to disorder categories is largely motivated by the failure of our current classification system to identify and align with advances in genetics and neuroscience (Simpson, 2012). The initiative proposes a series of domains such as negative valence systems (e.g., acute threat, loss), positive valence systems (e.g., reward valuation, habit), cognitive systems (e.g., attention, perception, memory), systems for social processes (e.g., affiliation, social communication), and arousal and regulatory systems (e.g., resting state activity). Each of these domains will be addressed at varying units of analysis, including genes, molecules, cells, circuits, physiology, behavior, self-reports, and paradigms. By evaluating multiple domains at various units of analysis, RDoCs will be better able to identify the effect of dysregulation in one domain upon the functioning of another, developing a more comprehensive understanding of the complexity and heterogeneity of symptom manifestation (Craske, 2012a).

Ultimately, the R-DoC approach is considered to have direct clinical applicability. The overall approach should help produce treatments that are more precisely targeted to underlying dysfunctions, that better identify subgroups of individuals who will respond to targeted interventions, and whose mechanisms are better understood as actual mediators of therapeutic change (Craske, 2012a). With this move to shift our study of psychopathology to a matrix of domains and units of analyses, this also encourages us as clinicians to similarly focus less on discrete diagnostic entities and more on the processes associated with underlying observed symptoms. This is what we are seeking to do in this book.

As the focus has begun to shift in our study of psychopathology, so has the implementation of psychological or psychiatric treatment. This shift is toward identifying and disseminating empirically supported principles of change (ESPs). ESPs refer to principles or techniques that are empirically demonstrated to be contributors to clinical improvement and can be applied in a flexible manner based on clinician judgment (e.g., Beutler, Clarkin, & Bongar, 2000; Beutler, Moleiro, & Talebi, 2002; Rosen & Davison, 2003). ESPs are thought to reflect "research-informed principles that cut across both different theories of change and variations that exist among different techniques" (Beutler et al., 2002, p. 1203). Notably, empirically supported treatments (ESTs), often either confusingly referring to specific treatment packages or sets of treatment techniques, are not the same things as ESPs. Different treatment packages or ESTs may actually rely on the same underlying ESPs, arguing that that they may not represent truly distinct treatment alternatives (Herbert, 2000; Rosen & Davison, 2003).

Notably, the shift in focus from ESTs to ESPs may provide clinicians with research-supported interventions that can be better integrated into treatment in a flexible manner that allows for individual variability, diversity of treatment setting, and the application of therapy nonspecifics (Beutler et al., 2002). Emphasizing principles of change over ESTs further minimizes the focus on trademarked therapy packages and potentially returns the focus to scientific mechanisms (Rosen & Davison, 2003). However, applying ESPs in practice can be challenging, as it assumes that the clinician possesses a high level of proficiency in both clinical knowledge and in the theory that guides the principles (Beutler et al., 2002). This, however, is beginning to change with the emergence of transdiagnostic treatment approaches, which focus on teaching ESPs. Within the context of a broad transdiagnostic model, therapists match specific treatment strategies to specific emotional, cognitive, behavioral, or functional domains that are most dysregulated for a given patient (Craske, 2012b). This type of personalized transdiagnostic approach may actually ease dissemination burdens and additionally may better personalize and improve patient outcomes. This focus on principles underlying change is also what we are seeking to do in this book.

FACILITATING RESILIENCE AND RECOVERY
FOLLOWING TRAUMATIC EVENTS

We find ourselves at an exciting crossroads. This crossroads reflects a shift in our scientific understanding of psychopathology following trauma exposure, moving toward understanding distinct and shared features within and across disorders, and a shift in our focus away from empirically supported treatments for trauma-related psychopathology toward understanding empirically supported principles that target specific underlying dysfunctions. In the case of Mora, we do not see a particular disorder or a particular intervention promoting recovery. Instead, we see a pattern of reactions to a life-threatening motor vehicle accident, in the broader context of a life and a culture, and a pattern of resilience, recovery, and posttraumatic growth following this horrific event.

Being at a crossroads is always an interesting place because it is here where older and newer ideas intermix. This "communication" will be seen across the chapters in this book, where sometimes authors refer to a disorder specifically, such as PTSD, while at other times they refer to trauma-related psychopathology in general (suggesting a range of symptoms that commonly co-occur after trauma exposure, such as lack of positive affect, reexperiencing of the traumatic event, avoidance of trauma reminders, anxious arousal). Similarly, authors may refer to specific name-branded treatment packages such as trauma-focused cognitive-behavioral therapy (TF-CBT), or to therapeutic principles such as addressing avoidance of the trauma memory. These variations simply reflect our field being at this crossroads. We have encouraged the authors to highlight key principles that promote either natural or therapeutic recovery or both.

As you read through this book, consider this: Mora exists, albeit as a combination of remarkable men and women who have shared their lives with us. In our research and in our clinical work, we see the effects of trauma on men and women every day. We see profound sorrow, shattered lives, horrendous memories invading every aspect of life, and an ever-present fear that this event or events could happen again. However, we also see men and women rising above their circumstances, putting their fear and sorrow behind them, and building new and, potentially, better lives for themselves. Resilience and recovery after trauma are possible—we see it everyday.

ACKNOWLEDGMENTS

Preparation of this chapter was supported in part by Grant Nos. R01MH066347 (Lori A. Zoellner, Principal Investigator) and R01MH066348 (Norah C. Feeny, Principal Investigator).

REFERENCES

Beutler, L. E., Clarkin, J. F., & Bongar, B. (2000). *Guidelines for the systematic treatment of the depressed patient.* New York: Oxford University Press.

Beutler, L. E., Moleiro, C., & Talebi, H. (2002). Resistance in psychotherapy: What conclusions are supported by research? *Journal of Clinical Psychology, 58,* 207–217.

Bonnano, G. A. (2004). Clarifying and extending the construct of adult resilience. *American Psychologist, 69,* 265–267.

Bradley, R., Greene, J., Russ, E., Dutra, L., & Westen, D. (2005). A multidimensional meta-analysis of psychotherapy for PTSD. *American Journal of Psychiatry, 162,* 214–227.

Brewin, C. R., Andrews, B., & Valentine, J. D. (2000). Meta-analysis of risk factors for posttraumatic stress disorder in trauma-exposed adults. *Journal of Consulting and Clinical Psychology, 68,* 748–766.

Calhoun, L. G., & Tedeschi, R. G. (2006). *Handbook of posttraumatic growth: Research and practice.* Mahwah, NJ: Erlbaum.

Clark, L. A., Watson, D., & Reynolds, S. (1995). Diagnosis and classification of psychopathology: Challenges to the current system and future directions. *Annual Review of Psychology, 46,* 121–153.

Craske, M. G. (2012a). The RDoC Initiative: Science and practice. *Depression and Anxiety, 29,* 253–256.

Craske, M. G. (2012b). Transdiagnostic treatment for anxiety and depression. *Depression and Anxiety, 29,* 749–753.

Elhai, J. D., Grubaugh, A. L., Kashdan, T. B., & Frueh, B. C. (2008). Empirical examination of a proposed refinement to DSM-IV posttraumatic stress disorder symptom criteria using the National Comorbidity Survey Replication data. *Journal of Clinical Psychiatry, 69,* 597–602.

Herbert, J. D. (2000). Defining empirically supported treatments: Pitfalls and possible solutions. *The Behavior Therapist, 23,* 113–122.

Insel, T. R., Cuthbert, B. N., Garvey, M. A., Heinssen, R., Pine, D., Quinn, K., et al. (2010). Research domain criteria (RDoC): Toward a new classification framework for research on mental disorders. *American Journal of Psychiatry, 167,* 748–751.

Institute of Medicine. (2007). *Treatment of PTSD: Assessment of the evidence.* Washington, DC: National Academies Press.

Janoff-Bulman, R. (2004). Posttraumatic growth: Three explanatory models. *Psychological Inquiry, 15,* 30–34.

Kessler, R. C., Chiu, W. T., Demler, O., & Walters, E. E. (2005). Prevalence, severity, and comorbidity of 12-month DSM-IV disorders in the National Comorbidity Survey Replication. *Archives of General Psychiatry, 62,* 617–628.

Kessler, R. C., Sonnega, A., Bromet, E., Hughes, M., & Nelson, C. (1995). Posttraumatic stress disorder in the National Comorbidity Survey. *Archives of General Psychiatry, 52,* 1048–1060.

King, L. A., King, D. W., Fairbank, J. A., Keane, T. M., & Adams, G. A. (1998). Resilience–recovery factors in post-traumatic stress disorder among female and male Vietnam veterans: Hardiness, postwar social support, and additional stressful life events. *Journal of Personality and Social Psychology, 74,* 420–434.

Linley, P. A., & Joseph, S. (2004). Positive change following trauma and adversity: A review. *Journal of Traumatic Stress, 17,* 11–21.

Litz, B. T. (2004). Has resilience to severe trauma been underestimated? *American Psychologist, 60,* 262; discussion, 265–267.

Marshall, G. N., & Schell, T. L. (2002). Reappraising the link between peritraumatic dissociation and PTSD symptom severity: Evidence from a longitudinal study of community violence survivors. *Journal of Abnormal Psychology, 111,* 626–636.

Miller, M. (2010, February). Potential combinations of the DSM PTSD diagnosis [SSCPNET Archive]. Retrieved February 27, 2010, from *http://bit.ly/jkf5vl.*

National Institute for Health and Clinical Excellence. (2005). *Post-traumatic stress disorder.* London: Royal College of Psychiatrists and British Psychological Society.

O'Donnell, M. L., Creamer, M., & Pattison, P. (2004). Posttraumatic stress disorder and depression following trauma: Understanding comorbidity. *American Journal of Psychiatry, 161,* 1390–1396.

Ozer, E. J., Best, S. R., Lipsey, T. L., & Weiss, D. S. (2003). Predictors of posttraumatic stress disorder and symptoms in adults: A meta-analysis. *Psychological Bulletin, 129,* 52–73.

Powers, M. B., Halpern, J. M., Ferenschak, M. P., Gillihan, S. J., & Foa, E. B. (2010). A meta-analytic review of prolonged exposure for posttraumatic stress disorder. *Clinical Psychology Review, 30,* 635–641.

Riggs, D. S., Rothbaum, B. O., & Foa, E. B. (1995). A prospective examination of symptoms of posttraumatic stress disorder in victims of nonsexual assault. *Journal of Interpersonal Violence, 10,* 201–214.

Rosen, G. M., & Davison, G. C. (2003). Psychology should list empirically supported principles of change (ESPs) and not credential trademarked therapies or other treatment packages. *Behavior Modification, 27,* 300–312.

Rosen, G. M., & Frueh, B. C. (2007). Challenges to the PTSD construct and its database: The importance of scientific debate. *Journal of Anxiety Disorders, 21,* 161–163.

Rothbaum, B. O., Foa, E. B., Riggs, D. S., Murdock, T., & Walsh, W. (1992). A prospective examination of post-traumatic stress disorder in rape victims. *Journal of Traumatic Stress, 5,* 455–475.

Smid, G. E., van der Velden, P. G., Gersons, B. P., & Kleber, R. J. (2012). Late-onset posttraumatic stress disorder following a disaster: A longitudinal study. *Psychological Trauma: Theory, Research, Practice, and Policy,, 4*(3), 312.

Simpson, H. B. (2012). The RDoC Project: A new paradigm for investigating the pathophysiology of anxiety. *Depression and Anxiety, 29,* 251–252.

Solomon, Z., Horesh, D., & Ein-Dor, T. (2009). The longitudinal course of posttraumatic stress disorder symptom clusters among war veterans. *Journal of Clinical Psychiatry, 70,* 837–843.

U.S. Department of Defense and Department of Veterans Affairs Clinical Practice Guideline Working Group. (2003). *Management of post-traumatic stress.* Washington, DC: VA Office of Quality and Performance.

Chapter 2

Acute Intervention

Richard A. Bryant *and* Angela Nickerson

Trauma affects a large proportion of the world's population. Traumatic events can range from mass violence and disasters, such as war, genocide, and natural disasters; to interpersonal trauma, including abuses and assaults; to accidental trauma encompassing motor vehicle accidents, workplace accidents, and injuries. Most people who are exposed to traumatic events experience psychological distress in the immediate aftermath. Key questions emerging after traumatic events include: How can we tell if people are going to get better on their own? To what extent should we intervene in the immediate aftermath of a traumatic event? Which interventions are most effective in these circumstances?

TRAUMA EXPOSURE AND PSYCHOLOGICAL DISTRESS

Epidemiological surveys undertaken in Western countries indicate that between 50 and 90% of the population are exposed to some type of traumatic event throughout their lifetime (Breslau et al., 1998; Kessler, Sonnega, Bromet, Hughes, & Nelson, 1995). Moreover, almost universal lifetime exposure to trauma is likely in conflict-ridden settings. Psychological distress is commonly experienced in the aftermath of trauma, with rates of posttraumatic stress disorder (PTSD) ranging widely across trauma type, population, and setting (e.g., de Jong, Mulhern, Ford, van der Kam, & Kleber, 2000; Galea et al., 2002; Rothbaum, Foa, Riggs, Murdock, &

Walsh, 1992; van Griensven et al., 2006). In addition to PTSD and acute stress disorder (ASD), a range of other psychological disturbances immediately following trauma have also been documented, including depression, anxiety, shock, and dissociation (Shalev, 2002).

Studies investigating the trajectory of psychological responses indicate that the high rates of psychopathology observed immediately after a trauma decline sharply in subsequent weeks and months (Galea et al., 2002; Riggs, Rothbaum, & Foa, 1995; Rothbaum et al., 1992; Shalev et al., 1998). Thus, while most people who experience a traumatic event initially experience psychological symptoms, the majority of trauma survivors evidence psychological adaptation with time. There remains, however, a significant minority who experience persistent distress. Given the wide variety of responses to traumatic events, it is important to consider the utility of early intervention following trauma.

IS EARLY INTERVENTION FOLLOWING TRAUMA HELPFUL?

As posttraumatic distress typically declines following trauma exposure, people have questioned the necessity, and indeed advisability, of offering psychological treatments in the immediate aftermath of a trauma. In the context of this debate, two major approaches have emerged in early intervention following trauma: universal interventions for all survivors and targeted interventions for people who are at high risk for long-term disorder.

Universal Interventions

Universal or "blanket" interventions are generally offered to all individuals exposed to a traumatic event. These approaches were developed on the basis of the assumption that intervention can both alleviate acute psychological symptoms and prevent the development of chronic psychological problems such as PTSD.

Debriefing Approaches

Psychological debriefing, and most popularly critical incident stress debriefing (CISD), has been the most widely used posttrauma intervention over the past three decades. CISD was originally designed to address posttrauma reactions in emergency personnel (Mitchell, 1983). Since its inception, however, it has been more widely applied to survivors of a diverse array of types of traumatic events (Adler et al., 2008; Jacobs, Horne-Moyer, & Jones, 2004; Nurmi, 1999; Saarni, Saari, & Hakkinen, 1999; Sacks,

Clements, & Fay-Hillier, 2001; Simms-Ellis & Madill, 2001; Townsend & Loughlin, 1998; Wee, Mills, & Koehler, 1999). This intervention typically consists of a single debriefing session, administered within several days of the trauma exposure, in which a facilitator normalizes the experiences of the trauma survivors, and survivors discuss their psychological, cognitive, and emotional reactions to the trauma. It has been argued that this promotes emotional processing in the trauma survivor, which helps with adaptation (Mitchell, 1983). Although CISD was initially designed to be implemented in groups (predominantly with emergency responders), it has since been more frequently applied to individual survivors. While this intervention is still often used as a stand-alone intervention (Bisson & Kitchiner, 2003), the developers have more recently argued that it should be undertaken in the context of a multimodal approach known as critical incident stress management (Mitchell & Everly, 1995).

CISD is widely reported as being well received among trauma survivors (Adler et al., 2008; Carlier, Voerman, & Gersons, 2000; Everly & Boyle, 1999; Small, Lumley, Donohue, Potter, & Waldenstrom, 2000). It is important to note, however, that much of the evidence supporting CISD is anecdotal in nature, and the positive reports regarding the intervention often do not translate into improved mental health outcomes in trauma survivors (Marchand et al., 2006; Small et al., 2000). Meta-analyses and reviews examining the overall impact of single-session debriefing approaches on psychological symptoms have generally indicated that CISD is ineffective in reducing psychological symptoms in trauma survivors (Bisson, Brayne, Ochberg, & Everly, 2007; Litz & Gray, 2002; McNally, Bryant, & Ehlers, 2003; Rose, Bisson, Churchill, & Wessely, 2001; van Emmerik, Kamphuis, Hulsbosch, & Emmelkamp, 2002). Furthermore, some studies indicated that CISD may even be harmful, potentially leading to worsened psychological symptoms (Bisson, Jenkins, Alexander, & Bannister, 1997; Mayou, Ehlers, & Hobbs, 2000). To explain these findings, theorists have suggested that CISD may (1) interfere with natural recovery processes, (2) force premature processing of the trauma without providing adequate follow-up care, (3) compromise the individual's use of his or her own coping resources, (4) exacerbate negative symptom interpretations, (5) occur too early following a trauma, (6) promote rumination, and/or (7) pathologize normal psychological distress (Bisson & Andrew, 2007; Bisson et al., 1997; Bryant, 2004; Ehlers & Clark, 2003). Overall, the universal application of single-session debriefing approaches in the immediate aftermath of a traumatic event is now considered to be contraindicated (Bisson & Kitchiner, 2003). This is reflected in international guidelines outlining best-practice interventions following trauma, including those developed by the National Institute for Clinical Excellence (2005) and the International Society for Traumatic Stress Studies (Foa, Keane, Friedman, & Cohen, 2009).

Mechanisms Underlying Posttraumatic Distress

The recent resultant shift away from universal interventions following trauma has raised many questions concerning the optimal means to manage psychological stress in the acute phase of trauma. In searching for ways to enhance resilience after trauma, considerable emphasis has been placed on identifying mechanisms that are associated with better outcomes and trying to implement strategies that build on these principles. For example, Hobfoll and colleagues (2007) outlined five major principles that enhance recovery and resilience in the acute phase after trauma, and that are informed by research evidence. These principles include promoting (1) a sense of safety, (2) calming, (3) a perception of self-efficacy, (4) connectedness, and (5) hope. In terms of safety, not surprisingly, trauma survivors who continue to experience threats to their safety show elevated posttraumatic stress reactions (de Jong et al., 2001; de Jong, Mulhern, Ford, van der Kam, & Kleber, 2000; Neria, Solomon, Ginzburg, & Dekel, 2000). Among people remaining in a context of potential threat, those who establish a perception of safety are less likely to develop PTSD than those who do not (Bleich, Gelkopf, & Solomon, 2003; Grieger, Fullerton, & Ursano, 2003). In relation to the principle of calming, multiple studies indicate that hyperarousal in the acute phase is predictive of subsequent PTSD, including heightened resting heart rate (Bryant, Harvey, Guthrie, & Moulds, 2000; Shalev, Sahar, et al., 1998), respiration rate (Bryant, Creamer, O'Donnell, Silove, & McFarlane, 2008), and panic attacks (Bryant & Panasetis, 2001). There is indirect evidence that factors that alleviate arousal in the acute phase may lessen the likelihood of subsequent PTSD, including natural levels of gamma-aminobutyric acid (Vaiva et al., 2004) and the administration of morphine in the immediate hours after trauma (Bryant, Creamer, O'Donnell, Silove, & McFarlane, 2009). Regarding perceptions of self-efficacy, numerous studies have found that the extent to which trauma survivors believe they have agency in influencing future outcomes impacts on adjustment (Benight, Cieslak, Molton, & Johnson, 2008; Benight & Harper, 2002). Concerning social connectedness, many reports indicate that positive social support is a buffer against protracted stress reactions following trauma (Norris, Friedman, & Watson, 2002). Finally, in relation to hope, it is posited that expectancy of recovery and positive outcomes results in better adaptation (Carver & Scheier, 1998).

Universal Interventions Facilitating Coping

On the basis of these principles, immediate interventions now focus on enhancing these factors in both individuals and communities after trauma. Specifically, most initial interventions aim to meet basic needs, increasing agency and control for survivors, and providing support following traumatic events. One approach that has attracted much attention in recent years is psychological first aid (PFA; Brymer et al., 2006; Raphael, 1977). PFA attempts to meet the broader psychosocial needs of the individual following a traumatic event by reducing arousal; ensuring safety; access to information, emotional support, and services; instilling hope; and enhancing knowledge about self-care strategies. This approach focuses on supporting trauma survivors in utilizing their own coping resources. While survivors may talk about their experiences if they wish, this approach discourages the purposeful elicitation of trauma experiences or related emotions (Bryant, 2004). Litz (2008) notes that in settings of mass trauma resources that are typically drawn on to promote recovery may be unavailable, and that a nonintrusive and nonprescriptive model of care may be beneficial in meeting survivors' practical needs. In contrast to CISD, PFA does not propose to prevent the development of psychological disorders; instead, this approach recognizes that the majority of individuals exposed to traumatic events will recover on their own, and aims to facilitate this process. The increasing popularity of PFA approaches is reflected in best-practice guidelines that have recommended this approach following exposure to trauma (Inter-Agency Steering Committee, 2007). It must be noted, however, that PFA remains largely untested, and further research is necessary to determine the extent of the utility of this approach following trauma. One issue that remains for the evaluation of PFA is the defined goal of the intervention. As it does not aim to prevent subsequent disorder, it is necessary to operationalize the expected outcomes so the effects can be assessed. For example, it may be possible to index the effects of PFA through controlled evaluations of such factors as help seeking, accessing social support, utilization of resources, and arousal levels.

Clinical Implications

For clinicians working with survivors in the immediate aftermath of traumatic events, theory and research indicate that interventions that require the individual to discuss the traumatic event and his or her reactions to it are not universally indicated. Instead, it is important to normalize posttraumatic stress responses, and to provide education regarding the common nature of psychological reactions in the aftermath of trauma, and the tendency of such symptoms to decline over time. Furthermore, the clinician should assist the survivor with practical and logistical difficulties, for example, by facilitating access to necessities such as shelter, food, clothing, and social support. If the survivor expresses the desire to discuss his or her experiences, this should be undertaken in a safe context, in a supportive manner, and preferably in a setting where the survivor has access to follow-up care.

Screening

The relative ineffectiveness of blanket intervention approaches, combined with the scarcity of mental health resources in many trauma-affected settings, underscores the importance of identifying people at risk of developing psychological disorders in the aftermath of traumatic events. The diagnosis of ASD (American Psychiatric Association, 1994) was developed to assist with the classification of those individuals who are (1) experiencing significant psychological difficulties in the initial wake of trauma, and (2) most likely to develop chronic posttraumatic stress reactions (Bryant, 2004, 2007b). Many of the diagnostic criteria for ASD are analogous to PTSD criteria including the presence of persistent reexperiencing symptoms (such as intrusive memories or nightmares), marked avoidance (such as avoidance of internal or external reminders of the trauma), and anxiety or hyperarousal symptoms (such as difficulty sleeping, hypervigilence, or exaggerated startle response) (American Psychiatric Association, 1994). There also exist two key differences between ASD and PTSD; first, ASD can be diagnosed within the first month following the trauma, and second, a diagnosis of ASD requires the presence of three dissociative symptoms, such as numbing, reduced awareness, depersonalization, derealization, or dissociative amnesia (Bryant, 2004). Prospective studies indicate that ASD is highly sensitive in predicting PTSD, such that the majority of individuals with a diagnosis of ASD following a traumatic event go on to develop PTSD (Bryant, 2011). In contrast, the diagnosis has attracted criticism for evidencing low levels of specificity—that is, most people who develop PTSD do not show adequate symptoms for a diagnosis of ASD in the acute aftermath of the trauma. A number of studies indicate that insisting on the presence of dissociation for a diagnosis of ASD is excessively limiting, and that many very distressed people do not actually display dissociation (Harvey & Bryant, 1998, 1999). It is for this reason that DSM-5 initiated significant changes to the diagnosis of ASD. The revised ASD diagnosis describes severe acute stress reactions rather than attempting to predict PTSD, as well as requiring at least nine out of a possible 14 symptoms without regard to any particular clusters (American Psychiatric Association, 2013; Bryant, Friedman, Spiegel, Ursano, & Strain, 2011). This change recognized the heterogeneity of acute stress response and reduced the emphasis placed on acute dissociation.

Considering the frequency of acute stress reactions following trauma, an important challenge is to distinguish those with transient distress from individuals who are likely to go on to develop PTSD. It is important to note that assessment in the days following the trauma may merely index acute levels of distress, which are likely to rapidly reduce in many individuals. Accordingly, the identification of high-risk individuals is likely to be most accurate some weeks following the trauma, after initial acute reactions have subsided (Bryant, 2007b). A key advantage to the early identification of psychopathology following trauma is that it allows for the application of targeted interventions that address trauma-related symptomatology in individuals unlikely to recover on their own, and to potentially prevent the development of chronic PTSD. It is also recommended that identification should not be limited to the ASD diagnosis for the reasons stated above. Instead, focusing on those with severe acute stress reactions (without requiring dissociative responses to be present) will more likely capture those individuals who are experiencing the early signs of a longer term posttraumatic stress response. At present we lack data concerning the optimal screening instruments to employ in the acute phase and what the appropriate cutoffs are. One of the limitations in our knowledge is the focus on PTSD to the relative neglect of other important posttraumatic conditions, such as depression, substance abuse, insomnia, and other anxiety disorders. One scale, the Posttraumatic Adjustment Scale, has been developed to identify people in the acute phase who will subsequently develop either PTSD or depression (O'Donnell et al., 2008); this novel approach looks beyond acute symptoms, and indexes pretrauma characteristics, aspects of the trauma itself, and response factors in the aftermath of the trauma. This 10-item scale is very brief to administer, and provides good sensitivity and specificity of subsequent PTSD (.82 and .84, respectively) and depression (.72 and .75, respectively).

Clinical Implications

These findings have important implications for clinicians working with trauma survivors. If one's goal is to identify recently trauma-exposed people who are at high risk for subsequent disorder and who are most in need of early intervention, a scale such as the Posttraumatic Adjustment Scale may be useful because it avoids some of the pitfalls associated with the ASD diagnosis. There are additional points the clinician can keep in mind to enhance the utility of early identification. The sooner one tries to identify someone as being at "high risk," the more likely one will mistake a transient stress reaction to be a precursor of subsequent disorder. Identifying who is high risk within several days of a trauma is difficult, and so it may be useful to delay it until a week has elapsed. The process of identifying those at risk should also take into account the level of ongoing stressors the individual is experiencing; elevated stress responses may be in reaction to ongoing difficulties (e.g., housing difficulties, separation from loved ones, physical pain), and one needs to understand these are common and understandable responses to current stress. Removal of these stressors often alleviates the acute stress reaction. It can be useful to ask the individual if his or her symptoms have worsened, maintained, or reduced since the traumatic event. Those who report relative diminishment of symptom severity may not require active intervention because natural recovery may be underway.

If severe stress reactions are persisting several weeks after the event, the individual is a good candidate for early intervention.

Targeted Interventions

In contrast to universal interventions other researchers have developed more circumscribed treatments designed to target those at risk of developing chronic PTSD following trauma. These interventions typically do not commence until several weeks following the trauma to allow for natural adaptation and symptom reduction (Bryant, 2007a). Most of these treatments draw on evidence-based, cognitive-behavioral interventions that are recommended to reduce chronic PTSD in trauma survivors (Foa et al., 2009; National Health and Medical Research Council Treatment Guidelines, 2007; National Institute of Clinical Excellence, 2005). Typically, these interventions are shortened to four or five treatment sessions and incorporate multiple complementary elements including psychoeducation, imaginal exposure, *in vivo* exposure, cognitive restructuring, anxiety management, and relapse prevention (Bryant, 2007b). They usually commence with a psychoeducation component, in which the patient is informed about psychological responses following traumatic events and factors that may maintain psychological distress. A second core aspect of this treatment is imaginal exposure therapy in which the patient relives the memory of the traumatic event, often repeatedly, to facilitate habituation and emotional processing. Typically, *in vivo* exposure therapy is included in these interventions, such that the patient exposes him- or herself to increasingly more anxiety-provoking situations to elicit fear habituation and reduce avoidance behaviors. Cognitive restructuring focuses on the identification, evaluation, and correction of maladaptive appraisals regarding the trauma. Some treatments also include an anxiety management component incorporating strategies such as controlled breathing and progressive muscle relaxation. Finally, treatment typically ends with a relapse prevention module, in which therapy gains are consolidated, skills are reviewed, and plans are made to address potential future trauma-related symptoms.

Research indicates that cognitive-behavioral therapy (CBT) is a promising intervention for the prevention of chronic PTSD among trauma survivors with acute posttraumatic stress or ASD symptoms (Bisson, Shepherd, Joy, Probert, & Newcombe, 2004; Bryant, Harvey, Dang, Sackville, & Basten, 1998; Bryant, Mastrodomenico, et al., 2008; Bryant, Moulds, Guthrie, & Nixon, 2003; Bryant, Sackville, Dang, Moulds, & Guthrie, 1999; Sijbrandij et al., 2007; van Emmerik, Kamphuis, & Emmelkamp, 2008). Furthermore, a review concluded that trauma-focused CBT was "possibly efficacious" for ASD (Ponniah & Hollon, 2008). It is important to note, however, that almost all of the treatment trials investigating the efficacy for CBT in treating symptoms of ASD and preventing the development of chronic PTSD have been undertaken with survivors of civilian trauma including motor vehicle accidents, assaults, and sexual assaults. Further studies should be conducted examining the extent to which this intervention is effective in reducing psychological distress and subsequent psychopathology in other groups before strong recommendations about the usage of this intervention can be made.

Clinical Implications

For individuals who are continuing to exhibit symptoms of ASD (or PTSD) several weeks following the trauma, cognitive-behavioral interventions may be indicated. This may prevent the development of chronic posttraumatic stress reactions, and assist the survivor with psychological adaptation in the aftermath of trauma. Findings from controlled treatment trials suggest that it is often wiser to delay CBT for at least a week after trauma exposure because this can allow the individual to allocate more resources to treatment as the immediate effects of the trauma subside. Many people experience a range of problems in the weeks after trauma, including physical pain, legal proceedings, or social upheaval, and therapy can function more efficiently if these distractions have alleviated. It is impossible to predict with 100% accuracy how any individual will respond to therapy; however, there are certain presentations that one should be aware of when planning exposure-based therapy in the initial weeks after trauma. People who present with marked avoidance or dissociation may be reluctant to engage in therapy that involves confronting their feared memories. Furthermore, it is likely that these individuals may not experience the required emotions during exposure. A thorough assessment should be undertaken of the possible reasons for the avoidance/dissociation before proceeding because dismantling avoidance behaviors shortly after trauma exposure may result in an exacerbation of symptoms in some people. The clinician also needs to be aware of patients who are displaying extreme catastrophic appraisals about their traumatic experience, and their response to it. There is evidence that people who engage in thinking styles characterized by defeat and hopelessness tend to do worse in CBT (Ehlers et al., 1998), and so these individuals often benefit from focused cognitive restructuring that targets this negative perspective.

Although there is ample evidence that early provision of CBT can be beneficial after trauma, it is apparent that it is not appropriate for all survivors. Furthermore, even in controlled trials approximately one-third of people do not respond optimally. Another limitation to the indicated interventions after trauma exposure is that a significant proportion of people who will develop PTSD will not be detected in the acute phase. Delayed-onset cases are reported in 15–30% of cases (Andrews, Brewin, Philpott, & Stewart, 2007). Others will simply not be ready for active treatment because of the competing demands of the acute posttraumatic phase. It is important to remember that many people will benefit more from active therapy several months after exposure than from early intervention. In a key study conducted in Israel, Shalev and colleagues (2012) randomized recently traumatized people to either exposure or cognitive therapy within a month after trauma, or to exposure therapy 5 months after trauma. All conditions resulted in comparable treatment gains, which underscores the idea that delaying treatment does not impair the person's capacity to benefit from CBT. Therefore if a clinician is concerned about any adverse effects of providing CBT in the acute phase (may occur in a small minority of cases), or believes the person will not be able to apply him- or herself sufficiently to therapy at this time, it may be wiser to delay treatment until he or she is better able to focus on the requirements of therapy.

Pharmacotherapy

In contrast to the emerging evidence for psychotherapy in the acute phase after trauma, there is very little evidence concerning psychopharmacology. Considering the fact that, for most people, psychological distress will alleviate in the weeks following exposure to a traumatic event, caution should be exercised when prescribing medication in the acute period. Prior to prescribing medication, it is important that a thorough psychiatric and medical history be obtained, including current medications, allergies, and the use of illicit drugs and alcohol. The majority of research evidence for medications relates to the treatment of chronic posttraumatic stress symptoms. Selective serotonin reuptake inhibitors (SSRIs), such as sertraline and paroxetine, are considered first-line medications for longer term posttraumatic stress responses (Ballenger et al., 2004). Tricyclic antidepressents (such as impipramine, amitriptyline, and doxepin) may also have some efficacy for posttraumatic stress, as well as depressive symptoms (e.g., Robert, Blakeney, Villarreal, Rosenberg, & Meyer, 1999).

In the Shalev treatment study cited above, 242 patients admitted through an emergency room who subsequently met criteria for either full or subsyndromal ASD were randomized to either prolonged exposure therapy, cognitive restructuring, wait list (who were then randomized to exposure therapy after 12 weeks), escitalopram (an SSRI), or placebo (Shalev et al., 2012). At the 9-month follow-up assessment, PTSD rates were comparable across exposure (21%) and cognitive restructuring (22%) conditions, relative to the much higher rates in the SSRI (42%) and placebo (47%) conditions. Considering that this is the first large controlled trial of pharmacotherapy for ASD, these findings do suggest that SSRIs in the acute phase may not be superior to placebo, and are certainly less effective than trauma-focused psychotherapy.

Clinical Implications

It is important to note that these medications have adverse side effects and should be carefully monitored. Benzodiazepines are commonly prescribed in the acute period following a traumatic event because they have utility in reducing arousal and facilitating sleep. Despite these advantages, benzodiazepines can be highly problematic because they are addictive if used in a prolonged manner. Furthermore, there is some evidence that they do not prevent the development of chronic PTSD (e.g., Gelpin, Bonne, Peri, Brandes, & Shalev, 1996). This pattern suggests that benzodiazepines should only be considered a short-term option for those patients with extreme arousal and whose sleep problems are distressing them. In terms of SSRIs or other medication commonly applied for chronic PTSD, this option should be reserved for patients who are not eligible for trauma-focused psychotherapy. The available evidence indicates that the major role of pharmacological agents in the acute phase is to reduce acute distress and sleep disturbance rather than secondary prevention, and that the latter goal is much better achieved by CBT.

Conclusions

In summary, evidence to date indicates that universal interventions such as CISD are unnecessary and ineffective in the immediate aftermath of traumatic events, as the majority of people exhibit natural declines in symptoms in the weeks following the trauma. Furthermore, some studies suggest that the application of treatments such as CISD that promote the disclosure of traumatic experiences may be detrimental to the mental health of some trauma survivors, potentially by interfering with natural coping mechanisms. Instead, research evidence points to the screening of trauma survivors in the weeks following the traumatic event for high levels of psychological distress such as ASD, which has been found to predict the subsequent development of chronic PTSD. This facilitates the identification of individuals most in need of intervention, who are unlikely to recover from traumatic events on their own. In such cases, studies to date suggest that short trauma-focused CBT interventions are indicated to reduce acute psychological distress and prevent the development of PTSD. The primary role of pharmacological approaches appears to be in reducing arousal in the acute phase posttrauma rather than longer term management. Further research is required to determine the extent to which this screening and intervention process is applicable across diverse populations.

PSYCHOLOGICAL RESPONSES TO TRAUMA: SPECIAL CONSIDERATIONS

In the DSM-5, a traumatic event is defined as "exposure to actual or threatened death, serious injury, or sexual violence . . . ". This definition allows for direct experiencing of an event, witnessing an event, learning about an event that occurred to a close friend or relative, or repeated or extreme exposure to adverse details of an event (American Psychiatric Association, 2013). This definition belies the vast heterogeneity of traumatic experiences and myriad factors that may vary from one trauma context to the next. For example, while most research investigating early intervention following traumatic events has been undertaken in Western settings, a disproportionate amount of trauma is likely to occur in settings in which persecution and conflict are ongoing. This reality underscores a major gap in knowledge regarding acute intervention following trauma as there is very little empirical data collected on treatment in the aftermath of trauma in war-torn and low-resource settings. It is unclear the extent to which findings from research undertaken with Western survivors of discrete trauma applies to such contexts, precluding evidence-based recommendations regarding best practices in these settings. Despite the limited empirical knowledge regarding the intervention following trauma across varied settings, it is important to note key themes that may impact on research and practice into early intervention.

Trauma Characteristics

While all subsumed under the broad umbrella term of *trauma*, different types of traumatic events vary across multiple dimensions. For example, the traumatic experience of a survivor of a nonfatal motor vehicle accident in a high-income country is likely to differ markedly from that of a political activist who has been imprisoned and tortured on multiple occasions in a conflict-ridden setting. Similarly, the experience of a war veteran who has survived multiple military tours will be far removed from that of an individual who has endured years of childhood neglect and abuse at the hands of a parent. While the variation in long-term psychological outcomes following trauma has been investigated (Cloitre et al., 2009; de Jong et al., 2001; Ehring & Quack, 2010; Steel et al., 2009), there has been little consideration of how types of traumatic events differentially impact on acute responses and early intervention. Litz (2008) notes that research evidence primarily supports the use of CBT to treat acute reactions in survivors of accidents, with less evidence being available for violence-related interventions, and no evidence specifically attesting to the efficacy of this intervention for mass trauma, disaster survivors, or terrorism. Psychological needs of trauma survivors (and thus indicated interventions) are likely to differ considerably. For example, for a survivor of a motor vehicle accident in a high-income setting, short-term trauma-focused CBT is likely to be very useful. In contrast, this intervention may need to be adapted for a recently tortured individual who is experiencing substantial living difficulties including scarcity of food and medical care and displacement from social resources. Without research evidence to guide the selection of early interventions in such settings, it is crucial to assess the individual needs of the trauma survivor to determine which type of intervention (if any) is likely to be useful at a particular time-point.

It is also important to consider the absence of evidence for early intervention treatments following mass violence and trauma in the context of international aid programs. In the aftermath of recent humanitarian emergencies, teams of mental health workers have entered affected countries with the intention of providing evidence-based, trauma-focused therapy immediately following a traumatic event, without consideration of existing systems of care and resources (Pupavac, 2001; van Ommeren, Saxena, & Saraceno, 2005). Silove (2005) notes that short-term trauma-focused interventions may have the greatest utility in the medium term, after immediate psychosocial needs are met, and with careful assessment of local capabilities and resources. Unfortunately, by this time, donor enthusiasm has often reduced, and corresponding funds for acute mental health problems depleted. There exists an urgent need to evaluate the efficacy of acute interventions in these settings to provide guidelines for government and nongovernment organizations regarding the type of treatments that should be implemented at various stages following an emergency.

Psychological Interventions and Posttrauma Resources

One of the most salient aspects of the posttrauma environment is the extent of the resources available to provide mental health services. In the context of mass trauma such as war, genocide, humanitarian emergencies, terrorism, and mass disasters, the demands of the situation may easily overwhelm available resources in high-resource contexts; in low-resource settings, there may be very limited or no infrastructure, health professionals, social services, or healthcare available to address the needs of a devastated population (Silove & Bryant, 2006). The available resources must be taken into consideration when planning early intervention following a large-scale traumatic event. First, in the case of any mass trauma, there are likely to be significant urgent psychosocial needs including food, water, shelter, safety, and reunification of family members. The Inter-Agency Steering Committee (2007) has developed guidelines to direct the efforts of government and nongovernment organizations in meeting these needs. It is likely that, in the context of large-scale trauma, these basic needs will supersede mental health needs, at least in the initial phases. Once these needs are met, and psychological distress becomes a key priority, it is important to consider the available resources on a context-by-context basis. For example, in a setting in which there are few trained health professionals, it may not be possible to implement an intervention requiring a high level of skill, experience, and/ or supervision. Although there is recent evidence that short trauma-focused treatments can be effectively disseminated via lay healthcare staff (e.g.,

Neuner et al., 2008), there may not be time to undertake extensive training programs in the immediate aftermath of a large-scale traumatic event. As such, practical and achievable goals should be set based on the available resources. For example, in the context of a developing country affected by disaster (e.g., Haiti earthquake, Sri Lanka/Indonesia tsunami, Pakistan earthquake) one should plan for interventions that are commensurate with the available resources rather than extrapolating from settings that enjoy better resourced mental health services. Trying to assist a community in which there are few mental health–trained personnel and literacy is low results in intervention goals that can be achieved by the limited resources available. This may involve focusing efforts on infrastructure rebuilding, social connections, returning people to work, and utilizing local religious coping rituals rather than attempting to introduce variations of a treatment that has been validated in Western contexts.

Identification of At-Risk Trauma Survivors

Another feature of early intervention in the context of ongoing stressors, such as civil conflict or mass disaster, is the problem of identifying those who are at high risk. In the context of ongoing threat or stress, the actual traumatic period may be very protracted, which raises significant challenges for identifying those who will suffer in the long term because survival mode will result in many people displaying stress reactions. In these contexts it is possible that the trajectory from acute reactions to chronic PTSD may vary from expected patterns. One key exemplar of a differential trajectory is delayed-onset PTSD. Delayed-onset PTSD is a rare response in civilian populations, although there is some evidence that it is more common in military contexts (for a review, see Andrews, Brewin, Philpott, & Stewart, 2007). Different processes may account for delayed presentations of stress reactions, including numbing responses that inhibit expression of distress (Horowitz & Solomon, 1975), preoccupation with more immediate needs (e.g., pain, relocation) that distract attention from one's symptoms (Andreasen, 2004), the increase of stressors in the posttrauma period that compound the initial stress response (Bryant & Harvey, 2002), or subsequent increases in demands on resources that are required to manage emotional responses and which then lead to increased distress (Grossman, Levin, Katzen, & Lechner, 2004). The difficulty in identifying people shortly after disaster was highlighted in a study on the trajectory of adaptation after Hurricane Katrina, which found that rates of PTSD actually *increased* over time following the hurricane (Kessler et al., 2008). Delays in rebuilding infrastructure, lack of housing, and loss of basic infrastructures resulted in increasing psychological strain, which led to rising rates of PTSD. These patterns underscore why early identification and intervention need to be considered in the context of demands on survivors and availability of resources.

Enhancing Resilience

Following communitywide exposure to traumatic events, resilience may be fostered by enhancing local resources and strengths. For example, in non-Western settings it is important to make use of local healing resources (Eisenbruch, de Jong, & van de Put, 2004). Cultural factors greatly influence mental health, highlighting the importance of culturally appropriate psychological interventions, which may be facilitated by the shared worldview between traditional practitioners and their patients (Crawford & Lipsedge, 2004; Hinton & Otto, 2006; Kleinman, 1988; Shankar, Saravanan, & Jacob, 2006). The utility of engaging and empowering local staff has also been highlighted (Eisenbruch et al., 2004). A strong criticism of the area of humanitarian aid is the lack of long-term and sustainable interventions designed specifically for the context in which the disaster or conflict occurred. Working with local healers to develop an intervention that both encompasses best-practice interventions and indigenous healing methods may allow for the long-term implementation of interventions after Western-based organizations have left the context. As such, early intervention programs must be targeted to the specific context in which the trauma has occurred, taking into consideration local expressions of distress. For example, after the 2004 Asian tsunami, millions of people were extremely distressed across the region in the immediate aftermath of the tragedy. In many of these settings the distress was expressed via somatic concerns, including neck pain, weakness of limbs, and breathing difficutlies. Many communities strategically used local monks to pray with survivors to address these concerns and to encourage adaptive interpretations of the somatic sensations. In other settings, the frequent nightmares about loved ones who had died in the tsunami were widely interpreted as indications that the deceased were suffering; again, the use of monks was widely employed to address these concerns. Recently, there has been a trend toward integration of local healing methods into Western treatments when working with minority groups in Western settings (e.g., Aguilera, Garza, & Muñoz, 2010; Hinton & Otto, 2006; Hinton, Pich, Chhean, Safren, & Pollack, 2006). While there is a need for further evaluation of these hybrid methods, they represent a promising avenue for adapting trauma-focused interventions to cross-cultural contexts.

Ongoing Threat

Another dimension upon which traumatic events may differ substantially is the extent to which the trauma survivor is exposed to a situation of ongoing threat. Research has documented the relative persistence of posttraumatic distress in the context of ongoing threat (de Jong et al., 2001; Hobfoll et al., 2007; Neria, Solomon, Ginzburg, Dekel, et al., 2000; Porter

& Haslam, 2005). Typical trajectories in which posttraumatic symptoms decline in the weeks following the trauma may thus not apply when the violence and trauma are ongoing. The sense of safety that facilitates post-traumatic adaptation (Bleich et al., 2003; Grieger et al., 2003) may be unavailable in such settings. This has significant implications for early intervention following traumatic events. An individual who has experienced a mugging in a high-income country where violent crime is relatively rare may be considered to be living in circumstances of objective safety following the trauma. In contrast, a refugee who has been exposed to multiple traumatic events in his home country, and is now displaced in a third country that is experiencing a civil war may face the very real prospect of regular exposure to traumatic events, and may be fearful for friends and family remaining in the country of origin. The promotion of a sense of safety is a primary priority in settings where trauma is ongoing (Hobfoll et al., 2007), and may surpass the importance of therapeutic intervention (Silove, Steel, & Psychol, 2006). Often this must take place at the collective level in the context of large-scale programs undertaken by government and nongovernment organizations. For example, public education initiatives, media announcements of safety, leaflets announcing government steps to increase safety and security, web delivery of facts to reduce the common misinformation that is often circulated in the aftermath of large-scale traumas, and, importantly, practical steps to resume normal activities in the community will contribute markedly to an enhanced sense of security. Individuals may also be able to promote a sense of safety by following guidelines such as those outlined in PFA. There is very little evidence regarding the potential efficacy of short-term trauma-focused therapies when threat is ongoing. Intuitively, it seems that such interventions are unlikely to be effective in the case of extreme danger such as ongoing war and regular trauma. However, several studies have suggested that they may be successfully undertaken in settings where there exist significant security concerns (e.g., Neuner et al., 2008, 2010; Neuner, Schauer, Klaschik, Karunakara, & Elbert, 2004). The type of early intervention implemented must thus be carefully matched to the context and driven both by research evidence and local needs.

Collective Effects of Trauma

When trauma occurs in the context of war, genocide, persecution, terrorism, or natural disaster, it is important to recognize the collective impact of these events on communities and populations, and to take these into account when planning early interventions. In some cases, the infrastructure to support relief and intervention efforts may be nonexistent or destroyed. What resources are available may be overwhelmed by the high level of need within the community (Hobfoll et al., 2007). Furthermore, the social, psychological, and spiritual impact of these events on a collective level may be devastating. Much research attests to the importance of the posttrauma environment in facilitating recovery from the mental health effects of these events. A safe, supportive setting with social connectedness provides the optimal environment for recovery (Silove & Bryant, 2006). In the case of mass violence, social and institutional structures that would be generally used to navigate the posttrauma environment may be unavailable. It is for this reason that the reunification of family members (who often act as key providers of mental health care after mass trauma) (de Jong, 2002)) to provide a helpful social environment within which recovery can begin is considered a high priority by many international organizations. This also suggests that individual-level early interventions that are designed in the context of discrete trauma in Western settings may be inadequate to address the impact of traumatic events at the level of the family, community, and population. It may be useful to implement collective interventions in the early aftermath of a traumatic event to facilitate the rebuilding and reconnection of those community and religious structures that may be beneficial throughout the healing process. The promotion of activities developed at a community level including religious and healing activities and rituals may promote a sense of collective efficacy (Hobfoll et al., 2007). Further research should be undertaken to determine the type of interventions that may be useful at a collective level, and to evaluate their efficacy in protecting individuals against the negative effects of trauma.

INNOVATIONS IN EARLY INTERVENTION RESEARCH

There are a number of research innovations in early intervention following traumatic events, focusing on both pharmacological and psychological processes. Both approaches have focused on secondary prevention in the immediate hours/days of the trauma as a means of limiting consolidation of the trauma memory. In terms of the pharmacological approach, one line of research has attempted to reduce noradrenergic activation from consolidating fear conditioning (Cahill, Prins, Weber, & McGaugh, 1994). An initial study found that propranolol, a beta-blocker that reduces adrenergic activation, may limit fear conditioning after trauma; this study found that participants given propanolol evidenced lower reactivity to trauma reminders 3 months after the trauma compared to a placebo condition; however, this did not result in reduced PTSD (Pitman et al., 2002). Another (uncontrolled) study indicated that the administration of propanolol immediately following a traumatic event was related to reduced PTSD after 2 months (Vaiva et al., 2003). Although these research findings are mixed, these studies accord with evidence that factors that diminish arousal shortly after trauma exposure may lessen the subsequent PTSD, including administration of morphine in the immediate hours after trauma (Bryant, Creamer, O'Donnell, Silove, & McFarlane, 2009; Holbrook, Galarneau, Dye, Quinn, & Dougherty, 2010; Sacks et al., 2001).

Other researchers have explored the role of very early administration of cortisol as a secondary prevention strategy. Several studies have observed that patients in medical settings who were administered cortisol developed fewer traumatic memories than those who were not (Schelling et al., 2001, 2004). Animal research has also shown that hydrocortisone given immediately after a stressor results in less displayed anxiety compared to the administration of placebo (Cohen, Matar, Buskila, Kaplan, & Zohar, 2008). A recent pilot randomized controlled trial investigated the impact of administering high-dose hydrocortizone within hours of trauma exposure and found that it resulted in less ASD and later PTSD than placebo (Zohar et al., 2011). Although this evidence is tentative, cortisol administration may serve a useful secondary prevention role.

A novel approach from a psychotherapeutic perspectives involves achieving extinction learning very soon after trauma exposure. This approach emerges from animal evidence that extinction training conducted after an hour of conditioning results in more effective fear reduction than extinction conducted after 72 hours later (Myers, Davis, & Kessler, 2006). Building on this, Rothbaum and colleagues (2012) provided exposure therapy in the emergency room, as well as two subsequent sessions 1 and 2 weeks later. This intervention resulted in greater treatment gains than an assessment-only control condition. This study is interesting for two reasons. First, the finding that participants did not report adverse effects of treatment challenges the notion that exposure therapy is not appropriate immediately after trauma. Second, it raises the possibility, similar to the pharmacological interventions, that by intervening within hours of a traumatic event we may be able to alter the intensity of the fear memory in a more effective manner, and thereby reduce subsequent ASD and PTSD. It is too early to make definitive conclusions about these interventions at this point but they provide promising opportunities that build on established neuroscience foundations.

Other medications that are sometimes prescribed for trauma survivors include low-dosage antipsychotics, mood stabilizers, and medications that reduce arousal by blocking noradrenaline (Pitman et al., 2002; Stanovic, James, & VanDevere, 2001; Vaiva et al., 2003).

SUMMARY AND CLINICAL RECOMMENDATIONS

This chapter has discussed early intervention approaches following exposure to traumatic events that can enhance psychological adaptation. Research evidence indicates that most individuals exposed to trauma exhibit acute distress reactions; however, for the majority, these decrease in the weeks and months following the trauma. It is important that this pattern be encouraged by (1) not interfering with individuals' or communities' natural coping strategies, and (2) minimizing obstacles to implementation of these strategies in the acute phase. A stepped-care method appears to represent a pragmatic approach in the wake of many traumatic events, in which uniform support is provided that facilitates natural recovery, followed by selective and targeted intervention of those who appear to be showing signs of longer-term problems. A problem with many early intervention paradigms that rely on early identification of those at risk is that we currently are not very good at identifying in the acute phase many people who will subsequently develop psychological problems. We also know that after people leave primary care or other settings shortly after trauma exposure, most will avoid mental health services. Accordingly, it is critical to have monitoring procedures in place to track trauma survivors and encourage help-seeking for those in need. In this sense, enhancing resilience involves both promoting resilience at the individual level and developing resilient systems. The latter requires educational, monitoring, assessment, and intervention procedures. Through creative approaches that aim to overcome barriers to care, perhaps future research will demonstrate how we can limit PTSD via secondary prevention.

REFERENCES

Adler, A. B., Litz, B. T., Castro, C. A., Suvak, M., Thomas, J. L., Burrell, L., et al. (2008). A group randomized trial of critical incident stress debriefing provided to U.S. peacekeepers. *Journal of Traumatic Stress, 21,* 253–263.

Aguilera, A., Garza, M. J., & Muñoz, R. F. (2010). Group cognitive-behavioral therapy for depression in Spanish: Culture-sensitive manualized treatment in practice. *Journal of Clinical Psychology, 66,* 857–867.

American Psychiatric Association. (1994). *Diagnostic and statistical manual of mental disorders* (4th ed.). Washington, DC: Author.

American Psychiatric Association. (2013). *Diagnostic and statistical manual of mental disorders* (5th ed.). Arlington, VA: Author

Andreasen, N. C. (2004). Acute and delayed posttraumatic stress disorders: A history and some issues. *American Journal of Psychiatry, 161,* 1321–1323.

Andrews, B., Brewin, C. R., Philpott, R., & Stewart, L. (2007). Delayed-onset posttraumatic stress disorder: A systematic review of the evidence. *Amercian Journal of Psychiatry, 164,* 1319–1326.

Ballenger, J. C., Davidson, J. R., Lecrubier, Y., Nutt, D. J., Marshall, R. D., Nemeroff, C. B., et al. (2004). Consensus statement update on posttraumatic stress disorder from the International Consensus Group on Depression and Anxiety. *Journal of Clinical Psychiatry, 65*(Suppl.), 55–62.

Benight, C. C., Cieslak, R., Molton, I. R., & Johnson, L. E. (2008). Self-evaluative appraisals of coping capability and posttraumatic distress following motor vehicle accidents. *Journal of Consulting and Clinical Psychology, 76,* 677–685.

Benight, C. C., & Harper, M. L. (2002). Coping self-efficacy perceptions as a mediator between acute stress response and long-term distress following natural disasters. *Journal of Traumatic Stress, 15,* 177–186.

Bisson, J., & Andrew, M. (2007). Psychological treatment of post-traumatic stress disorder (PTSD). *Cochrane Database Systematic Reviews,* Issue 3 (Article No. CD003388), DOI: 10.1002/14651858.CD003388.pub3.

Bisson, J. I., Jenkins, P. L., Alexander, J., & Bannister, C. (1997). Randomised controlled trial of psychological debriefing for victims of acute burn trauma. *British Journal of Psychiatry, 171,* 78–81.

Bisson, J. I., & Kitchiner, N. J. (2003). Early psychosocial and pharmacological interventions after traumatic events. *Journal of Psychosocial Nursing and Mental Health Services, 41,* 42–51.

Bisson, J. I., Shepherd, J. P., Joy, D., Probert, R., & Newcombe, R. G. (2004). Early cognitive-behavioural therapy for post-traumatic stress symptoms after physical injury: Randomised controlled trial. *British Journal of Psychiatry, 184*(Suppl.), 63–69.

Bleich, A., Gelkopf, M., & Solomon, Z. (2003). Exposure to terrorism, stress-related mental health symptoms, and coping behaviors among a nationally representative sample in Israel. *Journal of the American Medical Association, 290,* 612–620.

Breslau, N., Kessler, R. C., Chilcoat, H. D., Schultz, L. R., Davis, G. C., & Andreski, P. (1998). Trauma and posttraumatic stress disorder in the community: The 1996 Detroit Area Survey of Trauma. *Archives of General Psychiatry, 55,* 626–632.

Bryant, R. A. (2004). Acute stress disorder: Course, epidemiology, assessment, and treatment. In B. T. Litz (Ed.), *Early intervention for trauma and traumatic loss* (pp. 15–33). New York: Guilford Press.

Bryant, R. A. (2007a). Does dissociation further our understanding of PTSD? *Journal of Anxiety Disorders, 21,* 183–191.

Bryant, R. A. (2007b). Early intervention for post-traumatic stress disorder. *Early Intervention in Psychiatry, 1,* 19–26.

Bryant, R. A. (2011). Acute stress disorder as a predictor of posttraumatic stress disorder: A systematic review. *Journal of Clinical Psychiatry, 72,* 233–239.

Bryant, R. A., Creamer, M., O'Donnell, M., Silove, D., & McFarlane, A. C. (2008). A multisite study of initial respiration rate and heart rate as predictors of post-traumatic stress disorder. *Journal of Clinical Psychiatry, 69,* 1694–1701.

Bryant, R. A., Creamer, M., O'Donnell, M., Silove, D., & McFarlane, A. C. (2009). A study of the protective function of acute morphine administration on subsequent posttraumatic stress disorder. *Biological Psychiatry, 65,* 438–440.

Bryant, R. A., Friedman, M.J., Spiegel, D., Ursano, R., & Strain, J. (2011). A review of acute stress disorder in DSM-V. *Depression and Anxiety, 28,* 802–817.

Bryant, R. A., & Harvey, A. G. (2002). Delayed-onset posttraumatic stress disorder: A prospective evaluation. *Australian and New Zealand Journal of Psychiatry, 3,* 205–209.

Bryant, R. A., Harvey, A. G., Dang, S. T., Sackville, T., & Basten, C. (1998). Treatment of acute stress disorder: A comparison of cognitive-behavioral therapy and supportive counseling. *Journal of Consulting and Clinical Psychology,* 66, 862–866.

Bryant, R. A., Harvey, A. G., Guthrie, R. M., & Moulds, M. L. (2000). A prospective study of psychophysiological arousal, acute stress disorder, and posttraumatic stress disorder. *Journal of Abnormal Psychology, 109,* 341–344.

Bryant, R. A., Mastrodomenico, J., Felmingham, K. L., Hopwood, S., Kenny, L., Kandris, E., et al. (2008). Treatment of acute stress disorder: A randomized controlled trial. *Archives of General Psychiatry, 65,* 659–667.

Bryant, R. A., Moulds, M., Guthrie, R., & Nixon, R. D. (2003). Treating acute stress disorder following mild traumatic brain injury. *American Journal of Psychiatry, 160,* 585–587.

Bryant, R. A., & Panasetis, P. (2001). Panic symptoms during trauma and acute stress disorder. *Behaviour Research and Therapy, 39,* 961–966.

Bryant, R. A., Sackville, T., Dang, S. T., Moulds, M., & Guthrie, R. (1999). Treating acute stress disorder: An evaluation of cognitive behavior therapy and supportive counseling techniques. *American Journal of Psychiatry, 156,* 1780–1786.

Brymer, M., Layne, C., Pynoos, R., Ruzek, J. I., Steinberg, A., Vernberg, E., et al. (2006). *Psychological first aid; Field operations guide.* Washington, DC: U.S. Department of Health and Human Services.

Cahill, L., Prins, B., Weber, M., & McGaugh, J.L. (1994). ß-adrenergic activation and memory for emotional events. *Nature, 371,* 702–704.

Carlier, I. V., Voerman, A. E., & Gersons, B. P. (2000). The influence of occupational debriefing on post-traumatic stress symptomatology in traumatized police officers. *British Journal of Medical Psychology, 73*(Pt. 1), 87–98.

Carver, C. S., & Scheier, M. R. (1998). *On the self-regulation of behavior.* New York: Cambridge University Press.

Cloitre, M., Stolbach, B. C., Herman, J. L., van der Kolk, B., Pynoos, R., Wang, J., et al. (2009). A developmental approach to complex PTSD: Childhood and adult cumulative trauma as predictors of symptom complexity. *Journal of Traumatic Stress, 22,* 399–408.

Cohen, H., Matar, M. A., Buskila, D., Kaplan, Z., & Zohar, J. (2008). Early poststressor intervention with high-dose corticosterone attenuates posttraumatic stress response in an animal model of posttraumatic stress disorder. *Biological Psychiatry, 64,* 708–717.

Crawford, T. A., & Lipsedge, M. (2004). Seeking help for psychological distress: The interface of Zulu traditional healing and Western biomedicine. *Mental Health, Religion and Culture, 7,* 131–148.

de Jong, J. T. (2002). Public mental health, traumatic stress and human rights violations in low-income countries: A culturally appropriate model in times of conflict, disaster and peace. In J. de Jong (Ed.), *Trauma, war, and violence: Public mental health in socio-cultural context* (pp. 1–91). New York: Kluwer Academic/Plenum.

de Jong, J. T., Komproe, I. H., Van Ommeren, M., El Masri, M., Araya, M., Khaled, N., et al. (2001). Lifetime events and posttraumatic stress disorder in 4 postconflict settings. *Journal of the American Medical Association, 286,* 555–562.

de Jong, K., Mulhern, M., Ford, N., van der Kam, S., & Kleber, R. (2000). The trauma of war in Sierra Leone. *Lancet, 355,* 2067–2068.

Ehlers, A., & Clark, D. M. (2003). Early psychological interventions for adult survivors of trauma: A review. *Biological Psychiatry, 53*, 817–826.

Ehlers, A., Clark, D. M., Dunmore, E., Jaycox, L., Meadows, E., & Foa, E. B. (1998). Predicting response to exposure treatment in PTSD: The role of mental defeat and alienation. *Journal of Traumatic Stress, 11*, 457–471.

Ehring, T., & Quack, D. (2010). Emotion regulation difficulties in trauma survivors: The role of trauma type and PTSD symptom severity. *Behavior Therapy, 41*, 587–598.

Eisenbruch, M., de Jong, J. T., & van de Put, W. (2004). Bringing order out of chaos: A culturally competent approach to managing the problems of refugees and victims of organized violence. *Journal of Traumatic Stress, 17*, 123–131.

Everly, G. S. Jr., & Boyle, S. H. (1999). Critical incident stress debriefing (CISD): A meta-analysis. *International Journal of Emergency Mental Health, 1*, 165–168.

Foa, E. B., Keane, T. M., Friedman, M. J., & Cohen, J. A. (Eds.). (2009). *Effective treatments for PTSD: Practice guidelines from the International Society of Traumatic Stress Studies* (2nd ed.). New York: Guilford Press.

Galea, S., Ahern, J., Resnick, H., Kilpatrick, D., Buculvalas, M., Gold, J., et al. (2002). Psychological sequelae of the September 11 terrorist attacks in New York City. *New England Journal of Medicine, 346*, 982–987.

Gelpin, E., Bonne, O., Peri, T., Brandes, D., & Shalev, A. Y. (1996). Treatment of recent trauma survivors with benzodiazepines: A prospective study. *Journal of Clincial Psychiatry, 57*, 390–394.

Grieger, T. A., Fullerton, C. S., & Ursano, R. J. (2003). Posttraumatic stress disorder, alcohol use, and perceived safety after the terrorist attack on the Pentagon. *Psychiatric Services, 54*, 1380–1382.

Grossman, A. B., Levin, B. E., Katzen, H. L., & Lechner, S. (2004). PTSD symptoms and onset of neurologic disease in elderly trauma survivors. *Journal of Clinical Experimental Neuropsychology, 26*, 698–705.

Harvey, A. G., & Bryant, R. A. (1998). The relationship between acute stress disorder and posttraumatic stress disorder: A prospective evaluation of motor vehicle accident survivors. *Journal of Consulting and Clinical Psychology, 66*, 507–512.

Harvey, A. G., & Bryant, R. A. (1999). The relationship between acute stress disorder and posttraumatic stress disorder: A 2-year prospective evaluation. *Journal of Consulting and Clinical Psychology, 67*, 985–988.

Hinton, D. E., & Otto, M. (2006). Symptom presentation and symptom meaning among traumatized Cambodian refugees: Relevance to a somatically focused cognitive behavior therapy. *Cognitive and Behavioral Practice, 13*, 249–260.

Hinton, D. E., Pich, V., Chhean, D., Safren, S. A., & Pollack, M. H. (2006). Somatic-focused therapy for traumatized refugees: Treating posttraumatic stress disorder and comorbid neck-focused panic attacks among Cambodian refugees. *Psychotherapy: Theory, Research, Practice, Training, 43*, 491–505.

Hobfoll, S. E., Watson, P., Bell, C. C., Bryant, R. A., Brymer, M. J., Friedman, M. J., et al. (2007). Five essential elements of immediate and mid-term mass trauma intervention: Empirical evidence. *Psychiatry, 70*, 283–315.

Holbrook, T. L., Galarneau, M. R., Dye, J. L., Quinn, K., & Dougherty, A. L.

(2010). Morphine use after combat injury in Iraq and post-traumatic stress disorder. *New England Journal of Medicine, 362*(2), 110–117.

Horowitz, M. J., & Solomon, G. F. (1975). A prediction of delayed stress response syndromes in Vietnam veterans. *Journal of Social Issues, 31*, 67–80.

Inter-Agency Steering Committee. (2007). *IASC guidelines on mental health and psychosocial support in emergency settings.* Geneva: Author.

Jacobs, J., Horne-Moyer, H. L., & Jones, R. (2004). The effectiveness of critical incident stress debriefing with primary and secondary trauma victims. *International Journal of Emergency Mental Health, 6*, 5–14.

Kessler, R. C., Galea, S., Gruber, M. J., Sampson, N. A., Ursano, R. J., & Wessely, S. (2008). Trends in mental illness and suicidality after Hurricane Katrina. *Molecular Psychiatry, 13*, 374–384.

Kessler, R. C., Sonnega, A., Bromet, E., Hughes, M., & Nelson, C. B. (1995). Post-traumatic stress disorder in the National Comorbidity Survey. *Archives of General Psychiatry, 52*, 1048–1060.

Kleinman, A. (1988). *Rethinking psychiatry: From cultural category to personal experience.* New York: Free Press.

Litz, B. T. (2008). Early intervention for trauma: Where are we and where do we need to go? A commentary. *Journal of Traumatic Stress, 21*, 503–506.

Litz, B. T., & Gray, M. J. (2002). Early intervention for mass violence: What is the evidence? What should be done? *Cognitive and Behavioral Practice, 9*, 266–272.

Marchand, A., Guay, S., Boyer, R., Iucci, S., Martin, A., & St.-Hilaire, M. H. (2006). A randomized controlled trial of an adapted form of critical incident stress debriefing for victims of an armed robbery. *Brief Treatment and Crisis Intervention, 6*, 122–129.

Mayou, R. A., Ehlers, A., & Hobbs, M. (2000). Psychological debriefing for road traffic accident victims. Three-year follow-up of a randomised controlled trial. *British Journal of Psychiatry, 176*, 589–593.

McNally, R. J., Bryant, R. A., & Ehlers, A. (2003). Does early psychological intervention promote recovery from posttraumatic stress? *Psychological Science in the Public Interest, 4*, 45–79.

Mitchell, J. T. (1983). When disaster strikes . . . the critical incident stress debriefing process. *Journal of Emergency Medical Services, 8*, 36–39.

Mitchell, J. T., & Everly, G. S. Jr. (1995). Critical incident stress management: A new era in crisis inervention. *ESTSS Bulletin, 12*, 3–7.

Myers, K. M., Ressler, K. J., & Davis, M. (2006). Different mechanisms of fear extinction dependent on length of time since fear acquisition. *Learning and Memory, 13*(2), 216–223.

National Health and Medical Research Council. (2007). *The Australian Guidelines for the Treatment of ASD and PTSD.* East Melbourne, Victoria, Australia: Author. Available at *http://guidelines.acpmh.unimelb.edu.au.*

National Institute of Clinical Excellence. (2005). *Post-traumatic stress disorder (PTSD): The management of PTSD in adults and children in primary and secondary care.* London: Author. Available at *http://publications.nice.org. uk/post-traumatic-stress-disorder-ptsd-cg26.*

Neria, Y., Solomon, Z., Ginzburg, K., & Dekel, R. (2000). Sensation seeking, wartime performance, and long-term adjustment among Israeli war veterans. *Personality and Individual Differences, 29,* 921–932.

Neria, Y., Solomon, Z., Ginzburg, K., Dekel, R., Enoch, D., & Ohry, A. (2000). Posttraumatic residues of captivity: A follow-up of Israeli ex-prisoners of war. *Journal of Clinical Psychiatry, 61,* 39–46.

Neuner, F., Kurreck, S., Ruf, M., Odenwald, M., Elbert, T., & Schauer, M. (2010). Can asylum-seekers with posttraumatic stress disorder be successfully treated?: A randomized controlled pilot study. *Cognitive Behaviour Therapy, 39,* 81–91.

Neuner, F., Onyut, P. L., Ertl, V., Odenwald, M., Schauer, E., & Elbert, T. (2008). Treatment of posttraumatic stress disorder by trained lay counselors in an African refugee settlement: A randomized controlled trial. *Journal of Consulting and Clinical Psychology, 76,* 686–694.

Neuner, F., Schauer, M., Klaschik, C., Karunakara, U., & Elbert, T. (2004). A comparison of narrative exposure therapy, supportive counseling, and psycheducation for treating posttraumatic stress disorder in an African refugee settlement. *Journal of Consulting and Clinical Psychology, 72,* 579–587.

Norris, F. H., Friedman, M. J., & Watson, P. J. (2002). 60,000 disaster victims speak: Part II. Summary and implications of the disaster mental health research. *Psychiatry, 65,* 240–260.

Nurmi, L. A. (1999). The sinking of the *Estonia*: The effects of critical incident stress debriefing (CISD) on rescuers. *International Journal of Emergency Mental Health, 1,* 23–31.

O'Donnell, M. L., Creamer, M. C., Parslow, R., Elliott, P., Holmes, A. C., Ellen, S., et al. (2008). A predictive screening index for posttraumatic stress disorder and depression following traumatic injury. *Journal of Consulting and Clinical Psychology, 76,* 923–932.

Pitman, R. K., Sanders, K. M., Zusman, R. M., Healy, A. R., Cheema, F., Lasko, N. B., et al. (2002). Pilot study of secondary prevention of posttraumatic stress disorder with propanolol. *Biological Psychiatry, 51,* 189–192.

Ponniah, K., & Hollon, S. D. (2008). Empirically supported psychological interventions for social phobia in adults: A qualitative review of randomized controlled trials. *Psychological Medicine, 38,* 3–14.

Porter, M., & Haslam, N. (2005). Predisplacement and postdisplacement factors associated with mental health of refugees and internally displaced persons: A meta-analysis. *Journal of the American Medical Association, 294,* 602–612.

Pupavac, V. (2001). Therapeutic governance: Psycho-social intervention and trauma risk management. *Disasters, 25,* 358–372.

Raphael, B. (1977). The Granville train disaster: Psychological needs and their management. *Medical Journal of Australia, 1,* 303–305.

Riggs, D. S., Rothbaum, B. O., & Foa, E. B. (1995). A prospective examination of symptoms of posttraumatic stress disorder in victims of nonsexual assault. *Journal of Interpersonal Violence, 10,* 201–214.

Robert, R., Blakeney, P. E., Villarreal, C., Rosenberg, L., & Meyer, W. J. (1999). Imipramine treatment in pediatric burn patietns with symptoms of acute stress disorder: A pilot study. *Journal of the American Academy of Child and Adolescent Psychiatry, 38,* 873–882.

Rose, S. C., Bisson, J., Churchill, R., & Wessely, S. (2001). Psychological debriefing for preventing post traumatic stress disorder (PTSD). *Cochrane Database of Systematic Reviews,* Issue 3 (Article No. CD000560), DOI: 10.1002/14651858.CD000560.

Rothbaum, B. O., Foa, E. B., Riggs, D. S., Murdock, T., & Walsh, W. (1992). A prospective examination of post-traumatic stress disorder in rape victims. *Journal of Traumatic Stress, 5,* 455–475.

Rothbaum, B. O., Kearns, M.C., Price, M., Malcoun, E., Davis, M., Ressler, K. J., et al. (2012). Early intervention may prevent the development of posttraumatic stress disorder: A randomized pilot civilian study with modified prolonged exposure. *Archives of General Psychiatry, 72,* 957–963.

Saarni, H., Saari, S., & Hakkinen, U. (1999). Critical incident stress debriefing (CISD) in a shipping company. *International Maritime Health, 50,* 49–56.

Sacks, S. B., Clements, P. T., & Fay-Hillier, T. (2001). Care after chaos: Use of critical incident stress debriefing after traumatic workplace events. *Perspectives of Psychiatric Care, 37,* 133–136.

Schelling, G., Briegel, J., Roozendaal, B., Stoll, C., Rothenhausler, H. B., & Kapfhammer, H. P. (2001). The effect of stress doses of hydrocortisone during septic shock on posttraumatic stress disorder in survivors. *Biological Psychiatry, 50,* 978–985.

Schelling, G., Kilger, E., Roozendaal, B., de Quervain, D. J., Briegel, J., Dagge, A., et al. (2004). Stress doses of hydrocortisone, traumatic memories, and symptoms of posttraumatic stress disorder in patients after cardiac surgery: A randomized study. *Biological Psychiatry, 55,* 627–633.

Shalev, A. Y. (2002). Acute stress reactions in adults. *Biological Psychiatry, 51,* 532–543.

Shalev, A. Y., Ankri, Y., Israeli-Shalev, Y., Peleg, T., Adessky, R., & Freedman, S. (2012). Prevention of posttraumatic stress disorder by early treatment: Results from the Jerusalem Trauma Outreach and Prevention Study. *Archives of General Psychiatry, 69,* 166–176.

Shalev, A. Y., Freedman, S., Peri, T., Brandes, D., Sahar, T., Orr, S. P., et al. (1998). Prospective study of posttraumatic stress disorder and depression following trauma. *American Journal of Psychiatry, 155,* 630–637.

Shalev, A. Y., Sahar, T., Freedman, S., Peri, T., Glick, N., Brandes, D., et al. (1998). A prospective study of heart rate response following trauma and the subsequent development of posttraumatic stress disorder. *Archives of General Psychiatry, 55,* 553–559.

Shankar, B. R., Saravanan, B., & Jacob, K. S. (2006). Explanatory models of common mental disorders among traditional healers and their patients in rural south India. *International Journal of Social Psychiatry, 52,* 221–233.

Sijbrandij, M., Olff, M., Reitsma, J. B., Carlier, I. V., de Vries, M. H., & Gersons, B. P. (2007). Treatment of acute posttraumatic stress disorder with brief cognitive behavioral therapy: A randomized controlled trial. *American Journal of Psychiatry, 164,* 82–90.

Silove, D. (2005). The best immediate therapy for acute stress is social. *Bulletin of the World Health Organization, 83,* 75–76.

Silove, D., & Bryant, R. A. (2006). Rapid assessments of mental health needs after disasters. *Journal of the American Medical Association, 296,* 576–578.

Silove, D., Steel, Z., & Psychol, M. (2006). Understanding community psychosocial needs after disasters: Implications for mental health services. *Journal of Postgraduate Medicine, 52*, 121–125.

Simms-Ellis, R., & Madill, A. (2001). Financial services employees' experience of peer-led and clinician-led critical incident stress debriefing following armed robberies. *International Journal of Emergency Mental Health, 3*, 219–228.

Small, R., Lumley, J., Donohue, L., Potter, A., & Waldenstrom, U. (2000). Randomised controlled trial of midwife led debriefing to reduce maternal depression after operative childbirth. *British Medical Journal, 321*, 1043–1047.

Stanovic, J. K., James, K. A., & VanDevere, C. A. (2001). The effectiveness of risperidone on acute stress symptoms in adult burn patients: A preliminary retrospective pilot study. *Journal of Burns Care and Rehabilitation, 22*, 210–213.

Steel, Z., Chey, T., Silove, D., Marnane, C., Bryant, R. A., & van Ommeren, M. (2009). Association of torture and other potentially traumatic events with mental health outcomes among populations exposed to mass conflict and displacement: A systematic review and meta-analysis. *Journal of the American Medical Association, 302*, 537–549.

Townsend, C. J., & Loughlin, J. M. (1998). Critical incident stress debriefing in international aid workers. *Journal of Travel Medicine, 5*, 226–227.

Vaiva, G., Ducrocq, F., Jezequel, K., Averland, B., Lestavel, P., Brunet, A., et al. (2003). Immediate treatment with propanolol decreases posttrauamtic stress disorder two months after trauma. *Biological Psychiatry, 51*, 189–192.

Vaiva, G., Thomas, P., Ducrocq, F., Fontaine, M., Boss, V., Devos, P., et al. (2004). Low posttrauma GABA plasma levels as a predictive factor in the development of acute posttraumatic stress disorder. *Biological Psychiatry, 55*, 250–254.

van Emmerik, A. A. P., Kamphuis, J. H., & Emmelkamp, P. M. G. (2008). Treating acute stress disorder and posttraumatic stress disorder with cognitive behavioral therapy or structured writing therapy: A randomized controlled trial. *Psychotherapy and Psychosomatics, 77*, 93–100.

van Emmerik, A. A. P., Kamphuis, J. H., Hulsbosch, A. M., & Emmelkamp, P. M. G. (2002). Single session debriefing after psychological trauma: A meta-analysis. *Lancet, 360*, 766–771.

van Ommeren, M., Saxena, S., & Saraceno, B. (2005). Mental and social health during and after acute emergencies: Emerging consensus? *Bulletin of the World Health Organization, 83*, 71–75.

Wee, D. F., Mills, D. M., & Koehler, G. (1999). The effects of critical incident stress debriefing (CISD) on emergency medical services personnel following the Los Angeles civil disturbance. *International Journal of Emergency Mental Health, 1*, 33–37.

Zohar, J., Yahalom, H., Kozlovsky, N., Cwikel-Hamzany, S., Matar, M. A., Kaplan, Z., et al. (2011). High dose hydrocortisone immediately after trauma may alter the trajectory of PTSD: Interplay between clinical and animal studies. *European Neuropsychopharmacology, 21*, 796–809.

Chapter 3

Therapeutic Recovery

Edna B. Foa *and* Carmen P. McLean

Several cognitive-behavioral therapy (CBT) interventions for post-traumatic stress disorder (PTSD) have received empirical support, including prolonged exposure (PE; e.g., Foa, Dancu, et al., 1999, 2005; Powers, Halpern, Ferenschak, Gillihan, & Foa, 2010; Schnurr et al., 2007) therapy, cognitive processing therapy (CPT; Chard, 2005; Monson et al., 2006; Resick et al., 2008; Resick, Nishith, Weaver, Astin, & Feuer, 2002), cognitive therapy (e.g., Ehlers et al., 2003), and stress inoculation training (SIT; e.g., Foa, Dancu, et al., 1999). Eye movement desensitization retraining for PTSD has also been evaluated (e.g., Rothbaum, Astin, & Marsteller, 2005). Of these treatments, PE (Foa, Hembree, & Rothbaum, 2007) and CPT (Resick & Schnicke, 1993) are specifically recommended in the Veterans Administration (VA)/Department of Defense Clinical Practice Guidelines for PTSD at the highest level. PE is a specific exposure therapy program for PTSD that is comprised of two main components: *in vivo* exposure to trauma reminders and imaginal exposure to the memory of the traumatic event (revisiting), with processing of the revisiting experience. CPT is comprised of three core components: psychoeducation, written exposure, and cognitive therapy, and is designed to challenge maladaptive thoughts and feelings that prevent trauma survivors from coming to terms with their trauma experience. Because PE and CPT have demonstrated efficacy in a number of randomized controlled trials, we focus our discussion of therapeutic recovery on the underlying principles associated with these two treatments.

Although CBTs tested in clinical trials are effective in significantly reducing PTSD symptoms in the majority of patients, some do not benefit from treatment and others continue to experience residual symptoms (Bradley, Greene, Russ, Dutra, & Westen, 2005). Research attempting to delineate who will benefit from CBT and who will not has been disappointing, with different studies often finding different predictors (e.g., Hembree, Marshall, Fitzgibbons, & Foa, 2001; Iverson, Resick, Suvak, Walling, & Taft, 2011; Taylor et al., 2001; van Minnen, Arntz, & Keijsers, 2002). This is problematic because the lack of reliable predictors of better and worse outcomes prevents us from identifying who is a good candidate for a given treatment and who should receive an alternative or augmented treatment.

In this chapter, we summarize research on therapeutic recovery from PTSD and provide an overview of the factors that moderate or mediate therapeutic recovery. We start by describing broad principles found to be associated with therapeutic recovery and examine patterns of change during treatment. We then review factors that predict treatment outcome, dropout, and adherence, as well as factors that were found to be unrelated to outcome despite clinical lore about their impediment to recovery.

PROCESSES OF THERAPEUTIC RECOVERY

In their review of theories of PTSD, Cahill and Foa (2007) remind us that adequate theories of psychopathology, including PTSD, must address three key components: (1) the psychopathology of PTSD, including specific symptoms and associated features (e.g., trauma-related cognitions about the dangerous nature of the world and the incompetence of the self); (2) the natural course of posttrauma reactions, including why some people recover adequately while others do not; and (3) the demonstrated efficacy of several CBT programs in treating PTSD and associated symptoms (e.g., depression, generalized anxiety, guilt). Theories of PTSD that address at least some of the above criteria include conditioning theories (e.g., Keane, Zimering, & Caddell, 1985; Kilpatrick, Veronen, & Best, 1985), schema theories (e.g., Epstein, 1991; Horowitz, 1976, 1986; Janoff-Bulman, 1992; McCann & Pearlman, 1990), cognitive theory (e.g., Ehlers & Clark, 2000), emotional processing theory (EPT; Foa & Kozak, 1985, 1986), and multirepresentational theories, such as dual-representation theory (Brewin, Dalgleish, & Joseph, 1996; Brewin & Holmes, 2003) and the SPAARS model (Dalgleish, 1999, 2004). By emphasizing different psychological processes each of these theories has contributed to our understanding of PTSD development and recovery. For example, cognitive theories emphasize a reciprocal relationship between the trauma memory and appraisals of the trauma, and therefore cognitive therapy uses cognitive procedures to modify negative appraisals. Conditioning theories, in contrast, rely on principles of classical and operant conditioning to explain the development and maintenance of

PTSD, and therefore emphasize the role of exposure in modifying erroneous associations. Because EPT integrates concepts from contemporary learning models, information-processing models, and cognitive theories, it constitutes a particularly useful framework for discussing the mechanisms of therapeutic recovery in CBT.

EPT posits that fear is represented in memory as a cognitive structure that includes representations of the fear stimuli, fear responses, and their meaning; the structure is activated when a person is presented with information that matches the representations in the structure (Foa & Kozak, 1985, 1986). In a normal fear structure, the associations between the stimuli, responses, and meaning representations represent reality accurately (e.g., a battlefield is dangerous). In this context, activation of the fear structure would be adaptive, as it would promote self-protection. In contrast, a fear structure is pathological when the associations among its representations are erroneous (e.g., crowded supermarkets are dangerous). To explain PTSD, EPT posits that the traumatic memory is represented as a specific pathological fear structure that includes erroneous associations among representations of stimuli that occurred during and after the trauma, responses that occurred during the trauma, and their meaning.

A unique strength of EPT is that it employs the same mechanisms to explain both natural and therapeutic recovery (Cahill & Foa, 2007): activation of the fear structure and presentation of information that disconfirms the pathological elements in the structure. Accordingly, natural recovery following trauma occurs when the person confronts trauma-related thoughts and feelings, shares his or her experiences and reactions with others, and approaches trauma reminders in daily life. In contrast, those who avoid trauma-related stimuli, memories, thoughts, and feelings are at risk of developing PTSD because avoidance prevents the activation of the fear structure and confrontation with information that disconfirms the expected harm (e.g., being in crowded places and not being attacked) (Foa, Huppert, & Cahill, 2006). According to EPT, one of the goals is to help PTSD sufferers confront traumatic reminders and correct their erroneous cognitions. Consistent with EPT and other theoretical models of PTSD, the following empirically supported processes have been identified as playing an important role in both natural and therapeutic recovery: (1) emotional engagement (i.e., activation of the trauma memory); (2) habituation; (3) organization and elaboration of the trauma memory; and (4) changes in erroneous cognitions. We will examine each of these processes in turn and provide evidence for their relevance to therapeutic recovery.

Emotional Engagement

EPT as well as cognitive models of PTSD emphasize the role of emotional engagement in recovery. Specifically, as noted above, EPT posits that the fear structure must be activated in order to be modified. Similarly, Ehlers and Clark (2000) propose that reliving the trauma is necessary in order to identify idiosyncratic appraisals of the trauma and to facilitate elaboration (i.e., associations with thematically and temporally related experiences) and contextualization (i.e., integration into the context of preceding and subsequent experience) of the trauma memory. One technique to evoke emotional engagement is exposure, *in vivo* or imaginal, to trauma-related stimuli. *In vivo* exposure refers to real-life confrontation with feared, but objectively safe stimuli. Imaginal exposure typically includes revisiting and recounting the traumatic event including details about the event as well as associated thoughts, feelings, and physical sensations. Studies of PE suggest that indicators of emotional engagement such as facial fear expression (Foa, Riggs, Massie, & Yarczower, 1995) during the first session of imaginal exposure as well as peak anxiety ratings during imaginal exposure (Rauch, Foa, Furr, & Filip, 2004) are positively associated with treatment outcome. Conversely, factors that interfere with emotional engagement such as anger (Foa, Riggs, et al., 1995) and the use of benzodiazepines (van Minnen et al., 2002) hinder recovery. Thus, fostering appropriate emotional engagement is an important task for therapists providing CBT for PTSD. For example, in PE, standard procedures such as asking the patient to close his or her eyes and use the present tense when recounting the trauma narrative are used to promote access of an emotional connection to the trauma memory.

Habituation

EPT suggests that the gradual reduction (or habituation) of anxiety within and between exposure sessions are indicators of emotional processing, which is the mechanism underlying recovery. Foa and Jaycox (1999) proposed that habituation constitutes information that disconfirms patients' erroneous expectations that anxiety during exposure will persist indefinitely and they will "fall apart." Although reported fear typically declines from the beginning to the end of an exposure session, the role of within-session habituation in treatment outcomes has not been well supported in PTSD treatment research or the broader exposure therapy literature (see Craske et al., 2008, for a review). In contrast, evidence from several studies suggests that between-session habituation is associated with therapeutic recovery (Pitman, Orr, Altman, & Longpre, 1996a; Pitman et al., 1996b; Rauch et al., 2004; van Minnen & Foa, 2006; van Minnen & Hagenaars, 2002). Using cluster analysis, Jaycox, Foa, and Morral (1998) examined patterns of distress among female assault victims during PE. Three distinct patterns were observed: (1) patients exhibiting high distress in the first session, and a gradual decline in distress over subsequent sessions; (2) patients exhibiting high distress in the first session and no habituation across sessions; and (3) patients exhibiting moderate distress in the first session and no change across sessions. Patients in the first group showed superior posttreatment gains to those in both the second and third groups, supporting EPT's proposition that both emotional engagement and habituation are involved in recovery. Thus, while within-session reductions in fear are no longer considered critical for improvement (Foa et al., 2006), habituation across therapy appears to be important for treatment success.

Organization and Elaboration of the Trauma Memory

Foa and Riggs (1993) proposed that memories of traumatic events are more disorganized and fragmented than memories of nontraumatic events and that the trauma memories of victims with PTSD are especially disorganized and fragmented. A similar view was advanced by Ehlers and Clark (2000). In support of this proposition, Amir, Stafford, Freshman, and Foa (1998) found a significant relationship between organization and articulation of rape narratives and PTSD severity such that patients with more articulated narratives reported significantly lower PTSD severity. Accordingly, EPT proposes that therapeutic recovery involves organization and elaboration of the trauma memory (Foa & Jacox, 1999). Two treatment outcome studies have found evidence in support for this hypothesis. Foa, Molnar, and Cashman (1995) devised a qualitative coding system to compare the rape narrative from patients' first and last session of exposure therapy. They found that narratives at the end of treatment were longer, had lower percentages of actions and dialogues, and higher percentages of organized thoughts. Importantly, the degree of reduction in fragmentation and increase in organization from pre- to posttreatment were highly correlated with reduced PTSD and depression symptoms. Replicating the design of Foa and colleagues' (1995) study, van Minnen and colleagues (2002) found a decrease in references to external events (*actions* and *dialogues* plus details) and an increase in *thoughts* and *feelings* in trauma narratives from pre- to posttreatment; they also found a significant decrease in *disorganized thoughts*, supporting Foa and colleagues' findings that organization in trauma narratives is associated with positive outcome. No other studies have assessed the organization and elaboration of trauma memories before and after treatment. However, several studies have shown that trauma narratives are more disorganized among those with PTSD than those without PTSD (e.g., Halligan, Michael, Clark, & Ehlers, 2003; Jones, Harvey, & Brewin, 2007), while other studies have not found differences in trauma narrative organization (e.g., Gray & Lombardo, 2001). Discrepant results are likely the result of operationalizing organization and elaboration differently across studies (O'Kearney & Perrott, 2006).

Ehlers and Clark (2000), in their cognitive theory of PTSD, also suggest that poor contextualization and elaboration of traumatic memories within the autobiographical memory base contributes to overall PTSD severity and especially to reexperiencing symptoms. Thus, a key aim of

cognitive therapy (CT) for PTSD is to help patients create a coherent narrative of the trauma. There are three primary treatment techniques used in
CT that are designed to foster trauma narrative elaboration: writing out a
detailed account of the event, imaginal reliving of the event, and revisiting
the site of the trauma (Ehlers, Clark, Hackmann, McManus, & Fennell,
2005). While the therapeutic function of these techniques is similar to techniques used in PE, the emphasis in CT is on identifying "hot spots" (i.e.,
moments of greatest distress in the trauma) that can then be evaluated and
challenged through cognitive restructuring (CR).

Changes in Erroneous Cognitions

Several schools of thought propose that traumatic events profoundly alter
one's view of him- or herself, others, and the world. Beginning with schema
theories of trauma sequela (e.g., Epstein, 1991; Horowitz, 1976, 1986;
Janoff-Bulman, 1992; McCann & Pearlman, 1990) traumatic events are
thought to result in negative thoughts about self, others, and the world.
Although schema theories imply that trauma survivors acquire these negative beliefs, they do not attempt to explain the development of specific
posttraumatic psychopathology. Nevertheless, they influenced contemporary theories of PTSD such as EPT and cognitive theory of PTSD (e.g., Foa
& Riggs, 1993; Resick & Schnicke, 1993). EPT, for example, proposes
that PTSD symptoms are maintained, in part, by dysfunctional, unrealistic
perceptions that the world is *entirely* dangerous and the victim is *entirely*
incompetent. Accordingly, therapeutic recovery from PTSD involves correcting these negative trauma-related perceptions.

Results from several studies support the hypothesis that CBT for
PTSD is associated with changes in world and self-perceptions. Foa and
Rauch (2004) reported that following 9–12 weekly sessions of PE with and
without CR, female assault survivors showed significant and lasting reductions in negative cognitions about the self and the world, as measured by
the Posttraumatic Cognitions Inventory (PTCI; Foa, Ehlers, Clark, Tolin,
& Orsillo, 1999). Moreover, change in negative cognitions was associated with reduction of PTSD symptoms. Similar results were obtained by
Paunovic and Ost (2001) with a sample of torture survivors with PTSD
who received PE with and without CR, using the World Assumptions
Scale (WAS; Janoff-Bulman, 1992). Interestingly, there is no evidence that
patients with severe negative trauma-related cognitions benefit more from
treatment programs that include exposure and cognitive techniques compared with a treatment that includes exposure only. In fact, a study by
Moser, Cahill, and Foa (2010) suggested that patients with more severe
pretreatment trauma-related cognitions (and more severe pretreatment
PTSD symptoms) fared slightly worse in treatment combining exposure
and CR than in the exposure-alone group. However, a randomized control

trial comparing CT to wait list among patients with mixed-trauma PTSD showed that changes in PTSD symptom severity were correlated with changes in the negative beliefs (Ehlers et al., 2003). Highlighting the overlap in treatment mechanisms, both PE (with and without CR) and CT are associated with reductions in negative cognitions, although adding CR to PE may not be indicated for those with severe negative cognitions. Assuming that CR and PE operate through similar mechanisms, it may be that adding one to the other is therapeutically redundant. On the other hand, the unexpected finding that adding CR to PE leads to worse outcomes among those with severe negative cognitions should caution us against the "more is better" approach to treatment provisions and highlights the deficiency of our understanding of therapeutic mechanisms of recovery from PTSD.

PATTERNS OF THERAPEUTIC RECOVERY

A large body of research shows that effective treatment can lead to significant and lasting recovery from PTSD. PE has received the most empirical support through controlled studies conducted by independent researchers with a wide range of trauma populations. Currently, over 25 randomized controlled trials indicate that PE is effective in reducing the array of PTSD symptoms (e.g., Bryant et al., 2008; Cloitre et al., 2010; Foa, Dancu, et al., 1999; Gilboa-Schechtman et al., 2010; Ready, Gerardi, Backscheider, Mascaro, & Rothbaum, 2010; for a comprehensive review, see Cahill, Rothbaum, Resick, & Follette, 2009). To date, there are four randomized controlled trials demonstrating the efficacy of CPT for PTSD: three studies showing that CPT is superior to wait list (Monson et al., 2006; Resick & Schnicke, 1992) or minimal attention control (Chard, 2005), and one study showing that CPT is equivalent to PE (Resick et al., 2002). Not only are PE and CPT effective at reducing PTSD symptoms, but they have also been shown to reduce depression (e.g., Foa et al., 2005; Nishith, Nixon, & Resick, 2005), anxiety (e.g., Foa, Dancu, et al., 1999), anger (e.g., Cahill, Rauch, Hembree, & Foa, 2003), and guilt (e.g., Resick et al., 2002). In summary, PE and CPT have been consistently associated with a pattern of rapid symptom reduction and maintenance of large effect sizes over time (e.g., Foa et al., 2005; Resick et al., 2002; Taylor et al., 2003).

Much of the research on CBT for PTSD, including PE and CPT, has examined changes from pre- to posttreatment, reflecting an assumption that therapeutic change is gradual and linear. However, some theoretical models suggest that there may be specific points during therapy at which change accelerates, decelerates, or levels off (see Collins, 2006). Assessing outcomes frequently over the course of therapy allows us to examine patterns of treatment process more closely, which may help us better understand what facilitates and inhibits therapeutic recovery. A small number of studies have examined individual differences in patterns of response to PTSD treatment.

Using curve estimation techniques, Nishith, Resick, and Griffin (2002) examined the pattern of symptom change among women with PTSD receiving either PE or CPT. The results showed that a curvilinear pattern of initial symptom increase followed by rapid symptom decrease provided the best fit for the pattern of PTSD symptom reduction in both types of therapy. This curvilinear pattern may be explained by the way that patients with PTSD typically try to cope with PTSD symptoms by avoiding situations, thoughts, or feelings related to the trauma. When therapy is initiated, avoidance behaviors are reduced to promote processing of trauma-related feelings and thoughts, thereby causing a temporary rise in reexperiencing and arousal symptoms before subsequent amelioration of symptoms. In PE, the first imaginal exposure occurs during the third session, and in CPT patients begin writing the trauma narrative for homework after the third session. It stands to reason that reexperiencing and autonomic arousal may be higher during the initial exposures sessions, as patients approach previously avoided trauma-related material. Then, as patients successfully process traumatic reminders, these symptoms show an accelerated decline.

Although the curvilinear pattern of therapeutic recovery was found for both CPT and PE, it has been taken as further evidence that exposure therapy leads to increased distress and is therefore less tolerable and associated with greater risk of dropout than other treatment approaches. For example, Pitman and colleagues (1996b) argued that EMDR was better tolerated than exposure therapy because it was less anxiety-provoking and less likely to produce negative consequences. Does exposure therapy lead to patient decompensation or greater dropout? This question was examined directly in a study of 76 women with chronic PTSD receiving PE. The results showed that a minority of patients (10%) experienced a reliable exacerbation of PTSD symptoms and that this increase occurred after the introduction of imaginal exposure (Foa, Zoellner, Feeny, Hembree, & Alvarez-Conrad, 2002). This exacerbation was temporary and was closely followed by a significant and lasting decrease in symptoms. Furthermore, the subset of individuals who experienced initial symptom exacerbation benefited from treatment as much as those who did not report such exacerbation and were no more likely to drop out of therapy (Foa et al., 2002). A later meta-analysis of 25 controlled studies of CBT for PTSD found no difference in dropout rates among exposure therapy, CT, stress inoculation training, and EMDR (Hembree et al., 2003).

Patterns of symptom change were also examined in a sample of 60 veterans randomly assigned to receive either CPT immediately or after a 10-week delay (Macdonald, Monson, Doron-Lamarca, Resick, & Palfai,

2011). Although a curvilinear pattern was hypothesized for those in the immediate-treatment group, the observed pattern was one of decelerating decline across treatment. Those in the delayed condition showed a stable level of symptomatology. Findings suggest that CPT produces quick and maintained improvements in veterans.

Recent research has examined the phenomenon of "sudden gains," which refer to rapid, large decreases in symptoms from one session to the next. Sudden gains were first noted in the treatment of depression (Tang & DeRubeis, 1999), but have now been identified in a number of clinical disorders. Two studies have examined sudden gains during PTSD treatment. In a sample of women with assault-related PTSD receiving CPT, Kelly, Rizvi, Monson, and Resick (2009) found that 39.2% reported sudden gains. Those who experienced sudden gains demonstrated significantly greater reductions in PTSD symptom severity at posttreatment and these gains were maintained at 6-month follow-up. Similar results were reported in a study of PE, in which 52% of women with assault-related PTSD reported sudden gains, and gains were related to lower PTSD severity at posttreatment (Doane, Feeny, & Zoellner, 2010). This study examined the timing of sudden gains, and found that approximately one-half of the gains occurred between sessions 3–5 and the other half occurred between sessions 7–9. Identifying the presence and timing of sudden gains provides clues into which aspects of treatment incite therapeutic change, which may lead to increased treatment efficiency.

In summary, nonlinear patterns of recovery and sudden gains have been demonstrated in both PE and CPT. Sudden gains appear to be relatively common and reliably related with treatment success. Additional research on sudden gains in PTSD is needed to understand the therapeutic factors associated with the presence and timing of sudden gains, and the patient factors that might predict sudden gains. Studies on patterns of change during PTSD treatment indicate that a minority of patients receiving CPT and PE experience a temporary increase in symptoms, typically during the initial phase of therapy when patients are asked to approach trauma-related material that they have been avoiding. Concerns that exposure therapy retraumatizes patients and exacerbates their symptoms have not been empirically supported; exposure therapy is not associated with posttreatment symptom worsening and the dropout rate is comparable to that in other CBT programs.

PREDICTORS OF TREATMENT OUTCOME

Although the average patient receiving CBT for PTSD manifests marked improvement, many studies show that some patients do not show a significant response to treatment. As noted above, a minority of patients drop out before benefiting from treatment (Hembree et al., 2003). Furthermore, even among those who complete a standard course of treatment, some continue to meet diagnostic criteria for PTSD. Identifying predictors of good and poor outcomes will enable us to determine who is a good candidate for a given treatment and who should receive an alternative or augmented treatment.

Pretreatment PTSD Severity

A number of treatment studies have found that individuals with higher PTSD severity at intake tend to show poorer outcomes at posttreatment (e.g., Karatzias et al., 2007; Taylor et al., 2001; van Minnen et al., 2002). For example, Foa and colleagues (2013) found that women veterans and active-duty personnel (most of whom had sexual trauma) with higher PTSD severity at pretreatment, as measured by the Clinician-Administered PTSD Scale (CAPS; Blake, Weathers, Nagy, & Kaloupek, 1995), were more likely to continue to meet diagnostic criteria for PTSD (defined as a CAPS severity score ≥ 45) at posttreatment. This finding is consistent with other studies using the CAPS in individuals with mixed-trauma (Karatzias et al., 2007) and road traffic accident-related PTSD (Taylor et al., 2001). In the above studies, the decrease in PTSD symptoms was similar for those with high and low pretreatment PTSD severity. Thus, pretreatment PTSD severity does not seem to predict the degree of benefit from treatment. However, patients with high baseline PTSD may require additional sessions in order to achieve symptom levels comparable to those with lower baseline severity. In fact, patients who did not achieve an excellent response after eight sessions of PE (defined as at least a 70% reduction in self-reported PTSD severity) experienced further reductions in PTSD severity after up to four additional sessions (Foa et al., 2005).

Prior Traumatic Experiences

In contrast to the number of studies examining the effect of prior trauma on risk for PTSD development (e.g., Breslau, Peterson, & Schultz, 2008), studies examining the influence of prior trauma on treatment outcome are scarce. Among adult female survivors of sexual and nonsexual assault receiving PE, SIT, or PE plus SIT, Hembree, Street, Riggs, and Foa (2004) found that childhood trauma, but not prior adult trauma, was significantly related to higher PTSD severity at posttreatment, even when controlling for baseline PTSD severity. In contrast, in a trial comparing CT to wait list, no strong relationship between prior trauma and posttreatment PTSD severity was reported (Ehlers et al., 2005). However, in the later study, the authors did not differentiate between prior childhood and adult traumas. Perhaps growing up in an abusive and/or violent family results in strong negative perceptions of self and the world that interfere with one's ability to benefit from treatment that aims to change these perceptions.

Comorbid Affective States

Comorbid affective states, such as depression and anger, may interfere with emotional and cognitive processing of a traumatic event. Consistent with this hypothesis, some studies show that individuals with higher levels of anger benefit less from CBT for PTSD (e.g., Speckens, Ehlers, Hackmann, & Clark, 2006; Taylor et al., 2001). Similarly, a study on CBT group treatment for Vietnam veterans with PTSD found that higher levels of pretreatment anger were related to worse treatment outcomes (Forbes, Creamer, Hawthorne, Allen, & McHugh, 2003). In a small sample of female assault survivors, Foa and colleagues (1995) found that those with higher levels of anger at pretreatment tended to benefit less from PE than those who reported low levels of anger. In contrast, in a larger sample of female assault victims, pretreatment anger did not predict posttreatment PTSD symptom severity (Cahill et al., 2003). While results are inconsistent across studies, excessive anger may interfere with therapeutic recovery.

The effect of comorbid depression on PTSD treatment outcome is less clear. Some PTSD studies suggest that individuals with comorbid depression have worse outcomes (e.g., Foa et al., 2013; Forbes et al., 2003; Taylor et al., 2001), while other studies have found that depression has little or no effect on treatment outcome (e.g., Hagenaars, van Minnen, & Hoogduin, 2010; Resick & Schnicke, 1992). Among patients receiving either CPT or PE, Rizvi, Vogt, and Resick (2009) found that patients with higher depression and guilt showed greater improvement in PTSD symptoms from pre- to posttreatment. However, these patients also had greater PTSD symptom severity. Therefore this finding likely reflects greater response to treatment due to initial symptom severity. Inconsistent results on the role of depression on PTSD treatment outcome may relate to the different methods of assessing depression (i.e., self-report vs. interview) or to different samples. Given evidence that PE and CPT both lead to significant reductions in depression (e.g., Foa, Dancu, et al., 1999; Marks, Lovell, Noshirvani, Livanou, & Thrasher, 1998; Paunovic & Öst, 2001; Resick et al., 2002; Tarrier et al., 1999), the presence of comorbid depression should not be viewed as a contraindication to treatment. In cases where major depression is the primary disorder, or when patients are at a high risk for suicide, therapists must first provide crisis management and containment.

Use of Psychotropic Medication

The effect of concurrent psychotropic medication in CBT for PTSD has been examined in several studies. Most studies to date indicate that there is no benefit to adding antidepressant medication to CBT for anxiety disorders (Foa et al., 2005; Otto et al., 2003). Benzodiazepine use, on the other hand, has been found to potentially interfere with treatment outcome in panic disorder (e.g., Otto, Pollack, & Sabatino, 1996) and PTSD (van Minnen et al., 2002). An explanation for this finding could be that certain medications, namely benzodiazepines, hinder emotional engagement during treatment, which was found related to good outcome (e.g., Foa, Riggs, et al., 1995; Jaycox et al., 1998).

The Therapeutic Alliance

Meta-analytic studies of psychotherapy have consistently found a significant relationship between the therapeutic alliance and treatment outcomes (e.g., Martin, Garske, & Davis, 2000), and there is evidence that suggests that this finding extends to the treatment of PTSD. For example, among individuals with PTSD related to childhood sexual abuse, Cloitre, Stovall-McClough, Miranda, and Chemtob (2004) found that a higher patient-rated therapeutic alliance at the beginning of treatment (modified PE) was associated significantly with lower PTSD posttreatment. Similarly, Keller, Zoellner, and Feeny (2010) found that higher levels of alliance were positively associated with adherence to PE (e.g., session attendance, homework completion) and treatment completion. These results suggest that therapists' time and effort spent in the service of supporting a strong therapeutic bond may help patients adhere to and complete treatment.

Treatment Expectancy and Attendance

The degree to which patients perceive the rationale and approach to treatment as credible has been shown to predict treatment outcome in several PTSD treatment studies (Foa et al., 2011; Tarrier et al., 1999; Tarrier, Sommerfield, Pilgrim, & Faragher, 2000; Taylor et al., 2003). This finding highlights the importance of providing patients with a clear and compelling treatment rationale, which in turn may motivate the patient to adhere to treatment demands including homework assignments. Convincing patients through providing a clear rationale for how the treatment directly addresses their distressing symptoms is particularly important when treatment requires that patients change basic behavioral and emotional patterns, as is the case with PE. In PTSD we hypothesize that extensive avoidance is a key maintaining factor of the disorder and accordingly the main component of PE. We can hardly expect patients to give up their "protective" strategies if they do not understand why treatment demands that they experience discomfort or how this short-term discomfort will help them recover.

Some evidence suggests that treatment attendance, including the number of missed sessions, the length of time between sessions, and the overall duration of therapy are related to treatment outcome (Karatzias et al., 2007; Perconte & Griger, 1991; Tarrier et al., 2000). For example, Perconte and Griger (1991) found that veterans who benefited the most from a partial hospitalization program for PTSD attended sessions more often and participated more in treatment activities. In a randomized study comparing imaginal exposure and CT for PTSD, variables related to treatment adherence (e.g., number of missed sessions) were significantly related to changes in PTSD severity from pre- to posttreatment, regardless of treatment type (Tarrier et al., 2000). Data from a meta-analysis of treatment for PTSD showed that the rate of treatment completion was negatively associated with pretreatment–posttreatment effect size, raising the possibility that patients who do not improve tend to drop out (Bradley et al., 2005).

In summary, several moderators (pretreatment PTSD severity, high anger, perceived treatment credibility), and mediators (attendance, therapeutic alliance) have been associated with PTSD treatment outcome. Additional factors that have received mixed results include comorbid depression, prior traumatic experiences, and use of psychotropic medication.

PREDICTORS OF ADHERENCE AND DROPOUT

Findings on predictors of treatment dropout are less consistent than research on predictors of overall treatment outcome. It remains unclear whether pretreatment PTSD severity or comorbid affective states significantly impact the likelihood of attrition. Comorbid substance abuse has been more frequently associated with PTSD treatment dropout than other comorbid diagnoses, although dropout may be a consequence of factors other than exposure therapy per se. Clinically, the findings discussed in this section suggest that certain patient factors such as comorbid substance dependence require therapists to simultaneously address both the PTSD and the comorbid disorder to ensure successful outcome.

Pretreatment PTSD Severity

Greater PTSD severity has been associated with poor attendance and adherence with treatment procedures, such as homework (Burstein, 1986; Foa, Rothbaum, Riggs, & Murdock, 1991; Scott & Stradling, 1997), as well as treatment dropout (Bryant, Moulds, Guthrie, Dang, & Nixon, 2003; Marks et al., 1998; Zayfert et al., 2005), while others found no strong relationship between pretreatment PTSD severity and treatment adherence or dropout (Foa, Dancu, et al., 1999; Tarrier et al., 1999; Taylor et al., 2003). The fact that many of these studies had a small number of dropouts (e.g., 10 out of 72 patients; Tarrier et al., 1999) makes it difficult to identify factors that predict dropout.

Depression Severity

The role of depression in treatment dropout is mixed. High pretreatment depression was associated with dropout among PTSD patients in a clinical-practice setting (Zayfert et al., 2005) and among patients in a randomized trial of imaginal exposure with and without CR for PTSD (Bryant et al., 2003). In contrast, Taylor and colleagues (2003) found no differences between treatment completers and dropouts on measures of depression, guilt, or global functioning among patients with PTSD due to motor vehicle accidents. This discrepancy may be due to sample size (i.e., Taylor et al. may have lacked sufficient power) or the way in which treatment completion was defined (e.g., achievement of treatment goals vs. completion of sessions).

Comorbid Substance Abuse

Substance abuse has been associated with treatment dropout fairly consistently (e.g., van Minnen et al., 2002; Perconte & Griger, 1991; Riggs, Rukstalis, Volpicelli, Kalmanson, & Foa, 2003). For example, in a sample of women with PTSD and substance dependence, only 63% of the patients completed a minimum of 25% of the treatment sessions (Najavits, Weiss, Shaw, & Muenz, 1998). Similarly, in a sample of patients with PTSD and comorbid substance dependence receiving exposure therapy plus coping-skills training, almost one-third of the sample completed less than 25% of the sessions and nearly two-thirds completed fewer than 60% of the sessions (Brady, Dansky, Back, Foa, & Carroll, 2001). Although these dropout rates are considerably higher than those found in PTSD trials that exclude substance-dependent participants (e.g., Foa et al., 2005), there is evidence that dropout may not be due to exposure therapy per se. Specifically, in the Brady and colleagues (2001) study the majority of dropouts (75%; 18/24) occurred before exposure therapy was initiated.

Perceived Treatment Credibility

In addition to affecting overall treatment outcome, perceived treatment credibility appears to impact the probability of dropout from treatment. Taylor and colleagues (2003) asked patients to rate the credibility of treatment after assigning them to receive one of three types of CBT for PTSD: exposure therapy, eye movement desensitization and reprocessing (EMDR), and relaxation. Although dropout rates and participant-rated treatment credibility did not differ across treatments, there was a significant relationship between perceived treatment credibility and dropout. Similarly, Tarrier and colleagues (1999) found that patients who dropped out of treatment rated the therapy as less credible and were less motivated to follow treatment protocols than completers.

FACTORS UNRELATED TO OUTCOMES

While negative findings cannot provide clear conclusions, they may be informative. Below we summarize patient characteristics that were unrelated to the efficacy of therapy.

Patient Factors

Multiple Traumas

Many clinicians believe that treatment is most effective with survivors of discrete traumas such as rape, natural disaster, or motor vehicle accidents. In fact, trauma type bears no relationship to treatment outcome (Ehlers et al., 2005; van Minnen et al., 2002). Many of the first systematic studies of exposure therapy for PTSD were conducted with combat veterans who had experienced a variety of traumatic events. PE, for example, has been successfully applied to combat veterans (e.g., Rauch et al., 2009; Tuerk et al., 2011), as well as to survivors of chronic childhood sexual abuse and other chronic trauma (Foa, Dancu, et al., 1999; Foa et al., 2005; Gilboa-Schechtman et al., 2010).

Comorbid Personality Disorders

Personality disorders, particularly borderline personality disorder (BPD), have been thought to impede effects of treatment of anxiety disorders (Merrill & Strauman, 2004); however, research suggests that individuals with PTSD and comorbid BPD can also benefit from PTSD treatment. Feeny, Zoellner, and Foa (2002) reanalyzed data of 72 patients who received either PE, SIT, or their combination and found that women with BPD symptoms benefited as much from treatment as those without these symptoms. Indeed, patients with BPD symptoms evidenced significant improvement on PTSD symptoms, PTSD diagnostic status, depression, anxiety, and social functioning. Clarke, Rizvi, and Resick (2008) obtained similar findings in a trial comparing CPT and PE for PTSD; those with borderline personality characteristics were as likely to complete and benefit from these treatments as those without such characteristics. Similarly, Mueser and colleagues (2008) found that 27 patients with comorbid BPD benefited as much as 81 patients without BPD from receiving a (primarily cognitive) CBT at a community mental health center. These data indicate that patients with BPD features may not necessarily require more complicated and long-term treatments than those without such features. Again, in cases where patients have a high risk for suicide or recent self-injurious behavior (e.g., cutting) clinical judgment dictates that PTSD treatment should be delayed until these problems are managed.

Dissociation

The potential for dissociative symptoms to interfere with PTSD treatment has been discussed (Jaycox & Foa, 1996; Shalev, Bonne, & Eth, 1996), but not systematically studied. A recent study by Hagenaars and colleagues (2010) demonstrated that PE can effectively reduce not only PTSD symptoms, but also numbing, depersonalization, and depressive symptoms. In contrast to the authors' hypothesis, pretreatment levels of trait dissociation, depersonalization, numbing, and depressive symptoms were not related to improvement or dropout. In fact, patients with high levels of these dissociative symptoms showed a similar reduction of PTSD symptoms from pretreatment to posttreatment and from pretreatment to follow-up as patients with low levels of dissociative phenomena. In sum, there is no evidence to date that dissociative phenomena have predictive value with respect to treatment outcome.

Treatment Factors

Multicomponent Treatment Programs

There seems to be an assumption among clinical researchers that treatment programs that include multiple components will have superior outcome to treatments with fewer components. Accordingly, most evidence-based treatment programs for PTSD include several techniques such as exposure, relaxation, cognitive restructuring, and modeling (e.g., Blanchard et al., 2003). Following this belief, a number of studies have compared PE combined with other evidence-based treatments to PE alone. In a dismantling study, Foa, Dancu, and colleagues (1999) compared PE combined with SIT to each component treatment. Contrary to prediction, all three treatments performed equally well on most measures, although PE alone yielded larger effect sizes on severity of PTSD, depression, and anxiety at posttreatment and follow-up. Interestingly, more participants dropped out of the PE/SIT combination (27%) and SIT alone (27%) than PE alone (8%) or the wait-list condition (0%). Furthermore, in the intent-to treat sample, PE alone was superior to SIT and PE/ SIT on several outcome indices.

Three randomized-controlled trials (RCTs) have demonstrated that combining PE with cognitive restructuring (CR) does not enhance outcome (Foa et al., 2005; Marks et al., 1998; Paunovic & Öst, 2001). Similarly, a dismantling study by Resick and colleagues (2008) found no significant differences between the full CPT protocol and its constituent components, cognitive therapy–only, and written accounts among 150 adult women with PTSD. These findings in both PE and CPT suggest that combining separately efficacious treatments does not enhance treatment outcome for

PTSD. One exception to this conclusion is Bryant and colleagues' (2008) finding that adding CR to exposure therapy did improve outcome. However, the study design precludes conclusions about the benefit of adding CR to standard PE because processing, an integral part of PE, was intentionally excluded from the imaginal exposure condition. In an RCT among women with PTSD related to childhood abuse, Cloitre and colleagues (2010) examined the effects of adding eight additional sessions of skills training to address negative mood regulation prior to beginning PE. The results showed marginally significant results in favor of the treatment that included skills training, which does not provide compelling evidence for the utility of additional treatment components.

Taken together, the studies discussed above do not support the view that the number of treatment components is positively associated with outcome. Supplemental components such as those suggested by Becker and Zayfert (2001; e.g., readiness groups, dialectical behavioral therapy techniques) may be useful, but at present the usefulness of such interventions has not been empirically tested. At present, available data suggest that "simple" may be better.

Length of Imaginal Exposure and Within-Session Habituation

In their original formulation of emotional processing theory, Foa and Kozak (1986) hypothesized that activation of fear and within- and between-session habituation are indicators of emotional processing, that is, the essence of the therapeutic recovery. Based on this theory, the PE protocol developed by Foa and her colleagues specifies that imaginal exposure should last 45–60 minutes to allow for within-session habituation (e.g., Foa & Rothbaum, 1998). This length of the imaginal exposure was informed by research with other anxiety disorders (e.g., agoraphobia; Foa & Chambless, 1978) showing that anxiety levels typically decrease after approximately 50–60 minutes of imaginal exposure. Subsequent research did not find a relationship between within-session habituation and treatment outcome (van Minnen & Foa, 2006). If within-session habituation is not strongly associated with treatment outcome, it follows that the duration of imaginal exposure can be reduced without attenuating treatment efficacy. To examine this hypothesis, van Minnen and Foa compared patients who underwent 60 minutes of imaginal exposure to patients who received 30 minutes of imaginal exposure. Consistent with the hypothesis, despite greater within-session habituation achieved by patients who received 60 minutes, both groups benefited equally from treatment. It should be noted, however, that although within-session reductions in fear are no longer considered critical for improvement (Foa et al., 2006), habituation of fear may be important for patients who hold erroneous beliefs about the consequences of anxiety (e.g., that it will

be unbearable or will last forever) as it constitutes information that disconfirms their erroneous beliefs.

SUMMARY AND CLINICAL RECOMMENDATIONS

The last two decades were marked by great strides in our ability to amelio-
rate PTSD symptoms in many sufferers through the use of short-term CBT
programs. But some patients do not benefit from the existing treatments
and many remain symptomatic. Attempts to raise the success ceilings by
combining different programs have failed. One way to overcome this stand-
still is to examine the mechanisms involved in the existing treatments in
order to develop new, theoretically informed therapies that are more effective. To this end, we have examined emotional engagement, habituation,
organizing and elaborating the trauma memory, and changes in self- and
world perceptions. This examination led us to conclude that there is considerable overlap across treatment programs in the mechanisms that are
thought to mediate their outcome. Another strategy that can help inform
us about how to improve treatments is to identify variables that moderate
outcome. Similar to our examination of the process of change, our review
of the literature on predictors of treatment outcome has not helped us to
identify ways to improve treatment outcome.

An alternative approach to examining mechanisms and predictors
comes from translational research including subhuman biological studies
of extinction and behavior. For example, research examining the use of
pharmacological agents as adjuncts to exposure therapy has showed some
promise. Augmentation of exposure therapy with D-cycloserine has demonstrated benefit in some (e.g., Hofmann et al., 2006; Ressler et al., 2004),
but not all controlled trials for anxiety disorders (e.g., Guastella et al.,
2007; Storch et al., 2007), and preliminary data with PTSD showed no
evidence of differential efficacy from placebo (Heresco-Levy et al., 2002).
Methylene blue is another drug that is implicated in the facilitation of fear
extinction (Gonzalez-Lima & Bruchey, 2004) that is currently being tested
as an augmentation strategy with exposure therapy. Yet another promising
approach to examining mechanisms of change is to translate basic science
research on memory reconsolidation to enhance exposure therapy. Recent
evidence suggests that the pathological fear responses seen in PTSD may
be altered if corrective information is presented during a specific window
of time called the "reconsolidation period" during which the fear structure is labile (Monfils, Cowansage, Klann, & LeDoux, 2009; Schiller et
al., 2010). In general, we have not yet fully exploited findings from basic
research in psychopathology. Greater collaboration between clinical scientists and therapy researchers has the potential to produce more powerful
and more efficient treatments for PTSD.

REFERENCES

Amir, N., Stafford, J., Freshman, M. S., & Foa, E. B. (1998). Relationship between trauma narratives and trauma pathology. *Journal of Traumatic Stress, 11*(2), 385–392.

Becker, C. B., & Zayfert, C. (2001). Integrating DBT-based techniques and concepts to facilitate exposure treatment for PTSD. *Cognitive and Behavioral Practice, 8*(2), 107–122.

Blake, D. D., Weathers, F. W., Nagy, L. M., & Kaloupek, D. G. (1995). The development of a clinician-administered PTSD scale. *Journal of Traumatic Stress, 8*(1), 75–90.

Blanchard, E. B., Hickling, E. J., Devineni, T., Veazey, C. H., Galovski, T. E., Mundy, E., et al. (2003). A controlled evaluation of cognitive behaviorial therapy for posttraumatic stress in motor vehicle accident survivors. *Behaviour Research and Therapy, 41*(1), 79–96.

Bradley, R., Greene, J., Russ, E., Dutra, L., & Westen, D. (2005). A multidimensional meta-analysis of psychotherapy for PTSD. *American Journal of Psychiatry, 162*(2), 214–227.

Brady, K. T., Dansky, B. S., Back, S. E., Foa, E. B., & Carroll, K. M. (2001). Exposure therapy in the treatment of PTSD among cocaine-dependent individuals: Preliminary findings. *Journal of Substance Abuse Treatment, 21*(1), 47–54.

Breslau, N., Peterson, E.L., & Schultz, L.R. (2008). A second look at prior trauma and the posttraumatic stress disorder effects of subsequent trauma. *Archives of General Psychiatry, 65*(4), 431–437.

Brewin, C. R., Dalgleish, T., & Joseph, S. (1996). A dual representation theory of posttraumatic stress disorder. *Psychological Review, 103*(4), 670–686.

Brewin, C. R., & Holmes, E. A. (2003). Psychological theories of posttraumatic stress disorder. *Clinical Psychology Review, 23*(3), 339–376.

Bryant, R. A., Moulds, M. L., Guthrie, R. M., Dang, S. T., Mastrodomenico, J., Nixon, R. D. V., et al. (2008). A randomized controlled trial of exposure therapy and cognitive restructuring for posttraumatic stress disorder. *Journal of Consulting and Clinical Psychology, 76*(4), 695–703.

Bryant, R. A., Moulds, M. L., Guthrie, R. M., Dang, S. T., & Nixon, R. D. V. (2003). Imaginal exposure alone and imaginal exposure with cognitive restructuring in treatment of posttraumatic stress disorder. *Journal of Consulting and Clinical Psychology, 71*(4), 706–712.

Burstein, A. (1986). Treatment noncompliance in patients with post-traumatic stress disorder. *Psychosomatics, 27,* 37–40.

Cahill, S. P., & Foa, E. B. (2007). Psychological theories of PTSD. In M. J. Friedman, T. M. Keane, & P. A. Resick (Eds.), *Handbook of PTSD: Science and practice* (pp. 55–77). New York: Guilford Press.

Cahill, S. P., Rauch, S. A., Hembree, E. A., & Foa, E. B. (2003). Effect of cognitive-behavioral treatments for PTSD on anger. *Journal of Cognitive Psychotherapy, 17*(2), 113–131.

Cahill, S. P., Rothbaum, B. O., Resick, P. A., & Follette, V. M. (2009). Cognitive-behavioral therapy for adults. In E. B. Foa, T. M. Keane, M. J. Friedman, & J. A. Cohen (Eds.), *Effective treatments for PTSD: Practice guidelines from the International Society for Traumatic Stress Studies* (2nd ed., pp. 139–222). New York: Guilford Press.

Chard, K. M. (2005). An evaluation of cognitive processing therapy for the treatment of posttraumatic stress disorder related to childhood sexual abuse. *Journal of Consulting and Clinical Psychology, 73*(5), 965–971.

Clarke, S. B., Rizvi, S. L., & Resick, P. A. (2008). Borderline personality characteristics and treatment outcome in cognitive-behavioral treatments for PTSD in female rape victims. *Behavior Therapy, 39*, 72–78.

Cloitre, M., Stovall-McClough, K. C., Miranda, R., & Chemtob, C. M. (2004). Therapeutic alliance, negative mood regulation, and treatment outcome in child abuse-related posttraumatic stress disorder. *Journal of Consulting and Clinical Psychology, 72*(3), 411–416.

Cloitre, M., Stovall-McClough, K. C., Nooner, K., Zorbas, P., Cherry, S., Jackson, C. L., et al. (2010). Treatment for PTSD related to childhood abuse: A randomized controlled trial. *American Journal of Psychiatry, 167*(8), 915–924.

Collins, L. M. (2006). Analysis of longitudinal data: The integration of theoretical model, temporal design, and statistical model. *Annual Review of Psychology, 57*, 505–528.

Craske, M. G., Kircanski, K., Zelikowsky, M., Mystkowski, J., Chowdhury, N., & Baker, A. (2008). Optimizing inhibitory learning during exposure therapy. *Behaviour Research and Therapy, 46*, 5–27.

Dalgleish, T. (1999). Cognitive theories of posttraumatic stress disorder. In W. Yule (Ed.), *Post-traumatic stress disorders: Concepts and therapy* (pp. 193–220). New York: Wiley.

Dalgleish, T. (2004). Cognitive approaches to posttraumatic stress disorder: The evolution of multi-representational theorizing. *Psychological Bulletin, 130*, 228–260.

Doane, L. S., Feeny, N. C., & Zoellner, L. A. (2010). A preliminary investigation of sudden gains in exposure therapy for PTSD. *Behaviour Research and Therapy, 48*(6), 555–560.

Ehlers, A., & Clark, D. M. (2000). A cognitive model of posttraumatic stress disorder. *Behaviour Research and Therapy, 38*(4), 319–345.

Ehlers, A., Clark, D. M., Hackmann, A., McManus, F., & Fennell, M. (2005). Cognitive therapy for post-traumatic stress disorder: Development and evaluation. *Behaviour Research and Therapy, 43*(4), 413–431.

Ehlers, A., Clark, D. M., Hackmann, A., McManus, F., Fennell, M., Herbert, C., et al. (2003). A randomized controlled trial of cognitive therapy, a self-help booklet, and repeated assessments as early interventions for posttraumatic stress disorder. *Archives of General Psychiatry, 60*(10), 1024–1032.

Epstein, S. (1991). The self-concept, the traumatic neurosis, and the structure of personality. In D. Ozer, J. M. Healy Jr., & A. J. Stewart (Eds.), *Perspectives on personality* (Vol. 3, Part A, pp. 63–98). London: Jessica Kingsley.

Feeny, N. C., Zoellner, L. A., & Foa, E. B. (2002). Treatment outcome for chronic PTSD among female assault victims with borderline personality characteristics: A preliminary examination. *Journal of Personality Disorders, 16*(1), 30–40.

Foa, E. B., & Chambless, D. L. (1978). Habituation of subjective anxiety during flooding in imagery. *Behaviour Research and Therapy, 16*(6), 391–399.

Foa, E. B., Dancu, C. V., Hembree, E. A., Jaycox, L. H., Meadows, E. A., & Street, G. P. (1999). A comparison of exposure therapy, stress inoculation training, and their combination for reducing posttraumatic stress disorder in female assault victims. *Journal of Consulting and Clinical Psychology, 67*(2), 194–200.

Foa, E. B., Ehlers, A., Clark, D. M., Tolin, D. F., & Orsillo, S. M. (1999). The Posttraumatic Cognitions Inventory (PTCI): Development and validation. *Psychological Assessment, 11*(3), 303–314.

Foa, E. B., Hembree, E. A., Cahill, S. P., Rauch, S. A. M., Riggs, D. S., Feeny, N. C., et al. (2005). Randomized trial of prolonged exposure for posttraumatic stress disorder with and without cognitive restructuring: Outcome at academic and community clinics. *Journal of Consulting and Clinical Psychology, 73*(5), 953–964.

Foa, E. B., Hembree, E. A., & Rothbaum, B. O. (2007). *Prolonged exposure therapy for PTSD: Emotional processing of traumatic experiences: Therapist guide.* New York: Oxford University Press.

Foa, E. B., Huppert, J. D., & Cahill, S. P. (2006). Emotional processing theory: An update. In B.O. Rothbaum (Ed.), *Pathological anxiety: Emotional processing in etiology and treatment* (pp. 3–24). New York: Guilford Press.

Foa, E. B., & Jaycox, L. H. (1999). Cognitive-behavioral theory and treatment of posttraumatic stress disorders. In D. Spiegel (Ed.), *Efficacy and cost-effectiveness of psychotherapy* (pp. 23–61). Washington, DC: American Psychiatric Press.

Foa, E. B., & Kozak, M. J. (1985). Treatment of anxiety disorders: Implications for psychopathology. In A. H. Tuma & J. D. Maser (Eds.), *Anxiety and the anxiety disorders* (pp. 451–452). Hillsdale, NJ: Erlbaum.

Foa, E. B., & Kozak, M. J. (1986). Emotional processing of fear: Exposure of corrective information. *Psychological Bulletin, 99,* 20–35.

Foa, E. B., Molnar, C., & Cashman, L. (1995). Change in rape narratives during exposure therapy for posttraumatic stress disorder. *Journal of Traumatic Stress, 8,* 675–690.

Foa, E. B., Powers, M. B., Gillihan, S. J., Chow, B. K., Yasinski, C., Hembree, E. A., et al. (2013). *Predictors of outcome in prolonged exposure and present centered therapy for posttraumatic stress disorder.* Manuscript in preparation.

Foa, E. B., & Rauch, S. A. M. (2004). Cognitive changes during prolonged exposure versus prolonged exposure plus cognitive restructuring in female assault survivors with posttraumatic stress disorder. *Journal of Consulting and Clinical Psychology, 72*(5), 879–884.

Foa, E. B., & Riggs, D. S. (1993). Post-traumatic stress disorder in rape victims. In J. Oldham, M. B. Riba, & A. Tasman, *Annual review of psychiatry* (Vol. 12, pp. 273–303). Washington, DC: American Psychiatric Association.

Foa, E. B., Riggs, D. S., Massie, E. D., & Yarczower, M. (1995). The impact of fear activation and anger on the efficacy of exposure treatment for posttraumatic stress disorder. *Behavior Therapy, 26*(3), 487–499.

Foa, E. B., & Rothbaum, B. O. (1998). *Treating the trauma of rape: Cognitive-behavior therapy for PTSD.* New York: Guilford Press.

Foa, E. B., Rothbaum, B. O., Riggs, D. S., & Murdock, T. B. (1991). Treatment of posttraumatic stress disorder in rape victims: A comparison between cognitive-behavioral procedures and counseling. *Journal of Consulting and Clinical Psychology, 59*(5), 715–723.

Foa, E. B., Zoellner, L. A., Feeny, N. C., Hembree, E. A., & Alvarez-Conrad, J. (2002). Does imaginal exposure exacerbate PTSD symptoms? *Journal of Consulting and Clinical Psychology, 70*(4), 1022–1028.

Forbes, D., Creamer, M., Hawthorne, G., Allen, N., & McHugh, T. (2003). Comorbidity as a predictor of symptom change after treatment in combat-related posttraumatic stress disorder. *Journal of Nervous and Mental Disease, 191*(2), 93–99.

Gilboa-Schechtman, E., Foa, E. B., Shafran, N., Aderka, I. M., Powers, M. B., Rachamim, L., et al. (2010). Prolonged exposure versus dynamic therapy for adolescent PTSD: A pilot randomized controlled trial. *Journal of the American Academy of Child and Adolescent Psychiatry, 49*(10), 1034–1042.

Gonzalez-Lima, F., & Bruchey, A. K. (2004). Extinction memory improvement by the metabolic enhancer methylene blue. *Learning and Memory, 11*(5), 633–640.

Gray, M. J., & Lombardo, T. W. (2001). Complexity of trauma narratives as an index of fragmented memory in PTSD: A critical analysis. *Applied Cognitive Psychology, 15*(7), S171–S186.

Guastella, A. J., Dadds, M. R., Lovibond, P. F., Mitchell, P., & Richardson, R. (2007). A randomized controlled trial of the effect of D-cycloserine on exposure therapy for spider fear. *Journal of Psychiatric Research, 41*(6), 466–471.

Hagenaars, M. A., van Minnen, A., & Hoogduin, K. A. L. (2010). The impact of dissociation and depression on the efficacy of prolonged exposure treatment for PTSD. *Behaviour Research and Therapy, 48*(1), 19–27.

Halligan, S. L., Michael, T., Clark, D. M., & Ehlers, A. (2003). Posttraumatic stress disorder following assault: The role of cognitive processing, trauma memory, and appraisals. *Journal of Consulting and Clinical Psychology, 71*(3), 419–431.

Hembree, E. A., Foa, E. B., Dorfan, N. M., Street, G. P., Kowalski, J., & Tu, X. (2003). Do patients drop out prematurely from exposure therapy for PTSD? *Journal of Traumatic Stress, 16*(6), 555–562.

Hembree, E. A., Marshall, R. D., Fitzgibbons, L. A., & Foa, E. B. (2001). The difficult-to-treat patient with posttraumatic stress disorder. In M. J. Dewan & R. W. Pies (Eds.), *The difficult-to-treat psychiatric patient* (pp. 149–178). Arlington, VA: American Psychiatric Publishing.

Hembree, E. A., Street, G. P., Riggs, D. S., & Foa, E. B. (2004). Do assault-related variables predict response to cognitive behavioral treatment for PTSD? *Journal of Consulting and Clinical Psychology, 72*(3), 531–534.

Heresco-Levy, U., Kremer, I., Javitt, D. C., Goichman, R., Reshef, A., Blanaru, M., et al. (2002). Pilot-controlled trial of D-cycloserine for the treatment of posttraumatic stress disorder. *International Journal of Neuropsychopharmacology, 5*(4), 301–307.

Hofmann, S. G., Meuret, A. E., Smits, J. A. J., Simon, N. M., Pollack, M. H., Eisenmenger, K., et al. (2006). Augmentation of exposure therapy with D-cycloserine for social anxiety disorder. *Archives of General Psychiatry, 63*(3), 298–304.

Horowitz, M.J. (1976). *Stress response syndromes.* New York: Aronson.

Horowitz, M.J. (1986). *Stress response syndromes* (2nd ed.). Northvale, NJ: Aronson.

Iverson, K. M., Resick, P. A., Suvak, M. K., Walling, S., & Taft, C. T. (2011). Intimate partner violence exposure predicts PTSD treatment engagement and outcome in cognitive processing therapy. *Behavior Therapy, 42*(2), 236–248.

Janoff-Bulman, R. (1992). *Shattered assumptions: Towards a new psychology of trauma.* New York: Free Press.

Jaycox, L. H., & Foa, E. B. (1996). Obstacles in implementing exposure therapy for PTSD: Case discussions and practical solutions. *Clinical Psychology and Psychotherapy, 3*(3), 176–184.

Jaycox, L. H., Foa, E. B., & Morral, A. R. (1998). Influence of emotional engagement and habituation on exposure therapy for PTSD. *Journal of Consulting and Clinical Psychology, 66*(1), 185–192.

Jones, C., Harvey, A. G., & Brewin, C. R. (2007). The organisation and content of trauma memories in survivors of road traffic accidents. *Behaviour Research and Therapy, 45*(1), 151–162.

Karatzias, A., Power, K., McGoldrick, T., Brown, K., Buchanan, R., Sharp, D., et al. (2007). Predicting treatment outcome on three measures for post-traumatic stress disorder. *European Archives of Psychiatry and Clinical Neuroscience, 257*(1), 40–46.

Keane, T. M., Zimering, R. T., & Caddell, J. M. (1985). A behavioral formulation of posttraumatic stress disorder in Vietnam veterans. *Behavior Therapist, 8*(1), 9–12.

Keller, S. M., Zoellner, L. A., & Feeny, N. C. (2010). Understanding factors associated with early therapeutic alliance in PTSD treatment: Adherence, childhood sexual abuse history, and social support. *Journal of Consulting and Clinical Psychology, 78*(6), 974–979.

Kelly, K. A., Rizvi, S. L., Monson, C. M., & Resick, P. A. (2009). The impact of sudden gains in cognitive behavioral therapy for posttraumatic stress disorder. *Journal of Traumatic Stress, 22*(4), 287–293.

Kilpatrick, D. G., Veronen, L. J., & Best, C. L. (1985). Factors predicting psychological distress among rape victims. In C. Figley (Ed.), *Trauma and its wake* (pp. 113–141). New York: Brunner/Mazel.

Macdonald, A., Monson, C. M., Doron-Lamarca, S., Resick, P. A., & Palfai, T. P. (2011). Identifying patterns of symptom change during a randomized controlled trial of cognitive processing therapy for military-related posttraumatic stress disorder. *Journal of Traumatic Stress, 24*(3), 268–276.

Marks, I., Lovell, K., Noshirvani, H., Livanou, M., & Thrasher, S. (1998). Treatment of posttraumatic stress disorder by exposure and/or cognitive restructuring: A controlled study. *Archives of General Psychiatry, 55*(4), 317–325.

Martin, D. J., Garske, J. P., & Davis, M. K. (2000). Relation of the therapeutic alliance with outcome and other variables: A meta-analytic review. *Journal of Consulting and Clinical Psychology, 68*(3), 438–450.

McCann, I. L., & Pearlman, L. A. (1990). *Psychological trauma and the adult survivor: Theory, therapy, and transformation.* New York: Brunner/Mazel.

Merrill, K. A., & Strauman, T. J. (2004). The role of personality in cognitive-behavioral therapies. *Behavior Therapy, 35*(1), 131–146.

Monfils, M.-H., Cowansage, K. K., Klann, E., & LeDoux, J. E. (2009).

Extinction-reconsolidation boundaries: Key to persistent attenuation of fear memories. *Science, 324,* 951–955.

Monson, C. M., Schnurr, P. P., Resick, P. A., Friedman, M. J., Young-Xu, Y., & Stevens, S. P. (2006). Cognitive processing therapy for veterans with military-related posttraumatic stress disorder. *Journal of Consulting and Clinical Psychology, 74*(5), 898–907.

Moser, J. S., Cahill, S. P., & Foa, E. B. (2010). Evidence for poorer outcome in patients with negative trauma-related cognitions receiving prolonged exposure plus cognitive restructuring: Implications for treatment matching in posttraumatic stress disorder. *Journal of Nervous and Mental Disease, 198,* 72–75.

Mueser, K. T., Rosenberg, S. D., Xie, H., Jankowski, M. K., Bolton, E. E., Lu, W., et al. (2008). A randomized controlled trial of cognitive-behavioral treatment for posttraumatic stress disorder in severe mental illness. *Journal of Consulting and Clinical Psychology, 76*(2), 259–271.

Najavits, L. M., Weiss, R. D., Shaw, S. R., & Muenz, L. R. (1998). "Seeking safety": Outcome of a new cognitive-behavioral psychotherapy for women with posttraumatic stress disorder and substance dependence. *Journal of Traumatic Stress, 11*(3), 437–456.

Nishith, P., Nixon, R. D. V., & Resick, P. A. (2005). Resolution of trauma-related guilt following treatment of PTSD in female rape victims: A result of cognitive processing therapy targeting comorbid depression? *Journal of Affective Disorders, 86*(2–3), 259–265.

Nishith, P., Resick, P. A., & Griffin, M. G. (2002). Pattern of change in prolonged exposure and cognitive-processing therapy for female rape victims with posttraumatic stress disorder. *Journal of Consulting and Clinical Psychology, 70*(4), 880–886.

O'Kearney, R., & Perrott, K. (2006). Trauma narratives in posttraumatic stress disorder: A review. *Journal of Traumatic Stress, 19,* 81–93.

Otto, M. W., Hinton, D., Korbly, N. B., Chea, A., Ba, P., Gershuny, B. S., et al. (2003). Treatment of pharmacotherapy-refractory posttraumatic stress disorder among Cambodian refugees: A pilot study of combination treatment with cognitive-behavior therapy vs sertraline alone. *Behaviour Research and Therapy, 41,* 1271–1276.

Otto, M. W., Pollack, M. H., & Sabatino, S. A. (1996). Maintenance of remission following cognitive behavior therapy for panic disorder: Possible deleterious effects of concurrent medication treatment. *Behavior Therapy, 27*(3), 473–482.80028-1

Paunovic, N., & Öst, L. (2001). Cognitive-behavior therapy vs. exposure therapy in the treatment of PTSD in refugees. *Behaviour Research and Therapy, 39*(10), 1183–1197.

Perconte, S. T., & Griger, M. L. (1991). Comparison of successful, unsuccessful, and relapsed Vietnam veterans treated for posttraumatic stress disorder. *Journal of Nervous and Mental Disease, 179*(9), 558–562.

Pitman, R. K., Orr, S. P., Altman, B., & Longpre, R. E. (1996a). Emotional processing and outcome of imaginal flooding therapy in Vietnam veterans with chronic posttraumatic stress disorder. *Comprehensive Psychiatry, 37*(6), 409–418.

Pitman, R. K., Orr, S. P., Altman, B., Longpre, R. E., Poiré, R. E., & Macklin, M.

L. (1996b). Emotional processing during eye movement desensitization and reprocessing therapy of Vietnam veterans with chronic posttraumatic stress disorder. *Comprehensive Psychiatry, 37*(6), 419–429.

Powers, M. B., Halpern, J. M., Ferenschak, M. P., Gillihan, S. J., & Foa, E. B. (2010). A meta-analytic review of prolonged exposure for posttraumatic stress disorder. *Clinical Psychology Review, 30*(6), 635–641.

Rauch, S. A. M., Defever, E., Favorite, T., Duroe, A., Garrity, C., Martis, B., et al. (2009). Prolonged exposure for PTSD in a Veterans Health Administration PTSD clinic. *Journal of Traumatic Stress, 22*(1), 60–64.

Rauch, S. A. M., Foa, E. B., Furr, J. M., & Filip, J. C. (2004). Imagery vividness and perceived anxious arousal in prolonged exposure treatment for PTSD. *Journal of Traumatic Stress, 17*(6), 461–465.

Ready, D. J., Gerardi, R. J., Backscheider, A. G., Mascaro, N., & Rothbaum, B. O. (2010). Comparing virtual reality exposure therapy to present-centered therapy with 11 U.S. Vietnam veterans with PTSD. *CyberPsychology, Behavior and Social Networking, 13*(1), 49–54.

Resick, P. A., Galovski, T. E., Uhlmansiek, M. O., Scher, C. D., Clum, G. A., & Young-Xu, Y. (2008). A randomized clinical trial to dismantle components of cognitive processing therapy for posttraumatic stress disorder in female victims of interpersonal violence. *Journal of Consulting and Clinical Psychology, 76*(2), 243–258.

Resick, P. A., Nishith, P., Weaver, T. L., Astin, M. C., & Feuer, C. A. (2002). A comparison of cognitive-processing therapy with prolonged exposure and a waiting condition for the treatment of chronic posttraumatic stress disorder in female rape victims. *Journal of Consulting and Clinical Psychology, 70*(4), 867–879.

Resick, P. A., & Schnicke, M. K. (1992). Cognitive processing therapy for sexual assault victims. *Journal of Consulting and Clinical Psychology, 60*(5), 748–756.

Resick, P. A., & Schnicke, M. K. (1993). *Cognitive processing therapy for rape victims: A treatment manual.* Newbury Park, CA: Sage.

Ressler, K. J., Rothbaum, B. O., Tannenbaum, L., Anderson, P., Graap, K., Zimand, E., et al. (2004). Cognitive enhancers as adjuncts to psychotherapy: Use of D-cycloserine in phobic individuals to facilitate extinction of fear. *Archives of General Psychiatry, 61*(11), 1136–1144.

Riggs, D. S., Rukstalis, M., Volpicelli, J. R., Kalmanson, D., & Foa, E. B. (2003). Demographic and social adjustment characteristics of patients with comorbid posttraumatic stress disorder and alcohol dependence: Potential pitfalls to PTSD treatment. *Addictive Behaviors, 28*(9), 1717–1730.

Rizvi, S. L., Vogt, D. S., & Resick, P. A. (2009). Cognitive and affective predictors of treatment outcome in cognitive processing therapy and prolonged exposure for posttraumatic stress disorder. *Behaviour Research and Therapy, 47*, 737–743.

Rothbaum, B. O., Astin, M. C., & Marsteller, F. (2005). Prolonged exposure versus eye movement desensitization and reprocessing (EMDR) for PTSD rape victims. *Journal of Traumatic Stress, 18*(6), 607–616.

Schiller, D., Monfils, M., Raio, C. M., Johnson, D. C., LeDoux, J. E., & Phelps, E. A. (2010). Preventing the return of fear in humans using reconsolidation update mechanisms. *Nature, 463*, 49–53.

Schnurr, P. P., Friedman, M. J., Engel, C. C., Foa, E. B., Shea, M. T., Chow, B. K., et al. (2007). Cognitive behavioral therapy for posttraumatic stress disorder in women: A randomized controlled trial. *Journal of the American Medical Association, 297*(8), 820–830.

Scott, M. J., & Stradling, S. G. (1997). Client compliance with exposure treatments for posttraumatic stress disorder. *Journal of Traumatic Stress, 10*(3), 523–526.

Shalev, A.Y., Bonne, O., & Eth, S. (1996). Treatment for posttraumatic stress disorder: A review. *Psychosomatic Medicine, 58*(2), 165–182.

Speckens, A. E. M., Ehlers, A., Hackmann, A., & Clark, D. M. (2006). Changes in intrusive memories associated with imaginal reliving in posttraumatic stress disorder. *Journal of Anxiety Disorders, 20*(3), 328–341.

Storch, E. A., Merlo, L. J., Bengtson, M., Murphy, T. K., Lewis, M. H., Yang, M. C., et al. (2007). D-cycloserine does not enhance exposure–response prevention therapy in obsessive–compulsive disorder. *International Clinical Psychopharmacology, 22*(4), 230–237.

Tang, T. Z., & DeRubeis, R. J. (1999). Sudden gains and critical sessions in cognitive behavioral therapy for depression. *Journal of Consulting and Clinical Psychology, 67,* 894–904.

Tarrier, N., Pilgrim, H., Sommerfield, C., Faragher, B., Reynolds, M., Graham, E., et al. (1999). A randomized trial of cognitive therapy and imaginal exposure in the treatment of chronic posttraumatic stress disorder. *Journal of Consulting and Clinical Psychology, 67*(1), 13–18.

Tarrier, N., Sommerfield, C., Pilgrim, H., & Faragher, B. (2000). Factors associated with outcome of cognitive-behavioural treatment of chronic post-traumatic stress disorder. *Behaviour Research and Therapy, 38*(2), 191–202.

Taylor, S., Fedoroff, I. C., Koch, W. J., Thordarson, D. S., Fecteau, G., & Nicki, R. M. (2001). Posttraumatic stress disorder arising after road traffic collisions: Patterns of response to cognitive–behavior therapy. *Journal of Consulting and Clinical Psychology, 69*(3), 541–551.

Taylor, S., Thordarson, D. S., Maxfield, L., Fedoroff, I. C., Lovell, K., & Ogrodniczuk, J. (2003). Comparative efficacy, speed, and adverse effects of three PTSD treatments: Exposure therapy, EMDR, and relaxation training. *Journal of Consulting and Clinical Psychology, 71*(2), 330–338.

Tuerk, P. W., Yoder, M., Grubaugh, A., Myrick, H., Hamner, M., & Acierno, R. (2011). Prolonged exposure therapy for combat-related posttraumatic stress disorder: An examination of treatment effectiveness for veterans of the wars in Afghanistan and Iraq. *Journal of Anxiety Disorders, 25*(3), 397–403.

van Minnen, A., Arntz, A., & Keijsers, G. P. J. (2002). Prolonged exposure in patients with chronic PTSD: Predictors of treatment outcome and dropout. *Behaviour Research and Therapy, 40*(4), 439–457.

van Minnen, A., & Foa, E. B. (2006). The effect of imaginal exposure length on outcome of treatment for PTSD. *Journal of Traumatic Stress, 19*(4), 427–438.

van Minnen, A., & Hagenaars, M. (2002). Fear activation and habituation patterns as early process predictors of response to prolonged exposure treatment in PTSD. *Journal of Traumatic Stress, 15*(5), 359–367.

Zayfert, C., DeViva, J. C., Becker, C. B., Pike, J. L., Gillock, K. L., & Hayes, S. A. (2005). Exposure utilization and completion of cognitive behavioral therapy for PTSD in a "real world" clinical practice. *Journal of Traumatic Stress, 18*(6), 637–645.

Part II

RESILIENCE AND RECOVERY IN SPECIAL POPULATIONS

Chapter 4

Sociocultural and Ecological Views of Trauma

Replacing Cognitive–Emotional Models of Trauma

Stevan E. Hobfoll *and* Joop T. V. M. de Jong

It is the nature of science to continue to fit empirical findings into existing paradigms until the paradigm is no longer robust enough to explain the totality of findings (Kuhn, 1962; Popper, 1959). At that point what occurs is a paradigm shift, which is in part what is represented by the very nature of this volume, which shifts from casualty to resilience. However, to the extent that theories of trauma and trauma treatment remain within any one corridor of understanding, be it psychodynamic, cognitive, emotional, biological, or cultural, empirical findings will quickly outstretch theory. We argue that findings have outstripped the central cognitive–emotional paradigm within which trauma has been largely understood, and that the cognitive–emotional underpinning, although critical, must be incorporated within a greater biological and cultural whole (Bracken, Giller, & Summerfield; 1995; de Jong, 2002; Hobfoll, 1998; Miller & Rasmussen, 2010). We argue that this is nothing less than a paradigm shift.

The past two decades have seen a renaissance of research and clinical progress regarding the understanding and treatment of traumatic stress reactions. New treatments have been developed and found to demonstrate some of the highest levels of effectiveness of the treatment of any mental health disorders (Powers, Halpern, Ferenschak, Gillihan, & Foa, 2010). At the same time, theories of traumatic stress have remained stale and are no longer consistent with the existing literature. Only recently, several reviews have expanded to contain a contextualized approach that includes some understanding of biological processes, environmental conditions, and culture, to build on the omnipresent and limited cognitive–emotional model. That is, although the cognitive–emotional model has much to contribute, we know that cognitions and emotions are biologically and culturally biased, and follow rules set within that biology and those cultures. We have no "culturally competent" model of posttraumatic stress disorder (PTSD) (Hinton & Lewis-Fernandez, 2011; Osterman & de Jong, 2007), or even a culturally inclusive model.

On a wider scale, our focus on a dyadic psychotherapeutic or pharmacological approach has contributed to the large global treatment gap. Every year up to 30% of the population worldwide has some form of mental disorder (Chisholm et al., 2007). At least two-thirds of those people receive no treatment, especially in low- and middle-income countries that carry the brunt of disasters and armed conflict. The huge differences in service delivery between high- and low-income countries cannot be explained by variations in psychopathology or in prevalence figures. They can only be explained in terms of political, sociocultural, and contextual variables and need to be addressed with different models (de Jong, 2010).

WHAT MIGHT RESILIENCE AND NATURAL RECOVERY LOOK LIKE?

A major limitation of current models of natural recovery is their lack of inclusion of resilience and its omnipresent representation following trauma (Bonnanno, 2004; Bonanno, Galea, Bucciarelli, & Vlahov, 2007; Layne, Warren, Watson, & Shalev, 2007). We do not think the literature will be well served by a single definition of resilience. There is too little yet known, and too much variation in the natural course of resilience to suggest one single definition. For now, by resilience we mean four things. First, *for most of the emerging literature, resilience refers to people's ability to withstand the most negative consequences of stressful challenges, even of traumatic challenges.* This suggests a broad range of reactivity, but that those who are resilient will not experience what Antonovsky (1979) called "breakdown," or severe psychopathology or physical pathology.

A second view of resilience is one that we find more accurately focuses on resilience and has been advocated by Bonanno (2004). *This view of resilience is defined by those who, when faced with major or traumatic life challenge, either develop few or no symptoms of pathology, or who, perhaps after experiencing moderate symptoms, recover quickly.* This is not at all what the vast majority of studies of resilience have examined, as they have overwhelmingly studied the first definition—the lack of marked distress or pathology. The former definition, and the cognitive–emotional theories that guide them, compares the profoundly or clinically distressed with all others. The latter definition compares the hardly distressed group with all others, and this is a major difference with meaningful implications since it potentially predicts who is doing well.

A *third intriguing definition of resilience is the extent to which people remain vigorous, committed, and absorbed in important life tasks, even amid significant challenge* (Hobfoll, 2011; Hobfoll et al., 2012). This aspect of resilience challenges current thinking on PTSD and trauma responding more generally. In the first view of resilience, that taken in most of the literature, the interest is in who remains relatively free of depression, PTSD, and health problems in the face of stress and trauma. The second definition focuses on who does well, and the third definition focuses on who continues to thrive and function amid adversity. Note that we do not mean that thriving includes growing from the experience, although a few might experience traumatic growth. Rather, they continue to thrive as evidenced by their rich participation in the tasks of life.

The third way of viewing resilience represents an intriguing heuristic path and refers to who remains involved and committed in their life tasks, even if they might at the same time, or recently, have suffered from difficult emotions and health problems. That significant life challenges and losses result in psychological and physical illness and distress is not surprising. That people with more personal, social, and material resources, and who have a healthier life history, experience less such difficulty is important, but again not surprising. That people may experience distress and disease and nevertheless remain committed and absorbed in their life tasks as parents, partners, workers, citizens, and friends is remarkable and something we know little about. We think it is a potential next horizon for research on severe stress and trauma.

Finally, a fourth way of viewing resilience is by adopting an ecological perspective that focuses on context, rather than individuals. One may, in this manner, conceptualize ecological resilience as *those assets and processes existent on all social–ecological levels that have shown to have a relationship with positive outcomes after exposure to situations of mass distress*, as Tol and colleagues (2009) have described for children in armed conflict. We think that all four definitions are valid and heuristic, and that researchers and theorists just need to be clear about which definition they are using.

In this chapter, it is our aim to theorize on this and provide initial results from studies our research groups have conducted in international contexts, where people have survived and the resilient thrived, amid what has been decades of war, terrorism, economic and geographic upheaval, and military occupation, with little expectation of surcease from these environmental conditions. For example, in a study in four postconflict settings

60–90% of the population was exposed to a wide range of traumatic events and 8–25% to torture. Yet, the lifetime prevalence of PTSD varied from 16 to 37%, which indicates that despite the protracted exposure to political violence a majority of the population showed no psychopathology (de Jong et al., 2001). A meta-analysis of torture and other traumatic events showed the importance of broader socioecological factors, such that internally displaced populations and refugees had higher rates of PTSD than those who were permanently resettled in another country (Steel et al., 2009). The act of resettlement and its stability was a certain resiliency factor.

THE EVOLUTIONARY NATURE
OF NATURAL RECOVERY FROM TRAUMA

In terms of our evolutionary shaping, which occurred before the advent of larger collective culture, humans existed under constant traumatic threat and depended on tribal units for sustenance and protection. Until recently, and even now in many regions in the world, trauma was an expected event. Any understanding of the biological and cultural origins of how we are shaped to react to trauma and recovery must be first understood in those terms.

In an evolutionary sense, trauma responses must have some survival components, and therefore hold insights about resilience, or they would have long ago devastated the species. Only recently, and only for a segment of the world population, are people generally protected from a rather regular exposure to devastating trauma. This means our biology and our cultural heritage are loss- and trauma-sensitive. In one of the earliest attempts to quantify infant mortality, estimated in 1661, about 333 of 1,000 infants died before 5 years of age (Gaunt, 1939), a rate more than 30 times higher than the current rate of about 10 per 1,000. The murder rate in Oxford, England, in the 14th century has been estimated to be about 110 per 100,000, 10 times the U.S. rate today (Stone, 1983). Rape is also a common historical threat to women, and especially common as a weapon of war. Even today in the Congo, 48 women are estimated to be raped each hour and 400,000 women were estimated to be raped over a recent period of conflict (Peterman, Palermo, & Bredenkamp, 2011). Partner violence remains a universal problem even in conditions of peace. A large study among 24,000 women in 15 sites in Asia, Africa, Latin America, and Europe reported a lifetime prevalence of physical or sexual partner violence, or both, between 15 and 71%, with six sites having a prevalence rate between 50 and 75% (Garcia-Moreno, Jansen, Ellsberg, Heise, & Watts, 2006). Since interventions for rape or partner violence are hardly available in low- and middle-income countries, these vast numbers of survivors depend on natural recovery to overcome their plight.

APPLYING CONSERVATION OF RESOURCES THEORY
TO RESILIENCE AND NATURAL RECOVERY

Conservation of resources (COR) theory has mainly been left out of trauma theories, but research suggests that resource loss is probably the single best predictor of PTSD and the negative consequences of trauma (Hobfoll, 1998, 2001). COR is the single trauma theory that explains how events occurring long after the trauma exposure can predict PTSD. Moreover, it is one of the few trauma-related theories that makes predictions about resilience and natural recovery.

The basic tenet of COR theory is that individuals have a primary motivation to build, maintain, and protect the resources necessary to protect the self, the family, and the tribe. Many of these resources are primary to survival, such as curiosity, stamina, shelter, tools, family stability, and having attachments to a larger social group. Others are secondary to survival, and include status, jobs and social roles, and objects of status (e.g., warriors' feathers and Rolex watches). Trauma occurs when there is massive threat or loss of primary resources in ways that threaten the self, family, or tribe. But this also means that there must be biological systems built in to the species for recovery from such trauma. Although biological in base, such systems will have social, cognitive, and behavioral routes of expression. Hence, narrative reentry rituals for cleansing following trauma, action motivation, and counteraggression and retribution will also emerge. This suggests that most individuals will be endowed with the ability to endure trauma, and by extension that the family and tribe will develop rituals and practices that will facilitate that process.

COR theory next states a series of principles that aid our understanding of these processes. *The first principle is that resource loss is disproportionally more powerful than resource gain.* Because traumatic stressors are characterized by rapid and momentous loss of resources, this principle is made all the more salient in the case of trauma (Hobfoll, 1991). If we add a more social component, which we must for understanding trauma and resiliency, than we understand that such losses are even more fundamental to the family and tribe than to the individual, and this relates to the aforementioned concept of ecological resilience. This is because the family and the tribe exist based on the fulfillment of roles played by its group members. A given female of fertile age may be lost, but given that during band society when humans were being shaped, band size was perhaps from 30–60 individuals (Fried, 1975), the loss of three or four such females would be devastating to the band, and likewise for the loss of three or four hunter-warriors. Or in modern times, Rockers and colleagues (2010) showed that community characteristics such as village-level traumatic experiences and wealth inequality, as well as individual experiences, may be important determinants of posttraumatic stress in low-income countries, such as postwar Liberia. Resource loss is also more powerful than gain because few life circumstances can cause rapid or momentous increase of individual, family, or tribal resources, but traumatic circumstances could easily result in rapid and momentous loss of such resources. Put another way, the individual or group biological, social, emotional, or structural systems enjoy little or no value in preparing for rapid resource gain, but must have major, central components and attributes that prepare and protect against resource loss. These pathways, be they biological, cognitive, emotional, or social must be *central, powerful, innate, and ritualized.*

The second principle of COR theory is that people must invest resources in order to protect against resource loss, recover from losses, and gain resources. This means that those individuals and groups with greater pretrauma resource reservoirs, and who are able to sustain resources following the trauma, will be more resistant to the initial impact of traumatic events, and to the cascade of resource losses that nearly always follow the initial trauma events. So, resource investment is by its nature fundamental to resiliency.

It follows that individuals, families, and tribes will have natural and built-in response systems for posttrauma resource investment, and individual resilience must be consistent with ecological resilience. The principle social investment factor that has been studied is social support, with many studies showing that social support that is structurally present and functionally activated aids individual, family, and group resiliency following trauma (Brewin & Holmes, 2003). One of the greatest myths of cognitive research was Seligman's (1975) idea of "learned helplessness." Based on the study of rats that could not escape, it explained a situation that seldom occurs among humans. Rather, we can see a catalogue of circumstances where hope, optimism, and rebirth emerge, Phoenix-like from the ashes of even major trauma. Certainly on the familial and tribal–societal level, there is no evidence for learned helplessness. Even in refugee camps people will, despite current restraints, still be coping at some levels, and will respond more favorably as paths are open to them.

The third principle of COR theory is paradoxical. Although resource loss is more potent than resource gain, the salience of gain increases under situations of resource loss (Hobfoll, 1998; Wells, Hobfoll, & Lavin, 1999). This third principle is a primum mobile to an understanding of resiliency and natural recovery. The key element of this principle is that, as people experience resource loss, the significance of gain—which is otherwise minimal—increases substantially. Furthermore, gain spirals accelerate in speed when conditions have produced multiple or critical losses, and they substantially increase in magnitude of their impact because gain's impact generally increases in the face of loss. Thus, although resource gain that is fundamental to resilience and recovery is of low impact biologically, cognitively, emotionally, and culturally under low-loss circumstances, it becomes salient and more fast-paced under high-loss circumstances. This principle also has a clear evolutionary basis. Given that humans were historically on the edge of survival, when losses occurred their circumstances became dire. Their loss focus had to turn quickly to a gain focus, and efforts by the individual and social group had to rally and mobilize powerfully and quickly to forestall doom when circumstances became traumatic. This approach is fundamental to psychological first aid and rapid emergency response to disaster, such as occurs ideally as aid is mobilized after houses and possessions are massively destroyed by a war or a natural disaster, but of course such mobilization of resources is often only available in relatively wealthy regions.

SOME ILLUSTRATIVE STUDIES

In one of the first studies of resiliency trajectories in a situation of chronic trauma exposure, Hobfoll and his colleagues (2009) examined a group of 709 Israeli Jews and Arabs, living within Israel at two times during a period of widespread trauma exposure during 2004 and 2005. About 36% of participants exhibited either few symptoms of depression or PTSD or quickly recovered from symptoms, which was termed "resistance" and "resilience trajectories," respectively. Slightly more than half (54%) of participants showed moderate-to-high levels of symptoms of depression or PTSD, and 10.3% actually became more distressed as environmental trauma eased. This represented much lower levels of resilience and resistance than previously found in more single-trauma circumstances (Bonanno, 2004), indicating that the chronic stress situation sets an outside limit, or passageway, as we develop in this chapter, within which individual response trajectories were exhibited.

It was further found that being in the resilient or resistant group was predicted by being male, having higher income, being a member of the majority (Jewish) population, and having higher education. Having experienced less psychosocial resource loss and greater social support predicted more likely resilience or resistance, and resource loss was the best predictor of outcomes. As they found in prior studies (Hobfoll et al., 2007), reporting greater posttraumatic growth was related to being less resilient or becoming worse over time. That is, those who reported greater posttraumatic growth were more likely to increase in PTSD and depression over time, and also endorsed more violent opinions about using extreme methods to kill the enemy (Hobfoll et al., 2007).

In a second, three-wave study of 1,196 Palestinians living in the areas occupied by Israel in the 1967 War, we found that the passageways of resilience, meaning the ecological conditions that favor or limit reliance, were even more restricted (Hobfoll, Mancini, Hall, Canetti, & Bonanno,

2011). Indeed, if we did not markedly relax the definitions of what resilience included, few individuals would have been termed resilient. By far, the most common trajectory, as can be seen in Figure 4.1, was having moderate levels of PTSD and depression symptoms, and then doing somewhat better as the environmental situation improved, with less violence during the course of the study from 2007 to 2008. This trajectory was exhibited by about two-thirds of participants. It could be termed resilience in that given the environmental levels of trauma, individuals did not develop full-blown PTSD and depression, and they did improve as the situation became less traumatic, but most people were quite symptomatic. Other groups either remained chronically high on distress, or showed high initial distress with some recovery. Those who were less exposed to violence, who were younger, and who had greater social support were more likely to be in the most favorable trajectory. Again, experiencing low levels of psychosocial resource loss was the best predictor of people's outcomes.

It is possible that other predictors of resilience versus distress were simply not included in the study. However, most predictors used in other work were included, but were not represented in final models. Again, the passageways of distress indicated that most individuals were distressed, irrespective of the influence of individual differences, and that individual

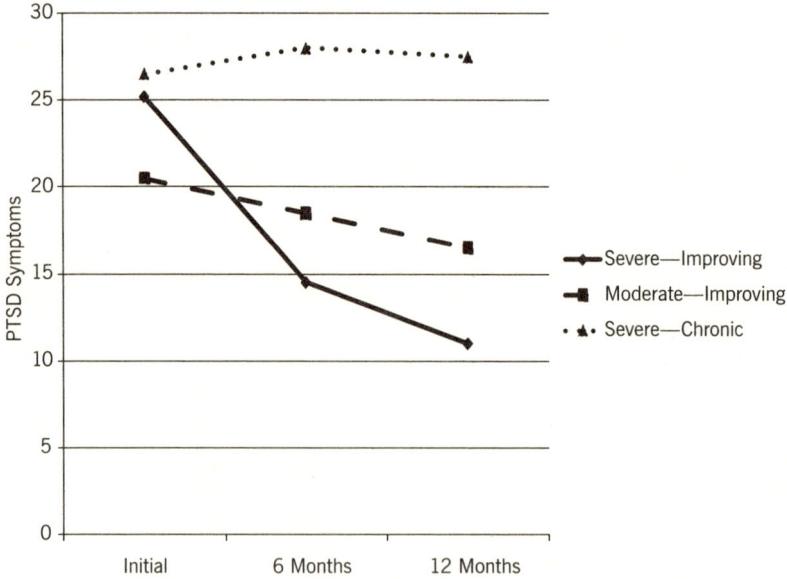

FIGURE 4.1. PTSD symptom trajectory classes in a prospective study of Palestinians during a period of occupation, war, and internecine violence.

differences only played a secondary role within the passageways dictated by the environment, a concept we will develop next.

CARAVAN PASSAGEWAYS
AS CORRIDORS OF NATURAL RECOVERY

Our literature focuses on individual effort and the individual as champion, victim, and patient. This is misleading, as resilience and natural recovery from trauma is most likely where the environmental conditions, present and past, have produced what Hobfoll (2010) has called *caravan passageways*, as illustrated by these prior studies. *Caravan passageways are the environmental conditions that support, foster, enrich, and protect the resources of individuals, families, organizations, communities, and societies, or that detract, undermine, obstruct, or impoverish people's resource reservoirs.*

Individuals and families are able to maintain and develop their resource caravans mainly out of circumstances that are beyond their and their families' control, as the concept of ecological resilience outlines (Tol et al., 2009). That is, the larger environmental conditions of neighborhood, the rule of law, and nation are the main conduits of caravan passageways (see Figure 4.2). From a wider socioecological perspective one

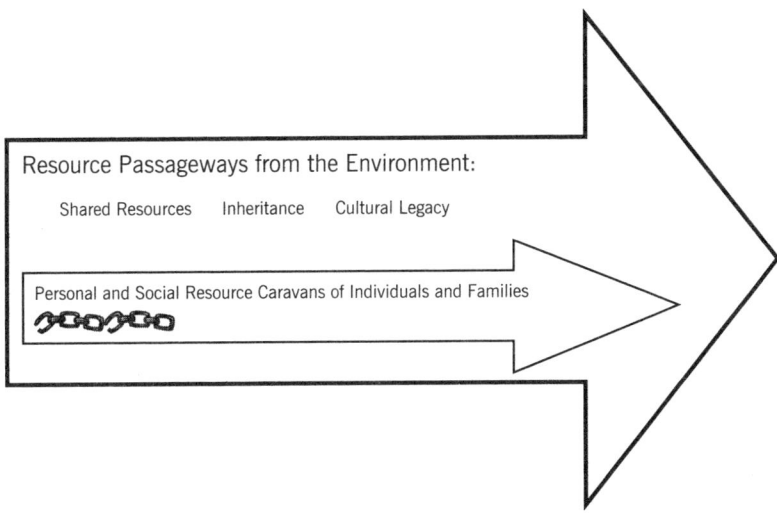

FIGURE 4.2. Resources are linked in resource caravans that are created, supported, and limited by resource passageways from the environment. From Hobfoll, Mancini, Hall, Canetti, and Bonanno (2011). Reprinted with permission from Elsevier.

may argue that the economic, diplomatic, political, criminal justice, human rights, military, health, and rural development sectors have to collaborate to promote peace or prevent the aggravation or continuation of violence (de Jong, 2010). The role played by family is itself large, but even here a positive family contribution usually exists where greater environmental conditions allow for this role. Environments differ in the degree to which they cover a wide variety of quality-of-life or social determinants such as physical safety, quality education, economies that encourage wealth or relative wealth, safe leisure activities, cleanliness of streets, the availability of good employment, the availability of quality medicine and psychological care, the degree of crowdedness, the extent of pollution, clean water, the availability of playgrounds, or green spaces. The environmental conditions are not something that is so much chosen, or created by the self or family, but are given mainly by circumstances of birth or geography.

Inheritance, cultural legacy, and geographic place are the principle mechanism by which material, social, and personal caravan passageways are created and preserved. This concept is important in arguing against the model of individualism, as the individual is hardly standing on his or her own two feet. Or said another way, self-efficacy is not produced substantially by efficacy of the self, but rather by pathways that nurture it. This inheritance is not only directly financial, although it is highly related to financial wealth. The first form of inheritance and cultural legacy that create these passageways is *social* and *cultural capital* (Putman, 2000). This takes the forms of linguistic style (i.e., speaking in an educated manner); access to certain jobs, schools, and social circles; and cultural practices representing status (Miller & McNamee, 1998). An additional form of inheritance and cultural legacy is through family processes, and is termed *inter vivos* transfers, meaning gifts between those living, including material, intellectual, and cultural transfers. These transfers are especially critical in terms of protection from trauma and being places in corridors of social safety. Thus, these *inter vivos* transfers include living in neighborhoods that have quality and safe schools, affordance to advanced education, aid in getting good jobs, and critical help in terms of providing a safety net for children that continues into their adult years.

How such passageways are inherited and transmitted across generations/transgenerationally and how they protect from trauma and support resiliency occurs on a broader community level is exemplified in school and neighborhood factors. Access to quality schools around the world is largely a function of family income, which allows access to good schools and in some parts of the world to any school. Hence, it is not surprising that the socioeconomic status (SES) of the school district and the typical class size are the best predictors of multiple school outcomes, and that poorer neighborhoods have larger average classroom size, making the problem doubly bad for low-income schools (Fowler & Walberg, 1991). Furthermore, these factors are directly and powerfully related to trauma exposure.

For example, the most dangerous neighborhoods in the United States tend to have the worst schools (Aizer, 2009; Kramer, 2000). As Kramer (2000) noted, poverty, inequality, and social exclusion, all structural social factors, are highly related to youth violence. Moreover, these same factors also were found to inhibit the positive influence of family and community resources toward reducing youth violence. Said another way, psychology has helped create a "fallacy of independence and autonomy," suggesting that individual and family efforts, rather than caravan passageways are key (Kramer, 2000). Nor is this merely a problem for the poor. A report by an all-party committee in Great Britain recently found that "opportunity hoarding" by the wealthiest classes made Great Britain one of the least socially mobile countries in Europe (Wintour, 2009). Seeing through such a lens helps explain the repeated cycle of mob violence and riots in the United Kingdom.

As Gallo and Matthews (2003) note, low-SES environments reduce individuals' reserve capacity to manage stress, and increase vulnerability to negative emotions and cognitions. Lower SES results in fewer resources and at the same time is linked to greater stressful experiences and fewer positive experiences in everyday life (Gallo, Bogart, Vranceanu, & Matthews, 2005). This can also be seen played out on the stage of disaster, as those who are poorer were both less likely to be resilient in the face of Hurricane Katrina and also less likely to be insured, which in turn was almost as highly related to psychological distress as was loss of loved ones (Lee, Shen, & Tran, 2009). This means that assistance and repair of these passageways, particularly at times of trauma, are critical intervention strategies.

TRAUMA AND MISSED FOCUS ON SOCIAL, ROLE, AND COMMUNITY CHARACTERISTICS IN AID OF RECOVERY

Because traumatic stress theories are based on experiential psychological platforms they, and the studies they generate, tend to ignore the familial, social, and structural aspects of trauma. Brewin and Holmes (2003) provide an excellent review of psychological theories of posttraumatic stress that we believe still encompasses the emphases of the field today. These theories only mention social context in the correlations with social support, are all cognitive–emotional theories, and are all carefully considered by Brewin and Holmes without regard to any disconfirming data or findings that would tend to argue against the theories from more social and ecological perspectives. That is, each theory does have evidence in its favor, but that the evidence is really partial, that many studies find that the theories do not hold, or that they hold partially, is never considered. This has much to do with the fact that the theories are all embedded in individually oriented clinical psychology and psychiatry, and are not set forth by individuals whose work is contextual, social, or anthropological. Moreover, we must remind ourselves that only 15% of the variance in psychotherapy can be ascribed to technique, 30% to universal therapist variables, 40% to contextual variables, and 15% to placebo (Asay & Lambert, 1999). Yet, in the course of our professional lives, we spend large amounts of time on learning therapeutic techniques and relatively little on handling contextual variables, which are not represented in these leading theories (de Jong, 2010).

Recent considerations in the social–anthropological literature on natural course of trauma reactivity and recovery often deemphasize or even reject PTSD as a concept. The argument that the trauma experience, especially at the time of the trauma (which is what all current theories posited by Holmes & Brewin, 2003, assert) is key is called into question by many community studies of trauma. This is illuminated by work by Ironson and her colleagues (1997) following the 1992 Hurricane Andrew in Florida. The main predictors of trauma reaction severity was rather unrelated to the cognitive–emotional or information-processing variables extant in most theories. Instead, the main factors were degree of material resource loss and length of time to receipt of insurance. These two variables were rather unrelated to the initial trauma experience. Many people only saw the destruction of their homes days and weeks after the hurricane when they returned from their evacuation. Length of time to insurance took months, and has to do with people's ability to activate and renew their life course. Likewise, long waiting periods for asylum status and posttraumatic living conditions predicts depression and PTSD among Iraqi asylum seekers, rather than trauma during the wars in Iraq (Laban, Komproe, Gernaat, & de Jong, 2008). Work by Galea and colleagues (2002) following the attacks on the World Trade Center on September 11, 2001, are also instructive. Consistent with memory and cognitive and emotional processing theories, peritraumatic reaction was a major predictor of outcomes. Inconsistent with such theories, however, was that loss of job and possessions was as large a predictor of PTSD as was any aspect of the experience that occurred at the time of the trauma. That is, loss of these resources was no less critical than the aspects of any of the theories that are posited by Brewin and Holmes (2003), and such losses were almost always known to individuals days and weeks after the initial trauma experience.

Similar findings that undermine emotional-processing and cognitive-processing theories are evidenced by work on Hurricane Katrina survivors. Adeola (2009) found that among the main predictors of post-Katrina distress was residency in the poorest parishes of New Orleans, having dependent children, unemployment, degree of property damage, and financial impacts sustained due to the disaster. Lee and colleagues (2009) found that among Katrina evacuees, not being insured, degree of home destruction, and human loss were the strongest predictors of posttrauma exposure distress. Desalvo and colleagues (2007) found that lack of property insurance, longer evacuation, and commuting distance to work in the post-Katrina period, and the inability to obtain quality new residences, were important predictors of PTSD symptoms. It is important to underscore that for most individuals, degree of home destruction and human loss were not personally witnessed, but facts obtained days or even weeks after the disaster. Likewise, several studies showed that in postconflict areas or among refugees, the period after the war or the human right violations is a more important predictor of psychopathology then the traumatic stress during the armed conflict. Miller and Rasmusssen (2010) argue that trauma-focused advocates tend to overemphasize the impact of direct war exposure on mental health, and fail to consider the contribution of stressful social and material conditions. These findings *require a revamping of our understanding of PTSD and trauma responding and recovery.*

Miller and Rasmussen (2010) found that indigenous expressions of distress were more closely tied to trauma exposure than were PTSD and more closely related to functional impairment than was PTSD. *Jigar khun* was a long-term kind of melancholy, which adults reported as more salient than intrusive images. *Asabi* is a blend of nervousness and anger that often leads to verbal and physical violence and self-beating. Likewise, researchers find dissociation in the form of spirit possession to be a common symptom in southern Ugandans who were exposed to trauma (Van Duijl, Nijenhuis, Komproe, Gernaat, & de Jong, 2010), among northern Ugandan former child soldiers being haunted by spirits called *Cen* (Akello, Richters, & Reis, 2009), and among southern Sudanese by spirits called *Jok Jok*. Furthermore, mass dissociative trance behavior was found among Bhutanese refugees in Nepal (Van Ommeren, Sharma, & Kromproe, 2001), in postwar Guinea Bissau (de Jong & Reis, 2010), in Mozambique (Igreja, 2008), and in Rwanda (Hagengimana & Hinton, 2009).

These behaviors often express themselves in epidemic forms of anxiety, which were observed in culture-bound syndromes such as *koro* in Southeast Asia or in what nowadays is termed "medically unexplained illness" or "idioms of distress." They are expressions of distress or panic molded by sociocultural factors, and bear resemblance to our "sick building syndrome," the mass epidemics in high schools around the globe, or the different syndromes among veterans from different war theaters (cf. Institute of Medicine, *http://veterans.iom.edu*). These epidemics share the following characteristics: (1) a high level of distress in a (sub)population; (2) culture-specific interpretations that make the threat plausible and credible; (3) the symptom and complaints spread primarily among people with an existing vulnerability for anxiety or prone to other vulnerability factors, and those sharing certain characteristics with others in the group; and (4) the symptoms are of short duration and mostly do not develop into chronic disorders (de Jong, 2010). It is quite obvious that these manifestations in so many different places on earth are expressions of (traumatic) stress that do not fit an exclusive PTSD paradigm, and more importantly challenge any theory of posttrauma reaction that does not include them as to how cognition, emotion, brain, context, and culture are interwoven.

The understanding of trauma, and now trauma resilience, is further undermined by the more recent emphasis on neuroscience. Even though we emphasized the biological basis of trauma responding, to think that brain imaging and cellular research will tell a complete story is quite illogical. The universality of neurobiology is challenged by research showing the bidirectional influence of culture and biology, as exemplified in the evolving and intriguing new domains of cultural neuroscience and neuroanthropology (Chiao, 2009; Dominguez Duque, Turner, Lewis, & Egan, 2010). Because the social and cultural fabric does not exist in the brain, it cannot be imaged or understood by neuroimaging, even as the brain must process this information. The cultural web exists outside of the brain and body.

It is our contention, that although these non-Western studies challenge the universality, and therefore the biology of PTSD and self-information processing and cognitive models, they also might shed light on Western samples when we open to the study of such concepts as shame, guilt, morality, spirituality, connectedness, and somatic responsiveness (Friedman, Resick, Bryant, & Brewin, 2011; Litz et al., 2009). That is, these models apply to the West and individualistic cultures, as well as to the East and more collectivist cultures. The bias of our models limits our understanding and study of the breadth of posttrauma findings. This means that PTSD does appear to be universal, as it has been found across highly diverse cultures, but at the same time it is not necessarily the central or focal response to trauma, especially as we move to non-Western and more collectivistic or sociocentric contexts (de Jong, 2005; Markus & Kitayama, 1991; Young, 1995). Since many ethnic subgroups in the West are also more collectivistic than individualistic, and Westernized without being Western, this may mean that models of trauma, PTSD, and recovery among many in the West also may challenge the dominant trauma models.

The focus on resilience also challenges basic assumptions of psychopathology. In our study of 1,196 Palestinians living in the area occupied by Israel following the 1967 War, we examined the extent to which PTSD and depression symptoms were related to people's degree of engagement in life's tasks. By "engagement," we meant the degree to which they persistently and pervasively participated in life tasks (e.g., work, parenting, social functioning), were committed to those tasks, and pursued them with vigor. Our models of psychopathology clearly would indicate that such engagement should be strongly inversely related to depression and PTSD.

When we examined the multiwave, prospective data, as can be seen in Figure 4.3, it can be noted that depression and PTSD were hardly related to engagement. This is open to several interpretations. First, it is possible that nonclinical samples are not debilitated, even when they have high levels of depression and PTSD symptoms. Second, it could be that depression and PTSD express themselves in different ways among Arabs than in Western samples. Third, resilience and psychopathology may coexist in a more pervasive fashion than we have assumed. But, all these interpretations challenge current theories of trauma reactivity and PTSD.

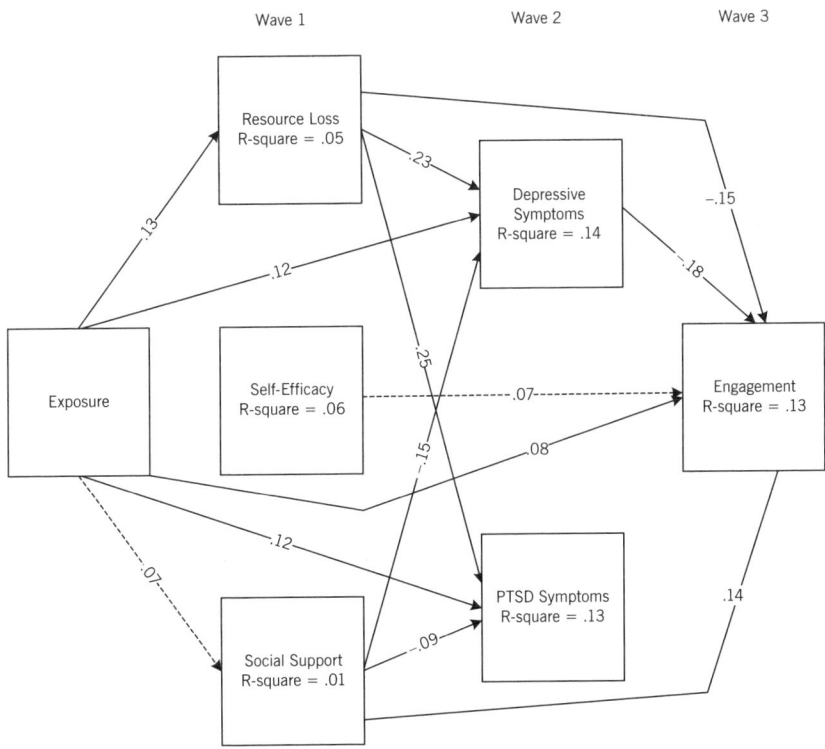

FIGURE 4.3. Multiwave study examining pathways between trauma exposure and engagement among Palestinians living in a period of occupation, war, and internecine violence. From Hobfoll, Mancini, Hall, Canetti, and Bonanno (2011). Copyright 2011 by Elsevier. Reprinted with permission.

THE PRIMACY OF ATTACHMENT AND ATTACHMENT
LOSS IN THE PSYCHOCULTURAL SPACE:
A NEW FOCUS FOR INTERVENTION

A place where the cognitive–emotional, brain, and biological models of trauma and culture may meet is the transactional space between the self and the "other." That is, rather than seeing an individualized self, with a separate psyche and biology, we might construct an idea more closely related to the idea of the socially nested self, in a sense removing the border between the self and others. This kind of thinking is supported by attachment theory, which asserts and finds that those who have close historical attachments, mental models of attachments, and actual attachments are more likely to be resilient and less likely to experience PTSD and other pathological responses to trauma (Ein-Dor, Doron, Solomon, Mikulincer, & Shaver, 2010). But even here we must broaden attachment theory to include attachment to cultural subgroups and larger social structure, all levels that have enormous potential for group, social, structural (e.g., building environments that encourage and enable attachment), and media intervention.

The resource losses most related to trauma and resilience can be grouped into a category that we might call "person-nested in family-nested in ethnic/social subgroup." This translates to an understanding of an attached self that is connected to the fabric of family and society. Society and family provide the defining framework for understanding trauma, outside of biological trauma of harm to the self. Furthermore, because safety is so integral to attachment from cradle to the grave, we can envision that attachments have a sustaining impact on the self and family structures. To the extent the trauma separates the individual from attachments to family, loved ones, home, and social role, it will be traumatic. To the extent these attachments are preserved or restored, trauma responses will be moderated and more short-lived.

Ethnic minority status has often been found to be a major risk variable for PTSD following trauma exposure (Beals et al., 2002; Galea et al., 2002; Kaniasty & Norris, 1993). These findings are typically explained by the presence of racism, and the social correlates of ethnic minority status, including poverty, lower education, and higher rates of single motherhood. But among Americans of Japanese ancestry, rates of PTSD among veterans are low (Friedman, Schnurr, Sengupta, Holmes, & Ashcraft, 2004) to nonexistent (Matsuoka & Hamada, 1991). Friedman and colleagues (2004) also found that the rates of lifetime PTSD were markedly lower for Americans of Japanese ancestry compared to whites, blacks, Hispanics, and Native Hawaiians. This was even more apparent for current PTSD (veterans were mostly in their 40s at the time of the study), which was only one-sixth of whites and Native Hawaiians, less than one-tenth of blacks, and less than one-fourteenth of Hispanics. For cultural factors to be so dominating strongly challenges peritraumatic, cognitive–emotional, and biological models that do not interweave culture as a major integrator of these other factors.

How might this change or expand treatment? We would especially see reattachment to family and the society and reintegration as key aspects if attachment were fundamental to trauma exposure and recovery. Obenchain and Silver (1992) developed a ceremony for the treatment of Vietnam War veterans, designed to address "sanctuary trauma, social isolation, and alienation." Not surprisingly, their treatment borrowed from the collectivist Native American rituals for returning warriors. Treatment would be more social, more societal, and more transitional from homecoming to employment to family reintegration.

SUMMARY AND CLINICAL RECOMMENDATIONS

Our arguments suggest a revision of theories of trauma reactivity and recovery. First, it appears that psychosocial resource loss around issues of safety and attachment are comingled and primary to trauma reactivity, including PTSD and depression. Furthermore, although PTSD appears to be universal, it is not the primary course of reactivity to trauma, it does not capture the diversity in trauma reactions around the globe, nor is it the primary pathological sequence. Rather, the resource passageways of a given culture and environment produce a pathway through which trauma reactivity and recovery follow, including on biological–brain levels. We therefore recommend more mixed-methods research into cultural expressions of distress and into sociocultural–ecological factors influencing resources losses and their impact on individuals, families, and communities.

All cultures produce and enact recuperative processes, and these tend to be consistent with cultural parameters. In the West, circa 20th and 21st century, psychotherapy with a cognitive–emotional emphasis is a culturally consistent pathway. However, because we have extrapolated from clinical populations we have wrongly emphasized, or overemphasized, individual–cognition–brain aspects of this process. Not only do these not accurately apply to nonclinical populations, we have made the mistake of thinking that because a model works in a clinical population in a given culture, that it is the accurate reflection of those processes, or the final solution for those who attempt to recover and find a new balance after extreme stress.

Said another way, if the cognitive–emotional–biological model was adequate, more individuals would develop clinical forms of PTSD with dysfunction, Americans of Japanese ancestry could not have near-zero levels of PTSD, and people in other cultures would express PTSD as the primary reactive response to trauma. Central to our argument, the fact that psychosocial resource loss, particularly around resources concerned with safety and attachment, is the strongest predictor or among the strongest predictors of PTSD and depression, does not fit with current cognitive–emotional models, particularly because these loss sequences are even major predictors if they signal loss weeks and months after the trauma exposure. Reactivity is integrally a function of the individual-nested in family-nested in tribe/group, and "nested" must be seen as meaning safety, attachment, and social role.

We therefore recommend that clinicians try to get more insight into passageways and systemic factors influencing the impact of distress in order to create synergy between external factors and community actors and their own clinical work.

In the end, it is important to incorporate the cognitive–emotional and the neurobiological models in a wider sociocultural context. This translates to more serious attempts to address the global prevention of extreme stress as well as multisectoral and interdisciplinary efforts inspired by the domains of global health, public mental health, and cultural psychology and psychiatry.

ACKNOWLEDGMENTS

This study was made possible, in part, by a grant from the National Institute of Mental Health (NIMH) (No. R01 MH073687) and a grant from the National Institutes of Health (NIH) to the Rush Center for Urban Health Equity (No. NIH-NHLBI 1P50HL105189). We also wish to thank Natalie Stevens, PhD, for her keen editorial assistance.

REFERENCES

Adeola, F. O. (2009). Mental health and psychosocial distress sequelae of Katrina: An empirical study of survivors. *Human Ecology Review, 16,* 195–210.

Aizer, A. (2009). Neighborhood violence and urban youth. In J. Gruber (Ed.), *The problems of disadvantaged youth: An economic perspective* (pp. 275–307). Chicago: University of Chicago Press.

Akello, G., Richters, A., & Reis, R. (2009). Coming to terms with accountability: Why the reintegration of former child soldiers in Northern Uganda fails. In P. Gobodo-Madikizela & C. Van Der Merwe (Eds.), *Memory, narrative, and forgiveness: Perspectives on the unfinished journeys of the past* (pp. 188–212). Newcastle upon Tyne, UK: Cambridge Scholars Publishing.

Antonovsky, A. (1979). *Health, stress, and coping.* San Francisco: Jossey-Bass.

Asay, T. R, & Lambert, M. J. (1999). The empirical case for the common factors in therapy: Quantitative findings. In M. A. Hubble, B. L. Duncan, & S. D. Miller (Eds.), *The heart and soul of change: What works in therapy* (pp. 23–55). Washington, DC: American Psychological Association.

Beals, J., Manson, S. M., Shore, J. H., Friedman, M., Ashcroft, M., Fairbank, J. A., et al. (2002). The prevalence of post traumatic stress disorder among American Indian Vietnam veterans: Disparities and context. *Journal of Traumatic Stress, 15,* 89–97.

Bonanno, G. A. (2004). Loss, trauma, and human resilience: Have we underestimated the human capacity to thrive after extremely aversive events? *American Psychologist, 59,* 20–28.

Bonanno, G. A., Galea, S., Bucciarelli, A., & Vlahov, D. (2007). What predicts psychological resilience after disaster?: The role of demographics, resources, and life stress. *Journal of Consulting and Clinical Psychology, 75,* 671–682.

Bracken, P. J., Giller, M. E., & Summerfield, D. (1995). Psychological responses to war and atrocity: The limitations of current concepts. *Social Science and Medicine, 40,* 1073–1082.

Brewin, C. R., & Holmes, E. A. (2003). Psychological theories of posttraumatic stress disorder. *Clinical Psychology Review, 23,* 339–376.

Chiao, J. Y. (2009). Cultural neuroscience: A once and future discipline. *Progress in Brain Research, 178,* 287–304.

Chisholm, D., Flisher, A. J., Lund, C., Patel, V., Saxena, S., Thornicroft, G., et al. (2007). Scale up services for mental health: A call to action. *Lancet, 370,* 1241–1252.

de Jong, J. T. V. M. (2002). Public mental health, traumatic stress, and human rights violations in low-income countries. In J. de Jong (Ed.), *Trauma, war, and violence: Public mental health in socio-cultural context* (pp. 1–91). New York: Kluwer Academic/Plenum.

de Jong, J. T. V. M. (2005). Deconstructing critiques on the internationalization of PTSD. *Culture, Medicine and Psychiatry, 29,* 361–370.

de Jong, J. T. V. M. (2010). Psychopathology. In J. de Jong & S. Colijn (Eds.), *Handbook of cultural psychiatry and psychotherapy* (pp. 401–421). Utrecht, The Netherlands: de Tijdstroom.

de Jong, J. T. V. M., Komproe, I. H., Van Ommeren, M., El Masri, M., Mesfin, A., Khaled, N., et al. (2001). Lifetime events and post-traumatic stress disorder in four post-conflict settings. *Journal of the American Medical Association, 286*(5), 555–562.

de Jong, J. T. V. M., & Reis, R. (2010). Kiyang-yang, a West-African postwar idiom of distress. *Culture, Medicine, and Psychiatry, 34,* 301–321.

De Salvo, K. B., Hyre, A. D., Ompad, D. C., Menke, A., Tynes, L. L., & Munter, P. (2007). Symptoms of posttraumatic stress disorder in a New Orleans workforce following Hurricane Katrina. (2007). *Journal of Urban Health: Bulletin of the New York Academy of Medicine, 84*(2), 142–152.

Dominguez Duque, J. F., Turner, R., Lewis, E. D., & Egan, G. (2010). Neuroanthropology: A humanistic science for the study of the culture–brain nexus. *Social Cognitive and Affective Neuroscience, 5*(2–3), 138–147.

Ein-Dor, T., Doron, G., Solomon, Z., Mikulincer, M., & Shaver, P. R. (2010). Together in pain: Attachment-related dyadic processes and posttraumatic stress disorder. *Journal of Counseling Psychology, 57,* 317–327.

Fowler, W. J., & Walberg, H. J. (1991). School size, characteristics, and outcomes. *Educational Evaluation and Policy Analysis, 13*(2), 189–202.

Fried, M. (1975). *The notion of the tribe.* New York: Cummings.

Friedman, M. J., Resick, P. A., Bryant, R. A., & Brewin, C. R. (2011). Considering PTSD for DSM-5. *Depression and Anxiety, 28,* 750–769.

Friedman, M. J., Schnurr, P. P., Sengupta, A., Holmes, T., & Ashcraft, M. (2004). The Hawaii Vietnam Veterans Project: Is minority status a risk factor for posttraumatic stress disorder? *Journal of Nervous and Mental Disease, 192,* 42–50.

Galea, S., Ahern, J., Resnick, H., Kilpatrick, D., Bucuvalas, M., Gold, J., et al. (2002). Psychological sequelae of the September 11 terrorist attacks in New York City. *New England Journal of Medicine, 346,* 982–987.

Gallo, L. C., Bogart, L. M., Vranceau, A., & Matthews, K. A. (2005). Socio-economic status, resources, psychological experiences, and emotional responses: A test of the reserve capacity model. *Journal of Personality and Social Psychology, 88,* 386–399.

Gallo, L. C., & Matthews, K. A. (2003). Understanding the association between socioeconomic status and physical health: Do negative emotions play a role? *Psychological Bulletin, 129,* 10–51.

Garcia-Moreno, C., Jansen, H. A. F. M., Ellsberg, M., Heise, L., & Watts, C. (on behalf of the WHO Multi-Country Study on Women's Health and Domestic Violence against Women Study Team). (2006, October). Prevalence of intimate partner violence: Findings from the WHO multi-country study on women's health and domestic violence. *Lancet, 368,* 1260–1269.

Gaunt, J. (1939). *Natural and political observations made upon the bills of mortality* (W. F. Willcox, Ed.). Baltimore: Johns Hopkins University Press.

Hagengimana, A., & Hinton, D. E. (2009). Ihahamuka, a Rwandan syndrome of response to the genocide. In D. E. Hinton & B. J. Good (Eds.), *Culture and panic disorder* (Rev. ed., pp. 205–229). Stanford, CA: Stanford University Press.

Hinton, D. E., & Lewis-Fernandez, R. (2011). The cross-cultural validity of post-traumatic stress disorder: Implications for DSM-5. *Depression and Anxiety, 28*(9), 783–801.

Hobfoll, S. E. (1991). Traumatic stress: A theory based on rapid loss of resources. *Anxiety Research: An International Journal, 4,* 87–197.

Hobfoll, S. E. (1998). *Stress, culture, and community: The psychology and philosophy of stress.* New York: Plenum Press.

Hobfoll, S. E. (2001). The influence of culture, community, and the nested-self in the stress process: Advancing conservation of resources theory. *Applied Psychology, 50,* 337–370.

Hobfoll, S. E. (2011). Conservation of resources theory: Its implication for stress. In S. Folkman (Ed.), *The Oxford handbook of stress, health, and coping* (pp. 127–147). New York: Oxford University Press.

Hobfoll, S. E., Hall, B. J., Canetti-Nisim, D., Galea, S., Johnson, R. J., & Palmieri, P. (2007). Refining our understanding of traumatic growth in the face of terrorism: Moving from meaning cognitions to doing what is meaningful. *Applied Psychology: An International Journal, 56,* 345–366.

Hobfoll, S. E., Johnson, R. J., Canetti, D., Palmieri, P. A., Hall, B. J., Lavi, I., et al. (2012). Can people remain engaged and vigorous in the face of trauma?: Palestinians in the West Bank and Gaza. *Psychiatry, 75*(1), 60–75.

Hobfoll, S. E., Mancini, A. D., Hall, B. J., Canetti, D., & Bonanno, G. A. (2011). The limits of resilience: Distress following chronic political violence among Palestinians. *Social Science and Medicine, 72,* 1400–1408.

Hobfoll, S. E., Palmieri, P. A., Johnson, R. J., Canetti-Nisim, D., Hall, B. J., & Galea, S. (2009). Trajectories of resilience, resistance and distress during ongoing terrorism: The case of Jews and Arabs in Israel. *Journal of Consulting and Clinical Psychology, 77,* 138–148.

Igreja, V. (2008). Gamba spirits, gender relations, and healing in post-civil war Gorongosa, Mozambique. *Journal of the Royal Anthropological Institute, 14,* 350–367.

Ironson, G., Wynings, C., Schneiderman, N., Baum, A., Rodriquez, M., Greenwood, D., et al. (1997). Post-traumatic stress symptoms, intrusive thoughts, loss, and immune function after Hurricane Andrew. *Psychosomatic Medicine, 59*(2), 128–141.

Kaniasty, K., & Norris, F. H. (1993). A test of the social support deterioration model in the context of natural disaster. *Journal of Personality and Social Psychology, 64,* 395–408.

Kramer, R. C. (2000). Poverty, inequality, and youth violence. *Annals of the American Academy of Political and Social Science, 567,* 123–139.

Kuhn, T. S. (1962). *The structure of scientific revolutions.* Chicago: University of Chicago Press.

Laban, C. J., Komproe, I. H., Gernaat, H. P. E., & de Jong, J. T. V. M. (2008). The impact of a long asylum procedure on quality of life, disability and physical health in Iraqi asylum seekers in The Netherlands. *Social Psychiatry and Psychiatric Epidemiology, 43,* 507–515.

Layne, C. M., Warren, J. S., Watson, P. J., & Shalev, A. Y. (2007). Risk, vulnerability, resistance, and resilience: Toward an integrative conceptualization of posttraumatic adaptation. In M. J. Friedman, T. M. Keane, & P. A. Resick (Eds.), *Handbook of PTSD: Science and practice* (pp. 497–520). New York: Guilford Press.

Lee, E. O., Shen, C., & Tran, T. V. (2009). Coping with Hurricane Katrina: Psychological distress and resilience among African American evacuees. *Journal of Black Psychology, 35,* 5–23.

Litz, B. T., Stein, N., Delaney, E., Lebowitz, L., Nash, W. P., Silva, C., et al. (2009). Moral injury and moral repair in war veterans: A preliminary model and intervention strategy. *Clinical Psychology Review, 29,* 695–706.

Markus, H. R., & Kitayama, S. (1991). Culture and the self: Implications of cognition, emotion and motivation. *Psychological Review, 98,* 244–253.

Matsuoka, J. K., & Hamada, R. (1991). The wartime and postwar experiences of Asian-Pacific American Vietnam veterans. *Journal of Applied Social Sciences, 16,* 23–36.

Miller, K. E., & Rasmussen, A. (2010). War exposure, daily stressors, and mental health in conflict and post-conflict settings: Bridging the divide between trauma-focused and psychosocial frameworks. *Social Science and Medicine, 70,* 7–16.

Miller, R. K., & McNamee, S. J. (1998). *The inheritance of wealth in America.* New York: Plenum Press.

Obenchain, J. V., & Silver, S. M. (1992). Symbolic recognition: Ceremony in a treatment of posttraumatic stress disorder. *Journal of Traumatic Stress, 5,* 37–43.

Osterman J. E., & de Jong, J. T. V. M. (2007). Cultural issues and trauma. In M. J. Friedman, T. M. Keane, & P. A. Resick (Eds.), *Handbook of PTSD: Science and practice* (pp. 425–446). New York: Guilford Press.

Peterman, A., Palermo, T., & Bredenkamp, C. (2011). Estimates and determinants of sexual violence against women in the Democratic Republic of the Congo. *American Journal of Public Health, 101,* 1060–1067.

Popper, K. R. (1959). *The logic of scientific discovery.* New York: Basic Books.

Powers, M. B., Halpern, J. M., Ferenschak, M. P., Gillihan, S. J., & Foa, E. B. (2010). A meta-analytic review of prolonged exposure for posttraumatic stress disorder. *Clinical Psychology Review, 30,* 635–641.

Putman, R. D. (2000). *Bowling alone: The collapse and revival of American community.* New York: Simon & Schuster.

Rockers, P. C., Kruk, M. E., Saydee, G., Tornorlah Varpilah, S., & Galea, S. (2010). Village characteristics associated with posttraumatic stress symptoms in post-conflict Liberia. *Epidemiology, 21*(4), 454–457.

Seligman, M. E. P. (1975). *Helplessness.* San Francisco: Freeman.

Steel, Z., Chey, T., Silove, D., Marnane, C., Bryant, R. A., & Van Ommeren, M. (2009). Association of torture and other potentially traumatic events with mental health outcomes among populations exposed to mass conflict and displacement: A systematic review and meta-analysis. *Journal of the American Medical Association, 302*(5), 537–549.

Stone, L. (1983). Interpersonal violence in English society, 1300–1980. *Past and Present, 101,* 22–33.

Tol, W. A., Jordans, M. J. D., Reis, R., & de Jong, J. T. V. M. (2009). Ecological resilience: Working with child-related psychosocial resources in war-affected communities. In D.Brom, R. Pat-Horenczyk, & J. Ford (Eds.), *Treating traumatized children: Risk, resilience, and recovery* (pp. 164–182). London: Routledge.

Van Dujil, M., Nijenhuis, E., Komproe, I. H., Gernaat, H. B. P. E., & de Jong, J. T. (2010). Dissociative symptoms and reported trauma among patients with spirit possession and matched healthy controls in Uganda. *Culture, Medicine, and Psychiatry, 34,* 380–400.

Van Ommeren, M., Sharma, B., & Komproe, I. H. (2001). Trauma and loss as determinants of culture-bound epidemic illness in a Bhutanese refugee community. *Psychological Medicine, 31*(7), 1259–1267.

Wells, J. D., Hobfoll, S. E., & Lavin, J. (1999). When it rains it pours: The greater impact of resource loss compared to gain on psychological distress. *Personality and Social Psychology Bulletin, 25,* 1172–1182.

Wintour, P. (2009, July). Britain's closed shop: Damning report on social mobility failings. *The Guardian.* Retrieved from *www.guardian.co.uk/society/2009/jul/21/all-party-report-on-social-mobility.*

Young, A. (1995). *The harmony of illusions: Inventing posttraumatic stress disorder.* Princeton, NJ: Princeton University Press.

Chapter 5

Children

John A. Fairbank, Ernestine C. Briggs,
Karen Appleyard Carmody, Johanna K. P. Greeson,
and Briana A. Woods

What facilitates resilience and successful adaptation in children exposed to trauma? How can clinicians help trauma-exposed children recover and heal? How do we minimize the sequelae associated with trauma exposure and alter developmental trajectories? In this chapter, we examine facets of resilience during critical developmental periods for children and adolescents exposed to trauma. We begin by delineating the prevalence of violence and trauma in childhood, the array of short- and long-term consequences, key conceptual and theoretical issues, and principles for designing prevention and intervention efforts that facilitate successful adaptation. We conclude with a discussion of the clinical implications for treatment and recovery.

PREVALENCE OF VIOLENCE AND TRAUMA

Among children and adolescents there are alarmingly high rates of exposure to violence and trauma. In a recent nationally representative sample of children and adolescents in the United States 0–17 years of age, 60.6% reported violence exposure in the past year (Finkelhor, Turner, Ormrod, & Hamby, 2009). Among these violence-exposed youth, 10% reported child maltreatment (i.e., physical abuse, emotional or psychological abuse, family abduction or custodial interference, and neglect), 6.1% reported sexual victimization, 38.7% reported two or more direct victimizations, and 10.9% reported five or more victimization experiences in the past year. In addition to high rates among national samples, studies have found similarly high prevalence in both urban and rural U.S. settings (e.g., 68% of children and adolescents in 11 rural western counties of North Carolina exposed to at least one traumatic event by age 16: Copeland, Keeler, Angold, & Costello, 2007; 82.5% of urban youth exposed to one or more traumatic event by age 23: Breslau, Wilcox, Storr, Lucia, & Anthony, 2004).

Specific groups may be at even higher risk for certain types of victimization experiences. For example, in the national sample described above, boys were more likely to be physically assaulted and physically bullied than girls, whereas girls were more likely to be sexually victimized (Finkelhor et al., 2009). Furthermore, 6- to 9-year-olds were more likely to be physically assaulted than younger and older youth, and 14- to 17-year-olds were more likely to be sexually assaulted and physically abused (Finkelhor et al., 2009).

CONSEQUENCES OF VIOLENCE EXPOSURE

The high prevalence of exposure has implications for both short- and long-term consequences across multiple domains of functioning (social, psychological, neurophysiological, and physical) and successful adaptation. Indeed, a growing body of research delineates patterns of increased risk among trauma-exposed youth for social and behavioral problems (interpersonal difficulties, conduct problems, delinquency, and antisocial behaviors), morbidity (e.g., posttraumatic stress disorder [PTSD], depression, substance use, health problems), and mortality (Briggs et al., 2013; Briggs, Thompson, Ostrowski, & Lekwauwa, 2011; Brown et al., 2009; Felitti et al., 1998). At the same time, some children demonstrate positive social, health, and developmental outcomes in the face of adversity or trauma (Luecken & Roubinov, 2012). Understanding the pathways to such adaptive outcomes has the potential to inform interventions with traumatized youth. Next, we explore theory and research on resilience in the lives of children and adolescents, particularly those exposed to maltreatment and other traumatic events.

RESILIENCE THEORY

Definition of Resilience

Resilience is often defined as "the process of, capacity for or outcome of successful adaptation despite challenging or threatening circumstances"

(Masten, Best, & Garmezy, 1990, p. 426). Thus, two conditions are required. First, an individual must be exposed to *adversity*, meaning negative experiences (e.g., poverty, parental psychopathology, violence, childhood maltreatment, and trauma) that have been statistically associated with adverse outcomes. Second, the individual must demonstrate *positive adaptation* following the adverse experience, frequently defined as successful accomplishment of stage-salient developmental tasks or competence in behavioral and social functioning (Luthar & Cicchetti, 2000; Masten, 2001).

Over four decades of research have sought to elucidate the observation that certain individuals demonstrate adaptive development in the face of adversity (e.g., Garmezy, 1974; Rutter, 1979; Werner & Smith, 1982). Initially, research focused on identifying factors (i.e., assets, resources, risks) that moderated associations between risk and adaptation. Within any given population, *assets* are "resources that enhance the likelihood of positive developmental outcomes, independent of risk status" (Yates & Masten, 2004), such as factors within an individual (e.g., coping skills) or within social relationships and organizations (e.g., good schools). *Risks* include "events or conditions that increase the probability of an undesired outcome in a group of people who have the risk factor" (Yates & Masten, 2004, p. 523). Notably, risk factors frequently co-occur, exerting a cumulative effect, such that the higher the number of risk factors, the more deleterious the outcome (Appleyard, Egeland, vanDulmen, & Sroufe, 2005; Sameroff, 2000).

Protective and vulnerability factors are conditions or processes that moderate the effect of risk or adversity on outcomes (Thomlison, 2004; Yates & Masten, 2004). That is, the effect of a protective or vulnerability factor is magnified under conditions of adversity. For example, children whose parents are unable to be supportive or sensitive to the child's need following a disclosure of sexual abuse may be less likely to weather the tides of sexual trauma. Similarly, a child with a behaviorally inhibited temperament or particularly sensitive physiological response system may be particularly vulnerable to developing PTSD following trauma. Yet, assets like the support and sensitivity received from teachers and supportive others at school and their actions to seek safety and treatment may moderate the long-term impact of his or her chronic maltreatment. Each of these factors can operate at the level of the individual, the family, the community, or the social context in which the individual resides. The preponderance of evidence can be summarized in a "short list" of characteristics or factors associated with resilience, as seen in Table 5.1.

In order to design effective interventions and policies to promote adaptation in children following adversity, we need to have not only a list of important factors but also an understanding of the processes through which these factors operate—that is, through which resilience is manifested.

TABLE 5.1. "Short List" of Resilience Factors

Individual
- History of positive adaptation (e.g., secure attachment in infancy, effective self-regulation, positive peer relationships)
- Good intellect and flexible problem-solving skills
- Self-regulation skills
- Positive beliefs about the self
- Appealing temperament/personality, appearance, and talents
- Belief that life has meaning

Family and close relationships
- Positive attachment relationships
- Effective parents and caregivers
- Stable and organized home environment
- Positive relationships with prosocial peers and romantic partners
- Connections to other competent and caring adults
- Supportive kinship networks
- Parents who are involved in education
- Socioeconomic advantages
- Spirituality, faith, and religious affiliations

Community
- Connections to prosocial organizations (e.g., clubs, sports)
- Available, quality social and health services
- Effective teachers and schools
- Safe and effective (i.e., high social cohesion) neighborhoods and communities

Note. From Masten (2001) and Masten, Cutuli, Herbers, and Reed (2009). Copyright 2001 by the American Psychological Association. Copyright 2009 by Oxford University Press. Adapted by permission.

Recent resilience research has focused on the processes underlying resilience that mediate positive, developmentally appropriate outcomes. What emerged from this research is the consistent finding that resilience can be expected, and even common, when basic human processes or adaptational systems (e.g., attachment and caregiving quality, self-regulatory systems) are operating well (Masten, 2001; Yates, Egeland, & Sroufe, 2003; Yates & Masten, 2004; see list in Table 5.2).

In essence, resilience functions as "ordinary magic" (Masten, 2001)—essentially, it is an outcome of normative processes operating under extreme conditions. When those basic functions are disrupted, competence following adversity is greatly challenged. Alternatively (and importantly, from an intervention perspective), preserving, supporting, or repairing these

TABLE 5.2. Basic Adaptational Systems for Resilience

- Attachment relationships
- Human intelligence and information processing (a human brain in good working order)
- Motivation to adapt and opportunities for agency (mastery motivation)
- Self-control and emotion regulation (self-regulation)
- Religious and cultural systems that nurture human development and resilience
- Schools and communities that nurture and support human development and resilience

Note. From Masten (2001). Copyright 2001 by the American Psychological Association. Adapted by permission.

systems may promote positive development following adversity (Yates & Masten, 2004). For example, with a child who has experienced abuse and been removed from the home, attempts to maintain connections with siblings and foster connections to support systems at school and efforts to encourage academic and social success may help a child adapt to and begin to address the challenges and traumatic experiences in his or her life. Thus, in the aftermath of trauma, the preservation and/or restoration of supportive relationships and resources is critical to promoting successful adaptation and minimizing developmental derailments.

These findings underscore the importance of conceptualizing resilience as a *process* of development as opposed to an *individual trait* or *characteristic residing in a particular child*. Early writings (scientific and popular) characterized children with resilient patterns of adaptation as "invulnerable," "invincible," or even "superhuman" (Masten, 2001). Rather than a permanent, static state of invulnerability, resilience should be considered as a relative or probabilistic state, which may change with shifting assets, risks, and adaptational systems. Indeed, individuals who have experienced major adversities may not exhibit consistently positive adjustment over the life course, and some fluctuation in functioning may be expected (see Luthar, Cicchetti, & Becker, 2000). To emphasize this point, Masten (1994) cautions against using the term "resiliency," as this implies a trait or personal attribute. Representing resilience as a trait increases the risk of stigmatizing traumatized children through interpretations (particularly by policymakers and the public) that children or individuals should simply "try harder" or "pull themselves up by their bootstraps" and "make themselves" resilient (Luthar & Cicchetti, 2000; Yates & Masten, 2004). From a clinical perspective, a thorough assessment of developmental history, assets, and risks within a child and his or her social ecology is critical to the development of a resilience-informed treatment plan. Moreover, ideally (however challenging practically), having a system of trauma-informed supports and services (e.g., case workers, resource parents, therapists) available to children across time (e.g., offering additional courses of treatment as new developmental issues arise) will be most helpful in promoting positive developmental trajectories.

Theory Behind Resilience

Three major theories influence the construct of resilience (Luthar et al., 2000; Yates et al., 2003). It is important to note that these theories are not uniquely associated with or applied to resilience (Luthar et al., 2000); rather, they are essential developmental theories that apply to many developmental concepts. This next section describes these theories in greater detail.

First, the assumption of a *triarchic framework* is key (Luthar et al., 2000). When considering resilience, protective and vulnerability factors are understood to operate at three levels: child (e.g., biology, personality), family (e.g., cohesion, quality of relationships), and larger social environment (e.g., culture, community). This multidimensional, multisystemic framework has informed much of the risk and resilience literature, emphasizing the need to examine resources across levels in order to best understand the processes influencing resilience in children and adolescents (Masten et al., 1990; Werner & Smith, 1982).

Building on this first theoretical perspective, the *ecological–transactional model* of development (Bronfenbrenner, 1977; Cicchetti & Lynch, 1993; Sameroff & Chandler, 1975) posits that the varying, nested levels within the child's ecology (e.g., child, caregiver/family, and environmental characteristics) mutually influence each other across time to shape the pathways of development. Factors within these ecological niches are thought to interact and transact with each other over time in ways that result in a balance or imbalance of risk factors and assets. It is the balance of negative and positive factors at a given time, and the history of previous experience and adaptation that result in the child's current experience and outcomes of development. Whichever way the hypothetical "scale" tips is thought to result in the child's overall experience or outcome. For example, an imbalance of risk factors (e.g., poverty, homelessness, exposure to domestic violence) without counteracting protective mechanisms (e.g., supportive caregivers, stable attachments, community-based resources) may result in maladaptation (such as depression, anxiety, or PTSD), whereas adaptation (such as positive behavioral and emotional functioning, positive peer relationships) may result from more protective mechanisms being in place.

Third, the *organizational perspective* on development (see Sroufe & Rutter, 1984; Yates et al., 2003) also underlies the process of resilience. The organizational perspective holds that development occurs in a hierarchical manner, such that developmental status at any age is built upon previous experience and competence (Sroufe & Rutter, 1984). Early childhood experiences and developmental accomplishments are carried forward in, and transformed by, later experiences and development (Egeland, Carlson,

& Sroufe, 1993). For example, competence in the stage-salient tasks of infancy and toddlerhood (e.g., secure attachment relationships, development of autonomy) serves as a strong base for competence in preschool and middle childhood tasks (e.g., self-regulation, effective peer relations, friendship formation; Egeland et al., 1993), even in the face of adversity. Conversely, those children without such firm foundations may be compromised in facing later challenges. In some respects, adaptation begets adaptation, whereas maladaptation begets maladaptation across development. The longer on any particular developmental path, the less likely it is for major shifts to occur (Sroufe, 1997; Yates et al., 2003). Yet dynamic transactions between the child and compensatory influences in the environment allow for change and "righting" of the developmental course (Sroufe, 1997). Taken together, these three guiding perspectives outline the role of multiple systems, the transactional nature of influences shaping development, and the importance of considering developmental history in defining resilience and developing strategies for prevention and intervention.

APPLYING THE THEORIES AND CONCEPTS
OF RESILIENCE TO CHILDHOOD TRAUMA

The empirical literature on resilience among children and adolescents following a traumatic event has largely been shaped by these three developmental theories. The emphasis in the literature has generally been on the *triarchic framework* or the ecological–transactional nature of modifiable risk and protective factors. These factors are frequently examined as moderators and mediators of the relations between trauma exposure and adaptation as well as independent predictors of positive adaptation among children and adolescents exposed to trauma. Current resilience research focuses not only on a child's individual traits and characteristics, but also on family and contextual factors (see Luthar et al., 2000). This is true of resilience research focused on traumatic events as well, which includes studies of individual, family, peer, school, and community risk and protective factors. In addition to examining factors at a variety of levels of children's social ecology, trauma and resilience research (outlined below) examines factors that promote adaptive functioning among children and adolescents exposed to a variety of traumatic events including domestic violence, physical abuse, sexual abuse, and community violence.

Domestic Violence

Among children exposed to domestic violence, research supports a range of risk and protective factors related to positive adaptation. At the individual level, research suggests easier temperament (measured by adaptability, intensity, approach, rhythmicity, and mood) often characterizes children who are successfully able to adapt in spite of the violence in their homes/families (i.e., children with nonclinical levels of internalizing and externalizing behaviors over time; Martinez-Torteya, Bogat, Von Eye, & Levendosky, 2009). At the family level, parenting style and behavior, as well as parental mental health are protective factors associated with resilience. In particular, high maternal control and authority and mother-rated parenting effectiveness are associated with lower externalizing behavior among children exposed to domestic violence (Levendosky & Graham-Bermann, 2000; Levendosky, Huth-Bocks, Shapiro, & Semel, 2003). Similarly, lower levels of maternal depression are also predictive of resilience among children exposed to domestic violence (Martinez-Torteya et al., 2009). Cultural expectations and beliefs about violence as well as available informal and formal supports, economic factors, and community resources are additional ecological factors that should be considered as part of the assessment and intervention. Understanding, for example, how poverty, high levels of conflict, excessive alcohol use, and childhood exposure to violence may interact with other cultural factors to predict domestic violence—albeit complicated—is important to developing effective intervention strategies. These many and varied factors underscore the role of assessment of these vulnerabilities and assets in order to address these issues comprehensively (e.g., providing treatment for maternal depression, training in effective parenting strategies in addition to trauma treatment for the child).

Physical Abuse

Among physically abused children, parental sensitivity (e.g., responsiveness) is associated with higher prosocial behavior and lower aggression (Haskett, Allaire, Kreig, & Hart, 2008). Furthermore, in a study examining intergenerational transmission of physical abuse, Dixon, Brown, and Hamilton-Giachritsis (2009) identified feelings of isolation and financial problems as risk factors for parents who were physically abused and continued the cycle of abuse with their children. Child physical abuse and domestic violence frequently co-occur, producing a potential "double whammy" of bad outcomes for children exposed to both (Moylan et al., 2010). From a clinical perspective, planned conjoint sessions with parents and children that promote parents' capability to respond supportively to their children and linkages and case management to address the social and concrete support needs of families may be beneficial with families with histories of physical abuse.

Sexual Abuse

Among children with a history of sexual abuse, research has documented relations between a number of risk and protective factors and child, adolescent, and adult adaptation, which differ by gender. At the individual level, religiosity and perceived health for females and emotional well-being for males tend to protect against negative outcomes including suicidal and self-injurious behaviors, substance use, sexual risk behavior, disordered eating behavior, delinquent behavior, and poor school performance (Chandy, Blum, & Resnick, 1996, 1997). At the family level, perceived caring from adults and living with both biological parents for females and maternal education and perceived caring from parents for males relate to positive adaptation (Chandy et al., 1996, 1997). In addition, satisfaction with caregiver emotional support related to the abuse incident is associated with resilience, including higher self-esteem, lower depression, fewer parent-reported internalizing problems, and fewer parent- and teacher-reported externalizing problems (Rosenthal, Feiring, & Taska, 2003). Looking specifically at protection against severe negative outcomes, a recent statewide survey demonstrated both family and contextual level factors, including family connectedness, perceived caring from teachers, perceived caring from other adults, and school safety significantly reduced the association between sexual abuse and suicidal ideation and suicide attempts among female and male students (Eisenberg, Ackard, & Resnick, 2007). Research examining childhood sexual abuse and adult adaptation suggests social support following the abuse predicted resilient outcomes in adulthood, particularly related to health status and psychological symptoms (Jonzon & Lindblad, 2006; Testa, Miller, Downs, & Panek, 1992). Taken together, a unifying theme across these studies indicates the need in clinical work with traumatized children to promote emotional support, such as through psychoeducation to family members and supportive others about the emotional needs of traumatized youth and coaching supportive others in how to provide support and enhance safety and stability following trauma.

Community Violence

Research suggests numerous factors at various levels may promote resilience among adolescents exposed to community violence, yet these factors are complex and differ depending on the outcome and population examined. At the individual level, emotion-focused and problem-focused coping predict fewer externalizing problems (Kliewer et al., 2006; McGee, 2003) and a sense of personal control protects against psychological problems (Rosenthal & Wilson, 2008) among children exposed to community violence. Furthermore, a sense of purpose and positive self-perceptions reduce the negative impact of community violence exposure on adaptive functioning for urban adolescents (Copeland-Linder, Lambert, & Ialongo, 2010; DuRant, Cadenhead, Pendergrast, Slavens, & Linder, 1994). For African American males, high academic competence and self-worth reduced the risk of later substance use following community violence exposure

(Copeland-Linder, Lambert, Chen, & Ialongo, 2011). Therapeutic interventions aimed at developing and modeling such skills and competencies (e.g., emotion-focused coping, problem-solving skills, positive self-perceptions) may support the healthy recovery of children from community violence. At the family level, factors such as parental monitoring and support are related to resilience; however, these associations are complex and depend on level of exposure. For example, research demonstrates that parental monitoring promotes resilience only among youth exposed to *low* levels of community violence (Ceballo, Ramirez, Hearn, & Maltese, 2003; Sullivan, Kung, & Farrell, 2004). Furthermore, while family support relates to fewer symptoms of distress among urban youth exposed to community violence (Howard, Budge, & McKay, 2010), general social support protects against mental health problems only under low levels of exposure (Hammack, Richards, Luo, Edlynn, & Roy, 2004). In addition, when examining academic outcomes, parental support does not buffer the impact of witnessing community violence on academic achievement (Henrich, Schwab-Stone, Fanti, Jones, & Ruchkin, 2004). In clinical and community settings, programs such as Strengthening Family Coping Resources (Kiser, Donohue, Hodgkinson, Medoff, & Black, 2010) and Strengthening Families Program (SFP; e.g., Spoth, Redmond, Shin, & Azevedo, 2004) that enhance parental monitoring, nurturing skills, and child management skills may be beneficial in preventing exposure to community violence and related sequelae (e.g., substance use, distress, poor academic functioning). Further research is needed to determine additional family-level sources of adaptation to facilitate resilience among children exposed to community violence.

At the school level, identification with school and teacher support is associated with resilience among children exposed to community violence (Ludwig & Warren, 2009; O'Donnell, Schwab-Stone, & Muyeed, 2002). The research on peer support is mixed, with some studies indicating peer support among urban youth exposed to community violence is associated with resilient outcomes (e.g., higher intentions to persist academically; Howard et al., 2010), whereas others suggest peer support is associated with nonadaptive outcomes (e.g., substance abuse, delinquency; O'Donnell et al., 2002). Thus, the types of peers or peer support provided may determine adolescents' outcomes. In summary, a variety of factors across ecological levels are associated with more positive outcomes for children and youth. Clinicians who are familiar with the research will be better prepared to target the appropriate interventions at the appropriate ecological levels.

FACILITATING RESILIENCE
THROUGH PREVENTION AND INTERVENTION

Resilience research holds many implications for the design of prevention and intervention strategies and policies. With an emphasis on strengths and positive outcomes along with modifiable factors and mechanisms that point to appropriate intervention targets, the construct of resilience is inherently geared toward prevention and intervention (Luthar & Cicchetti, 2000). Readers are cautioned, however, against making assumptions that children can "'make themselves' enduringly resilient" (Luthar & Cicchetti, 2000). For example, interventions focused on improving the child's coping skills in the absence of changing the child's environment or traumatic situations may fail (Luthar & Cicchetti, 2000). As emphasized by the ecological–transactional model, risk and protective factors function at multiple levels of the child's ecology (child, family, community). Thus, interventions that influence multiple levels of the child's ecology (e.g., Prinz, Sanders, Shapiro, Whitaker, & Lutzker, 2009; Saxe, Ellis, Fogler, Hansen, & Sorkin, 2005) are more likely to succeed.

Resilience theory and research point to three primary strategies for prevention and intervention (Masten, Cutuli, Herbers, & Reed, 2009). *Risk-focused strategies* aim to reduce children's exposure to risky or harmful experiences (e.g., screening for and treating postpartum depression and history of maltreatment or domestic violence in mothers of newborns). *Asset-focused strategies* seek to increase the amount or quality of resources available to children that promote development (e.g., educating parents about child development and effective parenting). *Process-focused strategies* focus on addressing the protective systems of development such as attachment relationships, self-regulation, and schools/communities (e.g., home visiting programs that enhance the quality of attachment relationships, treatments that build self-efficacy through graduated exposure to and mastery over challenges). Finally, since resilience is defined by successful achievement of stage-salient developmental tasks (e.g., secure attachment, adjustment to school), intervention targets change over time and across development (Shaffer & Yates, 2010). In early childhood, for example, interventions might focus on enhancing the infant–parent attachment relationship to promote/support early relationship and regulatory skills, whereas in middle childhood the focus may reach beyond the immediate household to relationships and opportunities outside the home (schools, peers, neighborhoods).

Taken together, work in this area underscores the need for comprehensive, developmentally appropriate prevention and intervention approaches, addressing multiple risks, assets, and processes to promote optimal outcomes for children and adolescents. Luthar and Cicchetti (2000) offer a set of guiding principles for designing resilience-based prevention and intervention strategies (see Table 5.3). These guidelines emphasize theoretical grounding, address both reduction in risk and promotion of strengths and resources at multiple levels of influence, and focus on developmentally and culturally appropriate practice. In addition, they highlight the value of evaluation and data-informed practice to promote intervention refinement, dissemination, and program sustainability. We next review several

TABLE 5.3. Principles for Designing Resilience-Based Prevention and Intervention Strategies

1. Interventions should be grounded in theory and research for the particular group being targeted by program, acknowledging transactional influences in human ecology, and addressing key modifiable factors.

2. Prevention and intervention efforts should focus not only on reducing negative outcomes or maladjustment, but also promoting positive adaptation or competence.

3. Interventions should not only reduce risk and vulnerability factors, but also build strengths and resources.

4. Strategies should work across multiple levels of influence, addressing salient vulnerability and protective processes.

5. Interventions should be developmentally informed, addressing developmentally appropriate issues for the target population.

6. Input from the target community should be considered to ensure cultural and contextual relevance of the intervention.

7. Consideration should be given to the long-term sustainability of the program within the community.

8. When possible, process and outcome data from comparison groups should be collected and compared with the intervention group, to determine the specific benefits of the intervention.

9. Documentation and ongoing evaluation are critical to guiding intervention development, refinement, and dissemination.

Note. From Luthar and Cicchetti (2000). Copyright 2000 by Cambridge University Press. Adapted by permission.

trauma-specific interventions that, through rigorous research and implementation science, meet these guidelines and promote resilience for children who have experienced trauma.

TRAUMA-SPECIFIC INTERVENTIONS FOR CHILDREN AND ADOLESCENTS

Over the last two decades, there has been a burgeoning of trauma-focused interventions for children and adolescents. Among these are several evidence-based and promising practices that are disseminated as part of the National Child Traumatic Stress Network (NCTSN; see *www.nctsn. org*), and include trauma-focused cognitive-behavioral therapy (TF-CBT; Cohen, Mannarino, & Deblinger, 2006), structured psychotherapy for adolescents responding to chronic stress (SPARCS; DeRosa et al., 2006), child–parent psychotherapy (CPP; Lieberman, Van Horn, & Ghosh Ippen, 2005), parent–child interaction therapy (PCIT; Eyberg, Boggs, & Algina, 1995; Hembree-Kigin & McNeil, 1995; Urquiza & McNeil, 1996), cognitive-behavioral interventions for trauma in schools (CBITS; Jaycox et al.,

2009; Kataoka et al., 2003), trauma-focused coping multimodality trauma treatment (Amaya-Jackson et al., 2003; March, Amaya-Jackson, Murray, & Schulte, 1998), trauma systems therapy (TST; Saxe et al., 2005), trauma adaptive recovery group education and therapy (TARGET-A; Ford & Russo, 2006), and alternatives for families (AF-CBT; Kolko & Swenson, 2002). Although the strategies used differ by the specific intervention, for the most part these interventions all include developing and improving supportive relationships, enhancing parental support and effectiveness, developing a sense of meaning, enhancing problem-solving and coping skills, and remediating factors in the social environment that perpetuate symptoms.

To illustrate how these factors may occur in treatment, we have selected a few interventions to highlight some of the elements commonly used in treatment to facilitate resilience and recovery. Among the evidence-based approaches for trauma exposure and sequelae, TF-CBT has the most evidence, demonstrating effectiveness in reducing PTSD, depression, shame, and trauma-related and general behavioral problems (Cohen et al., 2006; Silverman et al., 2008). TF-CBT is typically delivered in 12 to 20 sessions and is appropriate for children and adolescents ages 3 to 18 years. By working across multiple levels of the child's ecology (i.e., child, family), TF-CBT improves coping skills, self-regulation, and problem-solving skills, as well as enhances caregiver and parental effectiveness.

Coping Skills and Self-Regulation

Many trauma-focused interventions use components that address coping, relaxation, and affective modulation skills to enhance a child's ability to self-regulate and adapt. TF-CBT, for example, teaches youth to use relaxation techniques to reduce the physiological manifestations of stress and PTSD (e.g., increased adrenergic tone, startle response, hypervigilance, agitation), which can be especially problematic when traumatic reminders are experienced. Several relaxation strategies are taught, including focused breathing, mindfulness, meditation, and progressive muscle relaxation. The intervention also includes a specific focus on relaxation for children experiencing traumatic grief, as well as relaxation for parents.

Affective expression and modulation skills are also critical components that lead to successful adaptation and resilience. Children and adolescents who have experienced trauma learn how to identify, express, and manage their feelings more effectively, which in turn increases awareness and internal locus of control and decreases being overwhelmed by the strength of one's feelings. In essence, this approach trains children and adolescents to recognize the stimuli that may provoke negative emotions (e.g., feeling depressed or hopeless) and reduce physiological arousal via several techniques including relaxation and self-talk. This component is often multifaceted, and includes feelings identification, emotional expression, thought interruption, positive imagery, positive self-talk, enhancing the child's sense of safety, and social skills building. Feelings cards, thermometers, and other therapeutic aids facilitate awareness and help the child/adolescent more accurately gauge his or her reactions so that he or she can manage feelings more effectively. Some interventions also include skill-building components for caregivers (behavior management, emotional expression, affect management) to both teach and reinforce these skills.

Problem-Solving Skills

Given that chronic exposure to trauma often leads to the development of maladaptive coping responses, many trauma-focused interventions focus on enhancing problem-solving skills. For example, having very limited responses to uncertain or challenging situations may serve as a potential trigger for affect dysregulation. Although there may be slight variation across treatments, many include basic skills such as describing the problem, identifying possible solutions, considering likely outcomes of each solution, picking the solution most likely to achieve the desired outcome, and implementing that choice. SPARCS and TARGET, for example, include many of the aforementioned components and add a twist by emphasizing meaning (i.e., underlying beliefs and values—respect, justice, fairness, independence, and honesty) and tying meaning to both the goals and options components of problem solving to increase the likelihood of a prosocial desired outcome.

Parent and Caregiver Effectiveness

Many of the trauma-focused interventions (e.g., TF-CBT, AF-CBT, PCIT, TST) facilitate resilience by enhancing both caregiver support and their ability to respond to trauma-related emotional and behavioral problems. An array of parenting strategies are utilized including labeled praise, selective attention, effective time-out procedures, communication skills, and contingency reinforcement schedules (i.e., behavior charts).

Other interventions, such as CPP, an evidence-based treatment utilizing the parent–child relationship as the vehicle for young child improvement, focus on the dyadic relationship to facilitate resilience. Specifically, the goal of CPP is to support and strengthen the relationship between a child and his or her parent (or caregiver) in order to restore the child's sense of safety, attachment, and appropriate affect and improve the child's cognitive, behavioral, and social functioning. Regardless of the approach, the development of effective parenting skills promotes many of the aforementioned protective factors and reduces some of the aforementioned risk factors that serve as barriers to the child's healing process. For example, parents/caregivers learn how to maintain normal routines and consistent rules, set appropriate developmental expectations, improve responsiveness, remediate factors that threaten safety and stability, and enhance a sense of connectedness, which in turn promotes adaptive functioning in both the child and his or her adult caregiver.

SUMMARY AND CLINICAL RECOMMENDATIONS

Given the high rates of trauma exposure in both clinical and community populations of children, it is important for clinicians to be well versed in how to assess for trauma exposure and related symptoms (e.g., PTSD, depression, behavioral problems). It is equally important to understand the impact of trauma across multiple domains of functioning (e.g., social, behavioral, psychological, neurophysiological, and physical) and the factors that may either suppress (e.g., nurturing caregiver, prosocial activities, school-based resources) or exacerbate (e.g., ongoing violence, housing instability, parental substance use) symptom expression. Relevant individual, familial, and contextual risks and resources become particularly salient targets for intervention and treatment.

Protective factors that promote resilience in the clinical domain may take on many different forms including teaching effective parenting strategies; fostering the bonds of a secure attachment; enhancing a child's sense of purpose and meaning; teaching a variety of problem-solving, affect regulation, and coping skills; processing the trauma; addressing cognitive distortions; connecting the child and family to informal and formal resources; capitalizing on existing strengths; and mitigating factors within the environment that pose additional threat to the child's safety and well-being.

Many parents and caregivers may think that "forgetting" about the trauma or "moving on" are helpful steps in recovery; however, research and clinical experience has clearly demonstrated that gradually talking about the trauma is important in resolving symptoms and integrating the experience into the larger context of the child's life in an optimal way (Deblinger & Heflin, 1996; March et al., 1998). Additionally, linking problematic symptoms to trauma or violence exposure is another strategy for clinicians to help children and their caregivers learn about the impact of trauma (i.e., psychoeducation) as well as specific skills that facilitate coping, affect regulation, and management of trauma-related symptoms. For example, if the child has difficulty falling asleep, nightmares, or difficulty staying asleep, a clinician might work with the parent and child to build soothing and comforting rituals into bedtime routines. The clinician may also work with the parent to augment the child's sense of safety and security within the environment, as recovery can be thwarted by ongoing exposure to trauma, violence, and adversity. This sometimes means clinically addressing issues of ongoing violence, substance use, and other adversities such as persistent poverty, unsuitable housing conditions, and dangerous and threatening schools or neighborhoods.

Clearly, clinicians cannot tackle these tasks alone, but they can assist children and their families by supplementing effective interventions with case management services (e.g., coordinating treatment services, providing transportation, communicating with other providers), adjunctive interventions/services (e.g., prosocial activities, recreational programs, volunteer activities), or coordinating services/resources with community partners (e.g., social services, housing authority, legal aid, domestic violence shelters). Of course, these interventions must also be delivered in a manner that is culturally relevant, is sustainable, and leads to measurable outcomes. Certainly, ongoing evaluation is a critical step in developing, refining, implementing, and disseminating programs that foster healing, resilience, and recovery for children who have been exposed to trauma and violence.

Regardless of the type of trauma treatment selected, there are underlying principles that are important for new and experienced clinicians to consider as part of the therapy and recovery process. These concepts have been delineated in the Core Concepts of Child Trauma (CCCT) curriculum, a tool for accelerating and improving trauma-informed care. These core concepts include

> (a) enhancing practitioners empathic understanding of the nature of traumatic experiences from the child's and family's perspective, and the ways in which trauma and its aftermath influence their lives; (b) facilitating the development of clinical reasoning and clinical judgment in practitioners who work (or plan to work) with traumatized youth and families; (c) increasing practitioners' interest in, and readiness for, trauma-informed evidence-based practice (EBP), including training in specific EBPs; (d) providing a clinical practice- and clinical research-friendly conceptual framework that will facilitate clearer dialogue between practitioners and researchers of different theoretical orientations and professional disciplines; and (e) encouraging learners to systematically evaluate each case from multiple perspectives in ways that help them to better understand and address the unique circumstances, strengths, and needs of each client. (Layne et al., 2011, p. 245)

In conclusion, reactions to trauma and violence among children vary greatly; these responses are largely influenced by a host of risk and protective factors including child's temperament; the type, severity, and chronicity of the trauma or violence; the chronological age/developmental stage of the child at the time(s) of exposure; the availability of nurturing and supportive adults who can either emotionally protect or sustain the child; and neighborhoods or communities that are cohesive and effectively provide needed resources to support diverse resident needs. Thus, fostering recovery in the aftermath of trauma requires a multipronged approach that builds on the transactional nature of protective factors across multiple levels of the child's ecological context. Put simply, resilience-based prevention and clinical intervention efforts must be grounded in developmental theory, acknowledge the transactional nature of risk and protective factors, and recognize the impact that early traumatic experiences have on subsequent functioning and development.

REFERENCES

Amaya-Jackson, L., Reynolds, V., Murray, M., McCarthy, G., Nelson, A., Cherney, M., et al. (2003). Cognitive behavioral treatment for pediatric posttraumatic stress disorder: Protocol and application in school and commmunity settings. *Cognitive and Behavioral Practice, 10,* 204–213.

Appleyard, K., Egeland, B., & vanDulmen, M. H. M., & Sroufe, L. A. (2005). When more is not better: The role of cumulative risk in child behavior outcomes. *Journal of Child Psychology and Psychiatry, 46,* 235–245.

Breslau N., Wilcox H. C., Storr, C. L., Lucia, V., & Anthony, J. C. (2004). Trauma exposure and PTSD: A non-concurrent prospective study of youth in urban America. *Journal of Urban Health, 81,* 530–544.

Briggs, E. C., Fairbank, J. A., Greeson, J. K. P., Layne, C. M., Steinberg, A. M., Amaya-Jackson, L. M., et al. (2013). Links between child and adolescent trauma exposure and service use histories in a national clinic-referred sample. *Psychological Trauma: Theory, Research, Practice, and Policy, 5*(2), 101–109.

Briggs, E. C., Thompson, R., Ostrowski, S., & Lekwauwa, R. (2011). Psychological health, behavioral, and economic costs of child maltreatment. In J. W. White, Mary P. Koss, & Alan E. Kazdin (Eds.), *Violence against women and children: Vol. 1. Mapping the terrain* (pp. 77–97). Washington, DC: American Psychological Association.

Bronfenbrenner, U. (1977). Toward an experimental ecology of human development. *American Psychologist, 32,* 513–531.

Brown, D. W., Anda, R. F., Tiemeier, H., Felitti, V., Edwards, V. J., Croft, J. B., et al. (2009). Adverse childhood experiences and the risk of premature mortality. *American Journal of Preventive Medicine, 37,* 389–396.

Ceballo, R., Ramirez, C., Hearn, K. D., & Maltese, K. L. (2003). Community violence and children's psycholoical well-being: Does parental monitoring matter? *Journal of Clinical Child and Adolescent Psychology, 32,* 586–592.

Chandy, J. M., Blum, R. W., & Resnick, M. D. (1996). Gender-specific outcomes for sexually abused adolescents. *Child Abuse and Neglect, 20,* 1219–1231.

Chandy, J. M., Blum, R. W., & Resnick, M. D. (1997). Sexually abused male adolescents: How vulnerable are they? *Journal of Child Sexual Abuse, 6,* 1–16.

Cicchetti, D., & Lynch, M. (1993). Toward an ecological/transactional model of community violence and child maltreatment: Consequences for children's development. *Psychiatry, 56,* 96–118.

Cohen, J. A., Mannarino, A. P., & Deblinger, E. (2006). *Treating trauma and traumatic grief in children and adolescents.* New York: Guilford Press.

Copeland, W. E., Keeler, G., Angold, A., & Costello, E. J. (2007). Traumatic and posttraumatic stress in childhood. *Archives of General Psychiatry, 64,* 577–584.

Copeland-Linder, N., Lambert, S. F., Chen, Y., & Ialongo, N. S. (2011). Contextual stress and health risk behaviors among African American adolescents. *Journal of Youth and Adolescence, 40,* 158–173.

Copeland-Linder, N., Lambert, S. F., & Ialongo, N. S. (2010). Community violence, protective factors, and adolescent mental health: A profile analysis. *Journal of Clinical Child and Adolescent Psychology, 39,* 176–186.

Deblinger, E., & Heflin, A. H. (1996). *Treating sexually abused children and their non-offending parents: A cognitive behavioral approach.* Thousand Oaks, CA: Sage.

DeRosa, R., Habib, M., Pelcovitz, D., Rathus, J., Sonnenklar, J., Ford, J., et al. (2006). *Structured psychotherapy for adolescents responding to chronic stress.* Unpublished manual.

Dixon, L., Browne, K., & Hamilton-Giachritsis, C. (2009). Patterns of risk and protective factors in the intergenerational cycle of maltreatment. *Journal of Family Violence, 24,* 111–122.

DuRant, R. H., Cadenhead, C., Pendergrast, R. A., Slavens, G., & Linder, C. W. (1994). Factors associated with the use of violence among urban black adolescents. *American Journal of Public Health, 84,* 612–617.

Egeland, B., Carlson, E. A., & Sroufe, L. A. (1993). Resilience as process. *Development and Psychopathology, 5,* 517–528.

Eisenberg, M. E., Ackard, D. M., & Resnick, M. D. (2007). Protective factors and suicide risk in adolescents with a history of sexual abuse. *Journal of Pediatrics, 151,* 482–487.

Eyberg, S. M., Boggs, S. R., & James, A. (1995). Parent–child interaction therapy: A psychosocial model for the treatment of young children with conduct problem behavior and their families. *Psychopharmacology Bulletin, 31,* 83–91.

Felitti, V. J., Anda, R. F., Nordenberg, D., Williamson, D. F., Spitz, A. M., Edwards, V., et al. (1998). Relationship of childhood abuse and household dysfunction to many of the leading causes of death in adults: The Adverse Childhood Experiences (ACE) Study. *American Journal of Preventive Medicine. 14,* 245–258.

Finkelhor, D., Turner, H. A., Ormrod, R. K., & Hamby, S. L. (2009). Violence, abuse, and crime exposure in a national sample of children and youth. *Pediatrics, 124,* 1–14.

Ford, J. D., & Russo, E. (2006). Trauma-focused, present-centered, emotional self-regulation approach to integrated treatment for posttraumatic stress disorder and addiction: Trauma Adaptive Recovery Group Education and Therapy (TARGET). *American Journal of Psychotherapy, 60,* 335–355.

Garmezy, N. (1974). The study of competence in children at risk for severe psychopathology. In E. J. Anthony & C. Koupernik (Eds.), *The child in his family: Vol. 3. Children at psychiatric risk* (pp. 77–97). New York: Wiley.

Hammack, P. L., Richards, M. H., Luo, Z., Edlynn, E. S., & Roy, K. (2004). Social support factors as moderators of community violence exposure among inner-city African American young adolescents. *Journal of Clinical Child and Adolescent Psychology, 33,* 450–462.

Haskett, M. E., Allaire, J. C., Kreig, S., & Hart, K. C. (2008). Protective and vulnerability factors for physically abused children: Effects of ethnicity and parenting context. *Child Abuse and Neglect, 32,* 567–576.

Hembree-Kigin, T. L., & McNeil, C. (1995). *Parent–child interaction therapy.* New York: Plenum Press.

Henrich, C. C., Schwab-Stone, M., Fanti, K., Jones, S. M., & Ruchkin, V. (2004). The association of community violence exposure with middle-school achievement: A prospective study. *Journal of Applied Developmental Psychology, 25,* 327–348.

Howard, K. A. S., Budge, S. L., & McKay, K. M. (2010). Youth exposed to violence: The role of protective factors. *Journal of Community Psychology, 38,* 63–79.

Jaycox, L. H., Langley, A. K., Stein, B. D., Wong, M., Sharma, P., Scott, M., et al. (2009). Support for students exposed to trauma: A pilot study. *School Mental Health, 1*(2), 49–60.

Jonzon, E., & Lindblad, F. (2006). Risk factors and protective factors in relation to subjective health among adult female victims of child sexual abuse. *Child Abuse and Neglect, 30,* 127–143.

Kataoka, S., Stein, B. D., Jaycox, L. H., Wong, M., Escuerdo, P., Tu, W., et al. (2003). A school-based mental health program for traumatized Latino immigrant children. *Journal of the American Academy of Child and Adolescent Psychiatry, 42,* 311–318.

Kiser, L. J., Donohue, A., Hodgkinson, S., Medoff, D., & Black, M. M. (2010). Strengthening family coping resources: The feasibility of a multifamily group intervention for families exposed to trauma. *Journal of Traumatic Stress, 23,* 802–806.

Kliewer, W., Parrish, K. A., Taylor, K. W., Jackson, K., Walker, J. M., & Shivy, V. A. (2006). Socialization of coping with community violence: Influences of caregiver coaching, modeling, and family context. *Child Development, 77,* 605–623.

Kolko, D. J., & Swenson, C. C. (2002). *Assessing and treating physically abused children and their families.* Thousand Oaks, CA: Sage.

Layne, C. M., Ghosh Ippen, C., Strand, V., Stuber, M., Abramovitz, R., Reyes, G., et al. (2011). The core curriculum on childhood trauma: A tool for training a trauma-informed workforce. *Psychological Trauma: Theory, Research, Practice, and Policy, 3,* 243–252.

Levendosky, A. A., & Graham-Bermann, S. A. (2000). Behavioral observations of parenting in battered women. *Journal of Family Psychology, 14,* 80–94.

Levendosky, A. A., Huth-Bocks, A. C., Shapiro, D. L., & Semel, M. A. (2003). The impact of domestic violence on the maternal–child relationship and preschool-age children's functioning. *Journal of Family Psychology, 17,* 275–287.

Lieberman, A., Van Horn, P., & Ghosh Ippen, C. (2005). Toward evidence based treatment: Child–parent psychotherapy with preschoolers exposed to marital violence. *Journal of the American Academy of Child and Adolescent Psychiatry, 44,* 1241–1248.

Ludwig, K. A., & Warren, J. S. (2009). Community violence, school-related protective factors, and psychosocial outcomes in urban youth. *Psychology in the Schools, 46,* 1061–1073.

Luecken, L. J., & Roubinov, D. S. (2012). Pathways to lifespan health following childhood parental death. *Social and Personality Psychology Compass, 6,* 243–257.

Luthar, S. S., & Cicchetti, D. (2000). The construct of resilience: Implications for interventions and social policies. *Development and Psychopathology, 12,* 857–885.

Luthar, S. S., Cicchetti, D., & Becker, B. (2000). The construct of resilience: A critical evaluation and guidelines for future work. *Child Development, 71,* 543–562.

March, J. S., Amaya-Jackson, L., Murray, M. C., & Schulte, A. (1998). Cognitive-behavioral psychotherapy for children and adolescents with posttraumatic stress disorder after a single-incident stressor. *Journal of the American Academy of Child and Adolescent Psychiatry, 37*(6), 585–593.

Martinez-Torteya, C., Anne Bogat, G., Von Eye, A., & Levendosky, A. A. (2009). Resilience among children exposed to domestic violence: The role of risk and protective factors. *Child Development, 80,* 562–577.

Masten, A. S. (1994). Resilience in individual development: Successful adaptation despite risk and adversity. In M. Wang & E. Gordon (Eds.), *Risk and resilience in inner city America: Challenges and prospects* (pp. 3–25). Hillsdale, NJ: Erlbaum.

Masten, A. S. (2001). Ordinary magic: Resilience processes in development. *American Psychologist, 56*(3), 227–238.

Masten, A. S., Best, K. M., & Garmezy, N. (1990). Resilience and development: Contributions from the study of children who overcame adversity. *Development and Psychopathology, 2,* 425–444.

Masten, A. S., Cutuli, J. J., Herbers, J. E., & Reed, M. G. J. (2009). Resilience in development. In C. R. Snyder & S. J. Lopez (Eds.), *Oxford handbook of positive psychology* (pp. 117–131). Oxford, UK: Oxford University Press.

McGee, Z. T. (2003). Community violence and adolescent development. *Journal of Contemporary Criminal Justice, 19,* 293–314.

Moylan, C. A., Herrenkohl, T. I., Sousa, C., Tajima, E. A., Herrenkohl, R. C., & Russo, M. J. (2010). The effects of child abuse and exposure to domestic violence on adolescent internalizing and externalizing behavior problems. *Journal of Family Violence, 25,* 53–63.

O'Donnell, D. A., Schwab–Stone, M. E., & Muyeed, A. Z. (2002). Multidimensional resilience in urban children exposed to community violence. *Child Development, 73,* 1265–1282.

Prinz, R. J., Sanders, M. R., Shapiro, C. J., Whitaker, D. J., & Lutzker, J. R. (2009). Population-based prevention of child maltreatment: The U.S. Triple P System population trial. *Prevention Science, 10,* 1–12.

Rosenthal, B. S., & Wilson, W. C. (2008). Community violence and psychological distress: The protective effects of emotional social support and sense of personal control among older adolescents. *Adolescence, 43,* 693–712.

Rosenthal, S., Feiring, C., & Taska, L. (2003). Emotional support and adjustment over a year's time following sexual abuse discovery. *Child Abuse and Neglect, 27*, 641–661.

Rutter, M. (1979). Protective factors in children's responses to stress and disadvantage. In M. W. Kent & J. E. Rolf (Eds.), *Primary prevention in psychopathology: Vol. 3. Social competence in children* (pp. 49–74). Hanover, NH: University Press of New England.

Sameroff, A. J. (2000). Dialectical processes in developmental psychopathology. In A. Sameroff, M. Lewis, & S. Miller (Eds.), *Handbook of developmental psychopathology* (2nd ed,, pp. 23–40). New York: Kluwer Academic/Plenum Press.

Sameroff, A. J., & Chandler, M. J. (1975). Reproductive risk and the continuum of caretaker casualty. In F. D. Horowitz (Ed.), *Review of child development research* (Vol. 4, pp. 187–244). Chicago: University of Chicago Press.

Saxe, G. N., Ellis, B. H., Fogler, J., Hansen, S., & Sorkin, B. (2005). Comprehensive care for traumatized children: An open trial examines treatment using trauma systems therapy. *Psychiatric Annals, 35*, 443–448.

Shaffer, A., & Yates, T. M. (2010). Identifying and understanding risk and protective factors in clinical practice. In M. T. Compton (Ed.), *Clinical manual of prevention in mental health* (pp. 29–48). Washington, DC: American Psychiatric Publishing.

Silverman, W. K., Ortiz, C. D., Viswesvaran, C., Burns, B. J., Kolko, D. J., Putnam, F. W., et al. (2008). Evidence-based psychosocial treatments for children and adolescents exposed to traumatic events. *Journal of Clinical Child and Adolescent Psychology, 37*, 156–183.

Spoth, R., Redmond, C., Shin, C., & Azevedo, K. (2004). Brief family intervention effects on adolescent substance initiation: School-level growth curve analyses 6 years following baseline. *Journal of Counseling and Clinical Psychology, 72*, 535–542.

Sroufe, L. A. (1997). Psychopathology as an outcome of development. *Development and Psychopathology, 9*, 251–268.

Sroufe, L. A., & Rutter, M. (1984). The domain of developmental psychopathology. *Child Development, 55*, 17–29.

Sullivan, T. N., Kung, E. M., & Farrell, A. D. (2004). Relation between witnessing violence and drug use initiation in early adolescence: Parental monitoring and support as protective factors. *Journal of Clinical Child and Adolescent Psychology, 33*, 488–498.

Testa, M., Miller, B. A., Downs, W. R., & Panek, D. (1992). The moderating impact of social support following childhood sexual abuse. *Violence and Victims, 7*, 172–186.

Thomlison, B. (2004). Child maltreatment: A risk and protective factor perspective. In M. W. Fraser (Ed.), *Risk and resilience in childhood: An ecological perspective* (pp. 89–131). Washington, DC: NASW Press.

Urquiza, A. J., & McNeil, C. B. (1996). Parent–child interaction therapy: An intensive dyadic intervention for physically abusive families. *Child Maltreatment, 1*, 134–144.

Werner, E. E., & Smith, R. S. (1982). *Vulnerable but invincible: A study of resilient children*. New York: McGraw-Hill.

Yates, T. M., Egeland, B., & Sroufe, L. A. (2003). Rethinking resilience: A developmental process perspective. In S. S. Luthar (Ed.), *Resilience and vulnerability: Adaptation in the context of childhood adversity* (pp. 243–266). New York: Cambridge University Press.

Yates, T. M., & Masten, A. S. (2004). Fostering the future: Resilience theory and positive psychology. In P. A. Linley & S. Joseph (Eds.), *Positive psychology in practice* (pp. 521–533). Hoboken, NJ: Wiley.

Chapter 6

The Military

Brett T. Litz, Maria M. Steenkamp, *and* William P. Nash

Few life experiences place a greater strain on psychological, biological, social, and spiritual health than military service in wartime. Operationally deployed service members may regularly witness intense human suffering and cruelty, have their lives threatened, bear losses from violence, and be called upon to kill and maim others. What may be surprising is not that, for a subset of service members and veterans, exposure to warzone stress leads to chronic suffering and disabling mental disorders, but that the majority of men and women in uniform appear to survive these experiences relatively unscathed and asymptomatic. The decade since the beginning of the wars in Afghanistan and Iraq has witnessed significant advancements in research on the mental health consequences of wartime deployment and their treatment. Whereas most previous studies were retrospective, cross-sectional, and narrowly focused on posttraumatic stress disorder (PTSD), an increasing number of prospective, longitudinal, multimethod studies are assessing rates of psychological (e.g., Milliken, Auchterlonie, & Hoge, 2007; Smith et al., 2008) and neuropsychological (Vasterling et al., 2006) symptoms before, during, and after deployment. Treatment outcome research has also proliferated, including the testing of a promising new cognitive-behavioral treatment designed specifically to meet the unique needs of combat-exposed military populations (Gray et al., 2012; Steenkamp et al., 2010). In contrast, research on the *prevention* of PTSD and other psychological disorders—on promoting both *resilience* to and *recovery* from war-zone stress—has only recently become a mandate for the U.S. Department of Defense (DoD; e.g., Casey, 2011) and a major focus for mental health sciences (e.g., Meredith et al., 2011; Weinick et al., 2011).

In the context of prior wars, several decades of research focused on variables that were associated with risk for PTSD (e.g., Green, Grace, Lindy, Gleser, & Leonard, 1990). What is clear from this body of research is that PTSD does not have a single cause, but involves multiple interacting etiological pathways, which may differ across various populations (Vogt, King, & King, 2007). In any given person exposed to a potentially traumatic event, risk for developing PTSD is determined by the complex interaction over time of preexisting genetic and personality factors; the nature, intensity, and duration of stressor events; levels of perievent distress, dissociation, and loss of control; and the availability of postevent biological, psychological, social, and spiritual resources. As complex and poorly understood as the processes involved in conferring PTSD risk may be after decades of research, current understandings of the processes involved in resilience and recovery are even less well known. After all, a high level of resilience cannot simply be a low level of risk. That is, the forces operating within and between exposed persons that lead to positive mental health outcomes must be active and positive things in themselves, and not just the absence of negative carriers of risk. Because research about resilience and recovery among service members is so new, few, if any, compelling conclusions can yet be drawn about the factors that lead to positive outcomes following war-zone stressor exposures. Not only are data lacking to inform theoretical conceptions about the processes of resilience and recovery, but existing theoretical constructs are not yet well formed, particularly with respect to the breadth and range of severities of potentially damaging war-zone stresses. These considerations are not merely academic. Optimal public health programs in the military must include both methods to reduce risk and promote resilience and recovery.

It is no easy task to delineate risk and resilience variables among service members because of the rich diversity of individuals, military service variables, exposures, outcomes, and recovery contexts. To start, it is overly simplistic to categorize service members as either resilient (not developing PTSD) or nonresilient (developing PTSD) because service members and veterans display a range of adaptation strategies and outcomes that follow a dynamic course over time. In theory, outcomes span different levels of distress and impairment (no impairment, subclinical levels of impairment, and clinically diagnosable impairment), differ in duration (from quick remission to chronicity), and differ in the extent to which they are normative (e.g., high but expected levels of symptoms following intense combat). Service members' degree of resilience does not simply depend on the severity of their combat exposures, but on a complex interplay of biological, psychological, social, deployment, and event-related factors, of which the interacting char-acteristics and mechanisms remain poorly understood. Depending on the interplay of these factors over time, individuals may exhibit resilience and recovery to certain traumatic events but not to others, and may be resilient at one period of time but develop symptoms at another.

In this chapter, we consider the complexity of psychological outcomes to military deployment, and discuss the challenge of reconciling the intri-cacy with the goal of reliably predicting and modifying individual out-comes. We first describe the types of trauma exposure associated with mili-tary deployment, and the range of psychological reactions resulting from these events. We discuss ways in which these reactions can be theoretically conceptualized as falling on a continuum, rather than in the dichotomous categories PTSD, and as forming fluid trajectories, rather than static states. We then review factors known to correlate with "natural" resilience and recovery trajectories in the military, and consider how these natural resil-ience and recovery processes can be enhanced through formal psychologi-cal interventions, providing examples of current attempts to do so within the U.S. military. Last, we discuss ways of promoting "therapeutic" recov-ery in military personnel struggling with trauma-related symptoms.

TYPES OF COMBAT STRESSORS
AND STRESS OUTCOMES IN MILITARY PERSONNEL

Most service members will experience multiple traumatic events during their deployments (Hoge et al., 2004). Military deployment is stereotypi-cally associated with situations of threatened death (such as receiving fire or being ambushed), which correspond with the *Diagnostic and Statistical Manual of Mental Disorders* (5th ed.; DSM-5) examples of Criterion A traumas involving "exposure to war as a combatant or civilian, threatened or actual physical assault . . . torture, incarceration as a prisoner of war" (American Psychiatric Association, 2013, p. 274). There is increasing rec-ognition, however, that many of the events that are most subjectively trau-matic and impactful to service members may not necessarily involve threat of death or injury (Fontana & Rosenheck, 1999; King, King, Gudanowski, & Vreven, 1995). Indeed, life threat may be less distressing in military populations than in civilians, given that military training prepares service members for life-threatening conditions, and such traumas are a foresee-able part of war and may thus align with service members' professional expectations. The all-volunteer nature of the present-day military also ensures a self-selection of individuals drawn to the challenges and dangers of military service.

Instead, deployment experiences involving non-fear-based events may be more subjectively traumatic and may precipitate psychological symptoms for many service members. There are at least three types of non-fear-based highly aversive experiences. First, the death of close comrades, leaders, or other cared-for individuals, even if not witnessed, can be highly traumatic given the strength of the attachments that develop between service members during war (e.g., Davidovitz, Mikulincer, Shaver, Izsak, & Popper, 2007; Nash, 2007b). Loss of a colleague in combat is not uncommon in the current wars; among soldiers serving in Iraq in 2008–2009, 57% knew someone seriously injured or hurt and 45% had a member of their own unit become a casualty (Mental Health Advisory Team [MHAT] VI report, 2009). Normal grieving processes can be stymied by the deployment context, where there is little time to safely experience painful emotions and reflect on losses. Second, *moral injury,* stemming from carrying out or bearing witness to acts that violate deeply held moral beliefs and expectations, can provoke intense feelings of guilt and shame (see Litz et al., 2009). Examples of potentially morally injurious experiences include killing or seriously injuring others and participating in or witnessing cruel and inhumane actions. Among soldiers and Marines surveyed in Iraq, 52% reported shooting or directing fire at the enemy, 32% reported being directly responsible for the death of an enemy combatant, and 20% endorsed responsibility for the death of a noncombatant (Hoge et al., 2004). Third, service members will also be exposed to the aftermath of battle, witnessing horrific events during times when there might be no immediate threat to personal safety, for example, performing body-handling duties and seeing severely injured civilians. Body-handling duties in particular have been shown to result in high rates of PTSD (e.g., McCarroll, Ursano, & Fullerton, 1995). Of note, all of these experiences occur against a backdrop of sustained stress and hardship, such as constant exposure to threat, sleep deprivation, lack of privacy and typical comforts, and separation from natural support networks such as family and civilian friends (Nash, 2007b). Such "wear and tear" may deplete coping resources and increase the odds of adverse reactions to events to which the individual might have been resilient in other circumstances.

There is evidence that such different types of stressful deployment experiences may create different developmental pathways to psychopathology. For example, a study of troops serving in the current wars suggests that experiences associated with the aftermath of battle represent a separate developmental pathway to PTSD, one which is not mediated by perceptions of life threat, as is the case during combat (Renshaw, 2011). Research from the National Vietnam Veterans Readjustment Study (NVVRS) likewise showed that different deployment experiences (such as killing, experiencing life threat, or committing atrocities) differentially contributed to the development of PTSD (Fontana & Rosenheck, 1999; King et al., 1995).

Service members experience a range of psychological reactions to these traumas and losses, many of which will overlap with DSM-5-defined symptoms of PTSD and its comorbid disorders. Many of these responses are distinct from PTSD, including prolonged grief, loss of faith and meaning, dissociation, and changes in identity. For example, in factor-analytic studies service members' grief from the loss of a fellow soldier 30 years prior can be greater than even that of bereaved spouses whose partner died in the previous 6 months (Pivar & Field, 2004). In one study, loss of religious faith and meaning was more predictive of specialized Veterans Administration (VA) PTSD care utilization than severity of PTSD symptoms (Fontana & Rosenheck, 2004). Importantly, while fear conditioning models have been pivotal in informing conceptualizations of PTSD, because trauma-related symptoms extend beyond fear responses, causal mechanisms are more complex than can be accounted for by fear-conditioning models alone (McNally, 2003). However, non-fear-based trauma reactions have as yet received little empirical and theoretical attention. Basic and applied research in this area is needed if the range of posttrauma outcomes is to be fully understood (e.g., Do emotions such as guilt and shame extinguish similarly to emotions like fear?). Clinically, recent treatments such as adaptive disclosure have begun to focus explicitly on non-fear-based trauma reactions in service members and veterans (discussed below).

A CONTINUUM OF MILITARY STRESS REACTIONS SEVERITY: CROSS-SECTIONAL OUTCOMES

Just as there is heterogeneity in the *types* of combat traumas and peri-and postevent reactions, the *severity* of these reactions also vary. Indeed, service members' adaptation is best understood as falling on a continuum of severity of impact, rather than dichotomizing service members into those with and without a psychological disorder, for example. By contrast, a categorical approach to impact presupposes that those without diagnosable disorders are psychologically healthy and symptom-free; that everything to the left of mental illness is normative. This is related to the medical model that dictates somewhat arbitrary cutoffs and algorithms for determining whether suffering is deemed clinically diagnosable. As such, the absence of an assignment of a mental diagnosis may in some cases belie significant distress, dysfunction, and risk for morbidity, if not mortality. For example, psychological autopsy data following military suicides indicate that the majority of completed suicides did not meet criteria for a DSM-IV disorder at time of suicide (Hilton, Service, Stander, Werbel, & Chavez, 2008).

A categorical scheme is also not supported empirically. For example, latent class analyses of PTSD symptoms among civilians exposed to trauma confirm at least three groups: those without discernable PTSD, those with subclinical PTSD symptoms, and those meeting diagnostic criteria for PTSD (Ayer et al., 2011; Breslau, Reboussin, Anthony, & Storr, 2005).

In these studies, approximately 10% report clinically diagnosable levels of PTSD symptoms, whereas approximately one-third of individuals report intermediate, subclinical levels of PTSD symptoms. In Vietnam veterans, lifetime rates of subclinical PTSD are approximately 22% (Weiss et al., 1992). Taking such subclinical (or "subthreshold" or "partial") levels of PTSD into account is important for at least three reasons. First, subclinical symptoms have been shown to be associated with significant distress and impairment (e.g., Stein, Walker, Hazen, & Forde, 1997). Indeed, partial PTSD results in comparable levels of impairment and morbidity to full PTSD in some veteran (Weiss et al., 1992) and civilian (Zlotnick, Franklin, & Zimmerman, 2002) samples. Second, the extent to which subclinical levels of PTSD confer risk for subsequent PTSD (and thus represent an important marker of risk and an opportunity for secondary intervention) is a crucial clinical question and makes it an important phenomenological state in its own right. Third, taking into account subclinical levels of PTSD dramatically alters perceived rates of "resilience" in military populations; rates of resilience will be much higher when using PTSD/no-PTSD conceptualizations, as any service member not meeting diagnostic criteria for PTSD is presumed to be resilient, rather than possibly struggling with subclinical, yet still very impairing, levels of distress. This may result in misleadingly optimistic conclusions about service members' adjustment to deployment stress. As a concrete example, consider how the four-question Primary Care PTSD Screen (PC-PTSD; Prins et al., 2003) is currently being used by the DoD for screening service members immediately upon returning from war-zone deployments, and again 6 months later. Service members are considered "at risk for PTSD" only if they give positive responses to two or more of the four PC-PTSD screening questions included on mandatory DoD Post-Deployment Health Assessments (PDHA) and Post-Deployment Heath Reassessments (PDHRA; Hoge, Auchterlonie, & Milliken, 2006), so persons with only a single symptom, however severe, persistent, and disabling, may be told they are "good-to-go" and in need of no preventative care.

One recently developed military model used to conceptualize the breadth of psychological reactions to deployment-related stress is the U.S. Navy/Marine Corps' *stress injury continuum model* (see Nash, Steenkamp, Conoscenti, & Litz, 2011). The model has become the foundation for the Combat and Operational Stress Control doctrine, training, assessment, and intervention in the Marine Corps and Navy. The model views deployment stress reactions as wounds to the mind, body, and spirit, recognizing that the scope of these responses is broader than PTSD symptoms alone. These wounds, labeled "stress injuries," are conceptualized in terms of a continuum of distress or impairment, ranging in severity and persistence from "stress reactions," which are normal, common, and expectable responses to adversity, to "stress illnesses," which are less common but result in greater need for medical, spiritual, or mental health treatment in order to prevent long-term disability. The model includes adaptive coping and wellness (color coded green, as the "ready" zone); mild and reversible distress or loss of function (the yellow, "reacting" zone); more severe and persistent, yet subclinical, distress or loss of function (the orange, "injured" zone); and mental disorders arising from stress and unhealed stress injuries, such as PTSD (the red, "ill" zone). An advantage of this model is it provides a language and set of conceptual tools for matching interventions for resilience and recovery with the appropriate subsets of military populations, in a way that is usable by line military leaders at all levels. Compared to other models for promoting resiliency currently in use in the military, the stress continuum model provides a language and tool set for promoting psychological health—moving leftward along the stress continuum—that can be applied to any service member no matter where he or she lies on the stress continuum at any given point in time, and that can be adapted for use by military leaders, family members, chaplains, and medical and mental health professionals (Nash, 2011; Nash, Steenkamp, et al., 2011). As an example of its utility, the Arizona National Guard recently deployed a smartphone application for its members based on the stress continuum model.

A CONTINUUM OF ADAPTATION: LONGITUDINAL OUTCOMES

Because adjustment to trauma is fluid and involves varying symptom severity over time, there is increasing emphasis in the trauma field on conceptualizing posttraumatic outcomes in terms of longitudinal trajectories. In this context, resilience, for example, is not a static steady-state outcome, but an unfolding process. Several qualitatively distinct trajectories of posttrauma response have recently been proposed: *resistance, resilience, recovery, chronic impairment,* and *delayed distress* (Bonnano, 2004; Layne, Warren, Watson, & Shalev, 2007). *Resistance* refers to the maintenance of homeostasis after exposure to trauma or loss, with the development of no or few stress symptoms or impairment in functioning over time. In the model, there are two courses that reflect the ability of service members to bounce back from periods of stress reactions or injuries, namely resilience and recovery. The *resilience* course entails the development of mild-to-moderate symptoms, with a rapid return to baseline functioning; this is argued by Bonanno (2004) to be the most common long-term response to loss and trauma. *Recovery* involves an initial period of upheaval that dissipates more slowly in the weeks and months following the event, gradually returning to former levels of functioning (Bonanno, 2004). The *chronic impairment* course entails high, prolonged levels of distress and dysfunction. In the *delayed distress* trajectory, symptoms emerge over time after a period of apparent initial resilience or subclinical symptoms that worsen over time. Support for these trajectories has been documented in a number of civilian samples (e.g., Bonanno et al., 2008; deRoon-Cassini, Mancini, Rusch, & Bonanno, 2010; Norris, Tracy, & Galea, 2009). The trajectories have not yet been examined in service members exposed to combat stress, although Dickstein, Suvak, Litz, and Adler (2010) examined trajectories in a sample of peacekeepers deployed to Kosovo and found evidence for a resilient, recovery, and delayed trajectory.

RISK, RESILIENCE, AND RECOVERY FACTORS IN THE MILITARY

Deployment mental health outcomes have been shown to be influenced by a combination of predeployment, deployment, and postdeployment factors (e.g., King, King, Foy, Keane, & Fairbank, 1999); we briefly discuss some of the variables that have received the most empirical attention. In the military, the goal is to bolster the resources of service members and their families through training and preparatory activities provided by responsive and caring leaders. Leaders take responsibility for reducing the impact of modifiable risk factors and mitigating the impact of unavoidable stress exposures, and also ensure proper early care of stress injuries and illnesses so as to ensure a healthy fighting force. Generally, for service members, the core resilience factors entail training, leadership, and peer and family support.

Predeployment Factors

It is important to note that many of the predeployment factors that predict PTSD are not modifiable, such as genetic predisposition and trauma history. Twin studies of a Vietnam era cohort suggest that PTSD symptoms are moderately heritable (True et al., 1993) and that exposure to certain combat-related traumatic events also has a heritable basis (i.e., selection of one's environment, such as volunteering for military service, is partly determined by genetic factors; Lyons et al., 1993). There is also evidence that premilitary trauma exposure, in addition to directly impacting risk for PTSD, interacts with combat stressors to increase the likelihood of combat-related PTSD (Cabrera, Hoge, Bliese, Castro, & Messer, 2007; Iversen et al., 2008). Troops with a history of childhood adversity or abuse, for example, are more likely to develop combat-related PTSD (e.g., Zaidi & Foy, 1994).

Other predeployment variables are more amenable to modification. Two of the best-supported variables in promoting resilience in service members are psychological preparedness and self-efficacy, factors that are highly interrelated. Service members' confidence in their military skills and abilities is a robust predictor of their predeployment self-efficacy (Solberg, Laberg, Johnsen, & Eid, 2005), and high self-efficacy is in turn consistently linked to better posttrauma adjustment in both military and civilian populations (e.g., see Benight & Bandura, 2004, for a review; Solomon, Benbenishty, & Mikulincer, 1991). For example, service members returning from Iraq who perceived the demands of their in-theater duties to have exceeded their training and experience are at significantly greater risk of developing PTSD (Iversen et al., 2008). Prior training or past experience with a particular trauma have been repeatedly demonstrated to lead to better postevent outcomes (e.g., Perrin et al., 2007). This may be because training imposes a sense of control, familiarity, and predictability on various high-magnitude deployment experiences (e.g., Whealin, Ruzek, & Southwick, 2008), and can thus reduce anxiety during stressful events (Haglund, Nestadt, Cooper, Southwick, & Charney, 2007). As such, military training serves an important protective function by fostering psychological preparedness and self-efficacy. The more realistic the training, the more protective it is likely to be, and recent efforts have been made to develop highly realistic immersion trainings within the military. This point also underscores the important fact that numerous resilience-promoting processes are endemic to the military and do not involve direct involvement by mental health professionals.

Deployment Factors

Severity of combat exposure is an important predictor of both PTSD onset and course, with a number of studies demonstrating a dose–response relationship (e.g., Wolfe, Erickson, Sharkansky, King, & King, 1999). For example, sustaining bodily injury during the trauma is a major risk factor for the development of PTSD in veterans of war (Koren, Norman, Cohen, Berman, & Klein, 2005). Likewise, certain combat experiences, such as being a prisoner of war (POW), are associated with higher rates of PTSD. POWs have lifetime rates of PTSD of up to 96% (Sutker & Allain, 1996), with symptom severity being particularly related to extent of torture and weight loss while in captivity (Speed, Engdahl, Schwartz, & Eberly, 1989).

Two social variables have been shown to be of particular importance to mental health outcomes in military personnel: unit cohesion (i.e., social connectedness and bonding within the unit) and leadership. A large body of evidence from civilian studies indicates that strong social bonds are more common among resilient individuals than those who develop PTSD (see Charuvastra & Cloitre, 2008). In military populations, low unit cohesion is a risk factor for PTSD (Iversen et al., 2008), while high unit cohesion can mitigate deployment stress and may even offset the effect of prior (premilitary) life events on the subsequent development of combat-related PTSD (e.g., Brailey, Vasterling, Proctor, Constans, & Friedman, 2007). Effective military leadership has been shown to facilitate role clarity and meaning in unit members, to promote adaptive interpretations of stressful events in unit members, to enhance self-efficacy, and to foster a sense of pride and purpose about various sacrifices (e.g., Bartone, 2006; Britt, Davison, Bliese, & Castro, 2004). Both unit cohesion and leadership style are alterable and thus represent promising points of intervention, for example, training leaders in leadership styles that are most conducive to promoting mental health in troops.

Postdeployment Factors

Social support also continues to be an important protective variable upon return home from deployment. For instance, a study of National Guard veterans who served in Iraq and Afghanistan found that lower postdeployment social support predicted PTSD even after controlling for severity of combat exposure (Pietrzak, Johnson, Goldstein, Malley, & Southwick, 2009). Similarly, perceived negative homecoming reception and poor community support has also been shown to predict chronic PTSD (Koenen, Stellman, Stellman, & Sommer, 2003). Exposure to additional stressors following deployment is another risk factor for PTSD (King, King, Fairbank, Keane, & Adams, 1998). A recent study found an association between violent combat experiences and increased risk-taking behavior upon return home (Killgore et al., 2008); engaging in such unsafe behavior may also increase the likelihood of exposure to new traumatic events upon return home from deployment. Including family members in military mental health initiatives may help ensure positive homecomings and foster social support for returning veterans. In the absence of natural sources of support, the DoD and VA continue to make efforts to make formal psychological care available to all service members (discussed further below), while organizations such as the Veterans of Foreign Wars (VFWs) can serve a supportive function as well. Although these psychological health functions are the direct responsibility of military unit leaders, mental health professionals have an important role in educating service members (including reserve and National Guard members), their families, and other stakeholders regarding the best evidence-based or evidence-informed options open to them.

A CONTINUUM OF PREVENTION

In the military, the promotion of resilience and recovery, the prevention of stress injuries and illnesses, and the professional response to mental disorders, most notably PTSD, is a multifaceted process that is best conceived as a continuum. The Institute of Medicine Committee on the Prevention of Mental Disorders delineates three broad types of prevention interventions

(Mrazek & Haggerty, 1994). *Universal prevention* is the broadest application of prevention initiatives and such programs are delivered to entire populations, regardless of risk status. The aim is to improve the overall well-being and resilience of a given population, and/or to shift the population distribution of a disorder downward by addressing its underlying causes. *Selective prevention* targets individuals at heightened risk for developing a disorder, such as those who have recently experienced a traumatic event or those exhibiting known risk factors for PTSD. *Indicated prevention* is aimed at individuals who are already symptomatic and impaired but who do not yet meet diagnostic criteria for a disorder. More recently, the Institute of Medicine has recognized mental *health promotion* as another important category of intervention that can be applied irrespective of specific stressor exposures (National Research Council and Institute of Medicine, 2009).

Health Promotion and Universal Prevention in the Military

In recent years, the U.S. military has developed and broadly implemented a number of programs aimed at enhancing resilience in service members, including promoting mental wellness and growth and reducing rates of psychiatric disorders following deployment. The most notable example of this is the Army's Comprehensive Soldier Fitness (CSF) Program, a $125 million initiative, which is a health promotion and universal prevention approach designed to train soldiers and their families in mental "fitness" and resilience (Casey, 2011). It aims to decrease the incidence of stress pathologies in service members and to increase the number of service members who derive meaning and personal growth from their deployment (Cornum, Matthews, & Seligman, 2011). Based on principles of positive psychology, CSF consists of computerized assessment and learning modules completed by all soldiers designed to improve their emotional, social, family, and spiritual "fitness"; individualized computerized resilience training that is tailored to soldiers' relative strengths and weaknesses; and in-person training of noncommissioned officers in advanced resilience skills to facilitate the implementation of these principles with subordinates (Cornum et al., 2011). Despite its widespread implementation, there are currently no peer-reviewed, published outcome data available on CSF outcomes, and the mechanisms by which the intervention has its effects have not been clearly explicated.

Importantly, to justify their costs and the potential for unintended effects, military prevention programs need to demonstrate incremental validity over myriad natural and indigenous factors within the military that serve preventative functions (see Nash, 2007a). These include self-selection, intensive predeployment training, unit cohesion, family support, leadership, meaning and pride, and purpose developed from the military culture and ethos.

Selective and Indicated Prevention: Promoting Resilience in the Face of Stress Injury

A number of selective prevention interventions have also recently been developed for service members. For example, in the Army, battlemind psychological debriefing is an in-theater group-based method that occurs either in a time-drive fashion (at certain intervals during deployment, aimed at addressing the cumulative impact of deployment stressors), or an event-driven fashion (in response to a traumatic incident). Debriefings conducted by two facilitators aim to promote resilience by normalizing reactions, talking about emotions and events (though traumatic events are not recounted in detail), reinforcing the meaning of the unit's sacrifice, and psychologically preparing soldiers to return to duty (see Adler, Castro, & McGurk, 2009). No outcome data are as yet available for the efficacy of this intervention. A different battlemind debriefing is also delivered upon return from deployment, focusing on the transition from combat to home, encouraging peer support and the positive adaptation of occupational skills to the home environment, and stressing that traumatic deployment experiences occurred in the past and are not part of the individual's current experience (Adler, Bliese, McGurk, Hoge, & Castro, 2009). There is initial evidence that such battlemind debriefing is superior to standard stress education in reducing PTSD and depression symptoms among soldiers with high levels of combat exposure (Adler et al., 2009).

In terms of indicated prevention, in-theater combat stress control (CSC) teams have historically employed traditional forward military psychiatry principles to intervene with service members, especially those who are sufficiently distressed and impaired to be unable to perform their military duties. Based on the principles of PIES (proximity, immediacy, expectancy, and simplicity), these interventions normalize experiences and encourage restoration of function through simple and practical tools such as sleep, hygiene, and nutrition, delivered promptly and within close proximity of the unit, and with the expectation of return to the unit (see Ritchie, Schneider, Bradley, & Forsten, 2008). However, this approach has not been formally evaluated and evidence for its use is largely anecdotal (see Castro, Engel, & Adler, 2004).

The Navy and Marine Corps combat and operational stress control doctrine includes formalized psychological first aid principles for the indicated prevention (early intervention) of stress injuries. The model is called *combat and operational stress control first aid* (COSFA), and it differs from historical forward psychiatric early interventions in that it is based on the stress injury continuum model, and therefore includes a fundamental component of assessment to discriminate normal reactions following overwhelming experiences from those that confer significant risk for future illness, behavioral problems such as suicide or assault, or impairment of functioning in any sphere. COSFA interventions include both short-term responses to acute crises and longer-term interventions to promote healing and recovery of social connectedness, personal and collective competence, and self-confidence (see Nash, Krantz, Stein, Westphal, & Litz, 2011). As recently reviewed by Weinick and colleagues (2011), neither COSFA nor any other approach to indicated prevention in military settings has yet been empirically tested. However, the DoD is currently in the process of evaluating the effectiveness of COSFA as trained to small-unit leaders in marine ground combat units as part of the Marine Corps' Operational Stress Control and Readiness program.

Promoting Recovery and Rehabilitation: Interventions Targeting Military-Related PTSD

In a minority of service members, resilience and recovery resources are overwhelmed, leading to persistent serious mental health problems and associated functional impairment. Psychological treatment for deployment-related PTSD can occur either while the individual is still an active-duty service member (falling within the purview of the DoD) or, more commonly, when the individual has reentered civilian life as a veteran (falling within the purview of the Department of Veteran Affairs [VA]).

In the VA system, psychological treatments for veterans with PTSD have consisted mainly of applying protocols developed and tested on civilians, particularly female sexual assault survivors. To meet growing demands from the current wars, the VA initiated nationwide dissemination of two of these evidence-based PTSD psychotherapies, cognitive processing therapy (CPT) and prolonged exposure (PE; Karlin et al., 2010). Surprisingly, very few efficacy and effectiveness studies of PTSD exist in veterans. Effect sizes in PTSD randomized treatment trials targeting veterans with chronic PTSD (up until recently, usually conducted on Vietnam veterans decades after their service) have tended to be smaller relative to civilian trials (e.g., Monson et al., 2006; Schnurr et al., 2007). This may, at least in part, be attributed to the fact that the fear-conditioning and learning models underlying PTSD treatments may not sufficiently explain or address the diverse psychic injuries of war.

Efforts are also underway to disseminate PE and CPT within the DoD. For example, the Center for Deployment Psychology aims to train military and civilian clinicians to provide evidence-based mental health care to service members and their families through workshops, online trainings, and seminars. DoD-funded treatment outcome studies are also underway to evaluate the efficacy of these interventions, such as the South Texas

Research Organization Network Guiding Studies on Trauma and Resilience (STRONG STAR), a large multisite study developing and evaluating evidence-based early interventions for active-duty personnel and recently discharged veterans. Such efforts are particularly important when considering that no clinical trials of PTSD in active-duty veterans have been published.

There have also been recent attempts to develop PTSD treatments designed specifically for active-duty military populations, rather than seeking to simply overlay civilian treatment onto service members. One example of an evidence-based early intervention designed specifically for deployment-related PTSD is *Adaptive Disclosure* (AD). AD is an eight-session manualized early intervention program designed to foster willingness to engage with and disclose difficult deployment memories through a combination of imaginal exposure, cognitive restructuring, and meaning-making strategies (see Steenkamp et al., 2010). Imaginal exposure to the most pressing and frequently reexperienced deployment trauma forms the core of the treatment, but AD specifically includes techniques designed to address traumatic loss and moral conflict, in the form of "break-out" modules. In a program development and evaluation open trial of 44 in-garrison marines, AD was well tolerated and promoted significant reductions in PTSD, depression, negative posttraumatic appraisals, and increased posttraumatic growth (Gray et al., 2012).

In sum, as it becomes increasingly clear that deployment trauma-related problems extend beyond fear and anxiety to include highly chronic and debilitating levels of guilt, shame, grief, and dissociation (among others), treatments will need to be expanded to reflect the complexity of these outcomes. Treatments that honor and leverage the military ethos are also needed to ensure optimal acceptability and buy-in in this generally therapy-averse population.

SUMMARY AND CLINICAL RECOMMENDATIONS

War has a profound impact on everyone who deploys; the challenge for trauma researchers is to understand the myriad interacting factors that shape these changes, and to know how to adjust these factors as necessary to promote adaptive outcomes. Overall, the military trauma field is at a relatively early stage of empirical and theoretical development regarding predicting and modifying deployment mental health outcomes. Research from the current wars has lead to increased recognition of the wide-ranging nature and severity of psychological reactions to deployment, offering a more nuanced perspective than previous PTSD/no-PTSD conceptualizations. Some variables, such as social support and psychological preparedness, have relatively strong support for playing an important role in deployment outcomes. Though a number of such relevant variables have been consistently identified, they have not yet been translated into dependable risk algorithms for predicting individual outcomes. Furthermore, little attention has been paid to how to actually modify these variables in ways that reliably alter individuals' susceptibility to mental and behavioral health problems.

In the context of resilience and prevention, the most pressing questions that need to be addressed are: (1) prior to deployment, how best to assist leaders to identify those service members who may be susceptible to mental health difficulties (i.e., exhibit the most risk factors or fewest resilience factors) and how to intervene to decrease risk and improve resilience; (2) during deployment, considering that stress reactions are normative and widespread, how best to identify the minority of individuals who cross the threshold into stress injuries, making it difficult to recover on their own, and when and how to intervene to ensure recovery; and (3) after deployment, when and how best to treat those who have failed to recover and are demonstrating persistent difficulties. The enormous personal, societal, and economic costs associated with deployment-related PTSD create a compelling need for risk, resilience, and recovery research programs that address these questions. Their answers will likely entail a combination of providing universal psychoeducation and skills training, lasting throughout the deployment cycle, to ensure that all service members have the necessary knowledge and skills to increase the odds of being able to recognize difficulties when they arise (in self and others), and to react appropriately to these difficulties, either through effective application of learned coping strategies or through as-needed self-referral to formal interventions. More broadly, the success of these efforts will depend on a significant cultural shift in the military in which mental health problems are seen as legitimate injuries of war, and in which individuals feel able to seek additional support when needed.

REFERENCES

Adler, A. B., Bliese, P. D., McGurk, D., Hoge, C. W., & Castro, C. A. (2009). Battlemind debriefing and Battlemind training as early interventions with soldiers returning from Iraq: Randomization by platoon. *Journal of Consulting and Clinical Psychology, 77,* 928–940.

Adler, A. B., Castro, C. A., & McGurk, D. (2009). Time-driven battlemind psychological debriefing: A group-level early intervention in combat. *Military Medicine, 174,* 21–28.

American Psychiatric Association. (2013). *Diagnostic and statistical manual of mental disorders* (5th ed). Arlington, VA: Author.

Ayer, L., Danielson, C. K., Amstadter, A. B., Ruggiero, K., Saunders, B., & Kilpatrick, D. (2011). Latent classes of adolescent posttraumatic stress disorder predict functioning and disorder after 1 year. *Journal of the American Academy of Child and Adolescent Psychiatry, 50,* 364–375.

Bartone, P. T. (2006). Resilience under military operational stress: Can leaders influence hardiness? *Military Psychology, 18,* S131–S148.

Benight, C. C., & Bandura, A. (2004). Social cognitive theory of posttraumatic recovery: The role of perceived self-efficacy. *Behaviour Research and Therapy, 42,* 1129–1148.

Bonanno, G. A. (2004). Loss, trauma, and human resilience: Have we underestimated the human capacity to thrive after extremely aversive events? *American Psychologist, 59,* 20–28.

Bonanno, G. A., Ho, S. M. Y., Chan, J. C. K., Kwong, R. S. Y., Cheung, C. K. Y., Wong, C. P. Y., et al. (2008). Psychological resilience and dysfunction among hospitalized survivors of the SARS epidemic in Hong Kong: A latent class approach. *Health Psychology, 27,* 659–667.

Brailey, K., Vasterling, J. J., Proctor, S. P., Constans, J. I., & Friedman, M. J. (2007). PTSD symptoms, life events, and unit cohesion: Baseline findings from the Neurocognition Deployment Health Study. *Journal of Traumatic Stress, 20,* 495–503.

Breslau, N., Reboussin, B. A., Anthony, J. C., & Storr, C. L. (2005). The structure of posttraumatic stress disorder: Latent class analysis in 2 community samples. *Archives of General Psychiatry, 62,* 1343–1351.

Britt, T. W., Davison, J., Bliese, P. D., & Castro, C. A. (2004). How leaders can influence the impact that stressors have on soldiers. *Military Medicine, 169,* 541–545.

Cabrera, O. A., Hoge, C. W., Bliese, P. D., Castro, C. A., & Messer, S. C. (2007). Childhood adversity and combat as predictors of depression and post-traumatic stress in deployed troops. *American Journal of Preventive Medicine, 33,* 77–82.

Casey, G. W. (2011). Comprehensive soldier fitness: A vision for psychological resilience in the U.S. Army. *American Psychologist, 66,* 1–3.

Castro, C. W., Engel, C. C., & Adler, A. B. (2004). The challenge of providing mental health prevention and early intervention in the U.S. military. In B. T. Litz (Ed.), *Early intervention for trauma and traumatic loss* (pp. 301–318). New York: Guilford Press.

Charuvastra, A., & Cloitre, M. (2008). Social bonds and posttraumatic stress disorder. *Annual Review of Psychology, 59,* 301–328.

Cornum, R., Matthews, M. D., & Seligman, M. E. P. (2011). Comprehensive soldier fitness: Building resilience in a challenging institutional context. *American Psychologist, 66,* 4–9.

Davidovitz, R., Mikulincer, M., Shaver, P. R., Izsak, R., & Popper, M. (2007). Leaders as attachment figures: Leaders' attachment orientations predict leadership-related mental representations and followers' performance and mental health. *Journal of Personality and Social Psychology, 93,* 632–650.

deRoon-Cassini, T. A., Mancini, A. D., Rusch, M. D., & Bonanno, G. A. (2010). Psychopathology and resilience following traumatic injury: A latent growth mixture model analysis. *Rehabilitation Psychology, 55,* 1–11.

Dickstein, B.D., Suvak, M., Litz, B.T., & Adler, A.B. (2010). Heterogeneity in the course of posttraumatic stress disorder: Trajectories of symptomatology. *Journal of Traumatic Stress, 23,* 331–339.

Fontana, A., & Rosenheck, R. (1999). A model of war zone stressors and posttraumatic stress disorder. *Journal of Traumatic Stress, 12,* 111–126.

Fontana, A., & Rosenheck, R. (2004). Trauma, change in strength of religious faith, and mental health service use among veterans treated for PTSD. *Journal of Nervous and Mental Disease, 192,* 579–584.

Gray, M. J., Schorr, Y., Nash, W., Lebowitz, L., Lansing, A., Lang, A. J., et al. (2012). Adaptive disclosure: An open trial of a novel exposure-based intervention for service members with combat-related psychological stress injuries. *Behavior Therapy, 43,* 407–415.

Green, B. L, Grace, M. C., Lindy, J. D., Gleser, G. C., & Leonard, A. (1990). Risk factors for PTSD and other diagnoses in a general sample of Vietnam veterans. *American Journal of Psychiatry, 147,* 729–733.

Haglund, M. E. M., Nestadt, P. S., Cooper, N. S., Southwick, S. M., & Charney, D. S. (2007). Psychobiological mechanisms of resilience: Relevance to prevention and treatment of stress-related psychopathology. *Development and Psychopathology, 19,* 889–920.

Hilton, S. M., Service, D. B., Stander, V. A., Werbel, A. D., & Chavez, B. R. (2008). *Department of Navy Suicide Incident Report (DONSIR): Summary of findings, 1999–2007* (Report No. 09-15). San Diego, CA: Naval Health Research Center.

Hoge, C. W., Auchterlonie, J. L., & Milliken, C. S. (2006). Mental health problems, use of mental health services, and attrition from military service after returning from deployment to Iraq or Afghanistan. *Journal of the American Medical Association, 295,* 1023–1032.

Hoge, C. W., Castro, C. A., Messer, S. C., McGurk, D., Cotting, D. I., & Koffman, R. L. (2004). Combat duty in Iraq and Afghanistan, mental health problems, and barriers to care. *New England Journal of Medicine, 351,* 13–22.

Iversen, A.C., Fear, N. T., Ehlers, A., Hughes, J. H., Hull, L., Earnshaw, M., et al. (2008). Risk factors for post-traumatic stress disorder among U.K. armed forces personnel. *Psychological Medicine, 38,* 511–522.

Karlin, B. E., Ruzek, J., I., Chard, K. M., Eftekhari, A., Monson, C. M., Hembree, E. A., et al. (2010). Dissemination of evidence-based psychological treatments for posttraumatic stress disorder in the Veterans Health Administration. *Journal of Traumatic Stress, 23,* 663–673.

Killgore, W. D. S., Cotting, D. I., Thomas, J. L., Cox, A. L. McGurk, D., Vo, A. H., et al. (2008). Post-combat invincibility: Violent combat experiences are associated with increased risk-taking propensity following deployment. *Journal of Psychiatric Research, 42,* 1112–1121.

King, D. W., King, L. A., Fairbank, J. A., Keane, T. A., & Adams, G. A. (1998). Resilience-recovery factors in post-traumatic stress disorder among female and male Vietnam veterans: Hardiness, postwar social support, and additional stressful life events. *Journal of Personality and Social Psychology, 74,* 420–434.

King, D. W., King, L. A., Foy, D. W., Keane, T. M., & Fairbank, J. A. (1999). Posttraumatic stress disorder in a national sample of female and male Vietnam veterans: Risk factors, war-zone stressors, and resilience–recovery variables. *Journal of Abnormal Psychology, 108,* 164–170.

King, D. W., King, L. A., Gudanowski, D. M., & Vreven, D. L. (1995). Alternative representations of war zone stressors: Relationships to posttraumatic stress disorder in male and female Vietnam veterans. *Journal of Abnormal Psychology, 104,* 184–195.

Koenen, K. C., Stellman, J. M., Stellman, S. D., & Sommer, J. F. (2003). Risk factors for course of posttraumatic stress disorder among Vietnam veterans: A 14–year follow-up of American Legionnaires. *Journal of Consulting and Clinical Psychology, 71,* 980–986.

Koren, D., Norman, D., Cohen, A., Berman, J., & Klein, E. M. (2005). Increased PTSD risk with combat-related injury: A matched comparison study of injured and uninjured soldiers experiencing the same combat events. *American Journal of Psychiatry, 162,* 276–282.

Layne, C. M., Warren, J. S., Watson, P. J., & Shalev, A. Y. (2007). Risk, vulnerability, resistance, and resilience: Toward an integrative conceptualization of posttraumatic adaptation. In M. J. Friedman, T. M. Keane, & P. A. Resick (Eds.), *Handbook of PTSD: Science and practice* (pp. 497–520). New York: Guilford Press.

Litz, B. T., Stein, N., Delaney, E., Lebowitz, L., Silva, C., Maguen, S., et al. (2009). Moral injury and moral repair in war veterans: A preliminary model and intervention strategy. *Clinical Psychology Review, 29,* 695–706.

Lyons, M. J., Goldberg, J., Eisen, S. A., True, W., Tsuang, M. T., Meyer, J. M., et al. (1993). Do genes influence exposure to trauma?: A twin study of combat. *American Journal of Medical Genetics, 48,* 22–27.

McCarroll, J. E., Ursano, R. J., & Fullerton, C. S. (1995). Symptoms of PTSD following recovery of war dead: 13–15-month follow-up. *American Journal of Psychiatry, 152,* 939–941.

McNally, R. J. (2003). Progress and controversy in the study of posttraumatic stress disorder. *Annual Review of Psychology, 54,* 229–252.

Mental Health Advisory Team (MHAT) VI. (2009, May 8). Operation Iraqi Freedom 07–09. Retrieved August 16, 2011, from *www.armymedicine.army.mil/reports/mhat/mhat_vi/mhat_vi-oif_redacted.pdf.*

Meredith, L. S., Sherbourne, C. D., Gaillot, S., Hansell, L., Ritschard, H. V., Parker, A. M., et al. (2011). *Promoting psychological resilience in the U.S. military.* Santa Monica, CA: RAND Corporation.

Milliken, C. S., Auchterlonie, J. L., & Hoge, C. W. (2007). Longitudinal assessment of mental health problems among active and reserve component soldiers returning from the Iraq War. *Journal of the American Medical Association, 298,* 2141–2148.

Monson, C. M., Schnurr, P. P., Resick, P. A., Friedman, M. J., Yinong, Y., & Stevens, S. P. (2006). Cognitive processing therapy for veterans with military-related posttraumatic stress disorder. *Journal of Consulting and Clinical Psychology, 74,* 898–907.

Mrazek, P. J., & Haggerty, R. J. (1994). *Reducing risks for mental disorders: Frontiers for preventive intervention research.* Washington, DC: National Academy Press.

Nash, W. P. (2007a). Combat/operational stress adaptations and injuries. In C. R.

Figley & W. P. Nash (Eds.), *Combat stress injury theory, research, and management* (pp. 33–64). New York: Routledge.

Nash, W. P. (2007b). The stressors of war. In C. R. Figley & W. P. Nash (Eds.), *Combat stress injury theory, research, and management* (pp. 11–32). New York: Routledge.

Nash, W. P. (2011). U.S. Marine Corps and Navy combat and operational stress continuum model: A tool for leaders. In E. C. Ritchie (Ed.), *Combat and operational behavioral health* (pp. 107–119). Washington, DC: TMM Publications.

Nash, W. P., Krantz, L., Stein, N., Westphal, R. J., & Litz, B. (2011). Comprehensive soldier fitness, Battlemind, and the stress continuum model: Military organizational approaches to prevention. In J. I. Ruzek, P. P. Schnurr, J. J. Vasterling, & M. J. Friedman (Eds.), *Caring for veterans with deployment-related stress disorders: Iraq, Afghanistan, and beyond.* Washington, DC: American Psychological Association.

Nash, W. P., Steenkamp, M., Conoscenti, L., & Litz, B. T. (2011). The stress continuum model: A military organizational approach to resilience and recovery. In S. M. Southwick, B. T. Litz, D. Charney, & M. J. Friedman (Eds.), *Resilience and mental health: Challenges across the lifespan* (pp. 238–252). New York: Cambridge University Press.

National Research Council and Institute of Medicine. (2009). *Preventing mental, emotional, and behavioral disorders among young people: Progress and possibilities.* Committee on the Prevention of Mental Disorders and Substance Abuse Among Children, Youth, and Young Adults. Washington, DC: National Academies Press.

Norris, F. H., Tracy, M., & Galea, S. (2009). Looking for resilience: Understanding the longitudinal trajectories of responses to stress. *Social Science and Medicine, 68,* 2190–2198.

Perrin, M. A., DiGrande, L., Wheeler, K., Thorpe, L., Farfel, M., & Brackbill, R. (2007). Differences in PTSD prevalence and associated risk factors among World Trade Center disaster rescue and recovery workers. *American Journal of Psychiatry, 164,* 1385–1394.

Pietrzak, R. H., Johnson, D. C., Goldstein, M. B., Malley, J. C., & Southwick, S. M. (2009). Psychological resilience and postdeployment social support protect against traumatic stress and depressive symptoms in soldiers returning from Operations Enduring Freedom and Iraqi Freedom. *Depression and Anxiety, 26,* 745–751.

Pivar, I. L., & Field, N. P. (2004). Unresolved grief in combat veterans with PTSD. *Journal of Anxiety Disorders, 18,* 745–755.

Prins, A., Ouimette, P., Kimerling, R., Cameron, R. P., Hugelsofer, D. S., Shaw-Hegwer, J., et al. (2003). The primary care PTSD screen (PC-PTSD): Development and operating characteristics. *Primary Care Psychiatry, 9,* 9–14.

Renshaw, K., (2011). An integrated model of risk and protective factors for post-deployment PTSD symptoms in OIF/OEF era combat veterans. *Journal of Affective Disorders, 128,* 321–326.

Ritchie, E. C., Schneider, B., Bradley, J., & Forsten, R. D. (2008). Resilience and military psychiatry. In B. J. Lukey & V. Tepe (Eds.), *Biobehavioral resilience to stress* (pp. 25–42). Boca Raton, FL: CRC Press.

Schnurr, P. P., Friedman, M. J., Engel, C. C., Foa, E. B., Shea, M. T., Chow, B. K., et al. (2007). Cognitive behavioral therapy for posttraumatic stress disorder in women. *Journal of the American Medical Association, 297,* 820–830.

Smith, T. C., Ryan, M. A. K., Wingard, D. L., Slymen, D. J., Sallis, J. F., & Kritz-Silverstein, D. (2008). New onset and persistent symptoms of post-traumatic stress disorder self reported after deployment and combat exposures: Prospective population base U.S. military cohort study. *British Medical Journal, 366,* 366–371.

Solberg, O. A., Laberg, J. C., Johnsen, B. H., & Eid, J. (2005). Predictors of self-efficacy in a Norwegian battalion prior to deployment in an international operation. *Military Psychology, 17,* 299–314.

Solomon, Z., Benbenishty, R., & Mikulincer, M. (1991). The contribution of wartime, pre-war, and post-war factors to self-efficacy: A longitudinal study of combat stress reaction. *Journal of Traumatic Stress, 4,* 345–361.

Speed, N., Engdahl, B., Schwartz, J., & Eberly, R. (1989). Posttraumatic stress as a consequence of POW experience. *Journal of Nervous and Mental Disease, 177,* 147–153.

Stein, M. B., Walker, J. R., Hazen, A. L., & Forde, D. R. (1997). Full and partial posttraumatic stress disorder: Findings from a community survey. *American Journal of Psychiatry, 154,* 1114–1119.

Steenkamp, M. M., Litz, B. T., Gray, M., Lebowitz, L., Nash, W., Conoscenti, L., et al. (2010). A brief exposure-based intervention for service members with PTSD. *Cognitive and Behavioral Practice, 18,* 98–107.

Sutker, P. B., & Allain, A. N. (1996). Assessment of PTSD and other mental disorders in World War II and Korean Conflict POW survivors and combat veterans. *Psychological Assessment, 8,* 18–25.

True, W. R., Rice, J., Eisen, S. A., Heath, A. C., Goldberg, J., Lyons, M. J., et al. (1993). A twin study of genetic and environmental contributions to liability for posttraumatic stress symptoms. *Archives of General Psychiatry, 50,* 257–264.

Vasterling, J. J., Proctor, S. P., Amoroso, P., Kane, R., Heeren, T., & White, R. (2006). Neuropsychological outcomes of Army personnel following deployment to the Iraq War. *Journal of the American Medical Association, 296,* 519–529.

Vogt, D. S., King, D. W., & King, L. A. (2007). Risk pathways for PTSD: Making sense of the literature. In M. J. Friedman, T. M. Keane, & P. A. Resick (Eds.), *Handbook of PTSD: Science and practice* (pp. 99–115). New York: Guilford Press.

Weinick, R. M., Beckjord, E. B., Farmer, C. M., Martin, L. T., Gillen, E. M., & Acosta, J. D. (2011). *Programs addressing psychological health and traumatic brain injury among U.S. military servicemembers and their families.* Santa Monica, CA: RAND Corporation.

Weiss, D. S., Marmar, C. R., Schlenger, W. E., Fairbank, J. A., Jordan, B. K., Hough, R. L., et al. (1992). The prevalence of lifetime and partial posttraumatic stress disorder in Vietnam theater veterans. *Journal of Traumatic Stress, 5,* 365–367.

Whealin, J. M., Ruzek, J. I., & Southwick, S. (2008). Cognitive-behavioral theory and preparation for professionals at risk for trauma exposure. *Trauma, Violence, and Abuse, 9*, 100–113.

Wolfe, J., Erickson, D. J., Sharkansky, E. J., King, D. W., & King, L. A. (1999). Course and predictors of posttraumatic stress disorder among Gulf War veterans: A prospective analysis. *Journal of Consulting and Clinical Psychology, 67*, 520–528.

Zaidi, L. Y., & Foy, D. W. (1994). Childhood abuse experiences and combat-related PTSD. *Journal of Traumatic Stress, 7*, 33–42.

Zlotnick, C., Franklin, C. L., & Zimmerman, M. (2002). Does "subthreshold" posttraumatic stress disorder have any clinical relevance? *Comprehensive Psychiatry, 43*, 413–419.

Part III

FACILITATING NATURAL AND THERAPEUTIC RECOVERY

Modifiable Risk and Resilience Factors

Chapter 7

The Nature of Traumatic Memory and Trauma Recovery

Lori A. Zoellner, Frank J. Farach, Larry D. Pruitt, *and* Norah C. Feeny

"I check my rearview mirror and see Eric behind me, with his eyes closed, listening to his music and trying to ignore the debate between Jane and Peter about whose favorite pizza joint is better. The driver in front of me is getting into the left lane, which draws my attention back to the front. I don't know why he keeps changing lanes so much, and I decide to just move past him on the right. As I'm getting up beside him, he changes back into the right lane again. Now he's pulling back over. I don't understand, umm, so I swerve to the shoulder. And I could see a bridge and a streambed. And I'm not about to go in the streambed so I steer back into the traffic, and the back metal bar on his truck hits the front of my front wheel. It pops the front wheel and I lose control of the car and hit the center divider. First we rolled forward. Then sideways. Then onto the roof and everything is flying around. I get hit in the head with the floor jack and broken glass is everywhere. My, my, my, my car stops upside down and backwards, against the railing of the bridge. I'm hanging out the door."[1]

---

[1]This case represents a mixture of details from several clients whom we have seen in our clinical work. Case details have been altered to conceal client identities and any resemblance to a specific individual is purely coincidental.

As we look at the example of an individual's memory for a motor vehicle accident, it raises quesetions about what the nature of trauma memories is. Are they fragmented, incoherent, and with many missing pieces? Or, in contrast, are they fixed, indelible, almost photographic representations of what happened? And, most importantly for our purposes, how does their nature relate to recovery following trauma exposure? In this chapter, we explore what is thought about the nature of trauma memories and their relationship to recovery. Clearly, memory and memory-related impairments are at the very heart of psychological adjustment following trauma exposure. It is precisely these memory-related reexperiencing symptoms, vivid, intrusive, and unwanted thoughts and images of the traumatic event (e.g., reliving the accident), that make up some of the most upsetting, distressing, and persistent reactions for trauma survivors.

In this chapter, we explore how the storage and retrieval of traumatic memories facilitate both natural and therapeutic recovery following trauma exposure. Two key memory features are important to define when discussing traumatic memories. First, *storage strength* refers to how well the details of the event are learned while the event was actually happening. Information with higher storage strength is typically better integrated or associated with other memories and is responsible for the capacity to store unlimited information permanently. *Retrieval strength* refers to how well details of the event can be recalled at any point after the event. Information that is more accessible, primed, or activated in memory has a higher retrieval strength and is more easily recalled (Bjork & Bjork, 2006). Differentiating memory storage from retrieval is important because each process makes distinct contributions to the trauma survivor's experience of a traumatic memory. Both of these processes are explored with regard to traumatic memories.

STORAGE OF THE TRAUMATIC MEMORY

As with all memories, the characteristics of trauma memories are very specific to the individual and the circumstances of the event. Not surprisingly, people who have experienced the same incident generally do not have identical memories of it. Take the four people in the vehicle during the serious accident described above. The first, Eric, a passenger in the back seat, was sitting with his earphones in, listening to music with his eyes closed; he never saw the actual accident, only the aftermath. The second, Jane, was engaged in conversation with someone in the front and was immediately knocked unconscious when the accident happened; she only remembers the aftermath. The third, Carol, was driving the vehicle, saw the other vehicle driving erratically and took evasive action to no avail; she remembers the accident and its aftermath. The fourth, Peter, was in the passenger's front seat. He also saw the vehicle coming at them and saw the evasive action taken by the driver; he also remembers the accident and its aftermath. Whose memories are similar? Whose memories are different? Who is most likely to come out of the accident with chronic posttraumatic stress disorder (PTSD)? Who is not? It's the same accident, but with four very different circumstances, and four potentially different memories of that accident. To unravel this puzzle, we are going to discuss three key questions that must be considered when thinking about what information was likely stored: (1) What happened during the traumatic event?; (2) Where was attention directed during the event?; and (3) Who was experiencing the event?

What Happened during the Event?

Clearly, what is initially encoded in memory depends in part on the nature of the event. People sometimes experience physical or biological insult and injury during a traumatic event such as being hit in the head and knocked unconscious, loss of oxygen (e.g., strangulation), loss of blood (e.g., shock), or intoxicated by drugs (e.g., rohypnol or "roofies") or alcohol, producing a severely altered state of consciousness. These can adversely affect memory storage, making it less likely that details of the event will be stored. And, because these details have little or no storage strength, they most likely will not be retrievable. In fact, in our example above, it is much more likely that what little original memory the passengers may have had will become integrated with memories of being told what had happened. Thus, there are clear instances where there will be no initial storage strength because nothing was initially encoded. Information that is encoded is thought to undergo a physiological process known as *consolidation* in the initial hours after a memory is created. Consolidation involves neuronal, hormonal, molecular, and cellular mechanisms, operating in parallel, to concretize information into long-term storage (McGaugh, 2000). This process changes the neuronal structure of a memory from a state in which it is dependent on the hippocampus for construction and information integration, to an independent state, where it becomes largely stable (Squire & Alvarez, 1995). This process holds for fear-related memories as well, making use of chemical signals from the amygdala to attach specific, fear-related meaning to a memory (Pitts & Takahashi, 2011).

The severity of one's reaction to the event itself also affects what information is stored in memory. All other things being equal, the more emotional, stressful, and arousing one's reaction to an event, the better the key details of the memory will be encoded and remembered (Christianson, 1992). This likely has to do with a variety of factors, including the uniqueness and meaning of the event (e.g., Craik & Tulving, 1975; Kroll, 1972; Moscovitch & Craik, 1976; Titus & Robinson, 1973) as well as to an increased release of endogenous stress-responsive hormones and neuromodulators (see McGaugh, 1992). In general, high levels of stress hormones enhance memory, such that the more stressful an experience, the greater the storage strength for that event in memory. This suggests that the severity, duration, and proximity to a traumatic event (i.e., the "dose" of trauma exposure) are critical factors in determining vulnerability to the development of PTSD. From a parsimonious standpoint, the dose-dependent model of trauma exposure and subsequent PTSD is intuitive: the worse the traumatic event, the more severe the psychological reaction. Yet, many argue that it fails to fully capture the complexities of who will and will not develop PTSD, with event characteristics (e.g., Brewin, Andrews, & Valentine, 2000; Ozer, Best, Lipsey, & Weiss, 2003) and physiological arousal in the immediate aftermath of the trauma (e.g., Blanchard, Hickling, Galovski, & Veazey, 2002; Bryant, Harvey, Guthrie, & Moulds, 2000; Shalev et al., 1998) being only modest predictors of who will develop PTSD. Thus, event "dosage" and the severity of one's reaction may affect storage of the traumatic memory but do not fully capture who is likely to develop PTSD.

Although some researchers suggest that memories encoded during high level of stress, such as traumatic memories, are longer lasting and more easily retrieved (e.g., Shobe & Kihlstrom, 1997), others suggest that extremely high levels of stress may create a type of memory that is stored and processed completely differently from nontraumatic memories (e.g., Brewin, 2001; Brewin, Dalgleish, & Joseph, 1996; van der Kolk, 1996; van der Kolk, Burbridge, & Suzuki, 1997; van der Kolk & Fisher, 1994; van der Kolk & Kadish, 1987). If correct, this implies that our understanding of normal memory functioning may not apply to traumatic memories. Specifically, it is argued that an overstimulation occurs at the time of the traumatic event or shortly thereafter that interferes with the normal processing of traumatic memories (e.g., Pitman, 1988). This view is often extended to argue that traumatic memories are processed differently than memories of other types of events, in a separate memory storage system.

These dual-processing theories posit that trauma memories are separate from the individual's overall memory network, disproportionately characterized by sensory aspects, and lack a coherent verbal representation. Additionally, they allow for the possibility of *traumatic amnesia*, the inability to recall a traumatic memory—often for years or decades—despite its initial storage. Much evidence for traumatic amnesia, however, can either be simply explained with more parsimonious explanations, such as forgetting or not thinking about the trauma for a long time, or methodological flaws (see Lynn, Knox, Fassler, Lilienfeld, & Loftus, 2004; McNally, 2003a, 2003b). Furthermore, although these dual-representation theories have strong intuitive appeal, their greater complexity makes them more difficult to test empirically, as it is difficult to ascertain if the memory loss seen could be better accounted for by lack of initial encoding or normal forgetting processes (Lynn et al., 2004; McNally, 2003a, 2003b, 2004; Zoellner & Bittinger, 2004). This is not saying that traumatic amnesia is not possible, just that alternative explanations have to be carefully considered (see Schacter, Norman, & Koutstaal, 1997). Indeed, this is a area of controversy and well beyond the scope of this chapter. Regardless, both sides of this argument suggest that traumatic memories are strongly encoded. In general, all other things being equal, the more severe the experience of the traumatic event, the greater its storage strength. Certain aspects of traumatic memories ought to be well remembered.

Finally, memory of infantile trauma exposure merits brief comment. How does the child's developing brain affect the encoding of a traumatic event? From birth to the early to mid-20s, the child and adolescent brain, including key memory systems, is rapidly developing (e.g., Nelson, 1995). As in adulthood, memory for events during childhood itself appears to be good (e.g., Peterson, 1999; Peterson & Bell, 1996; Peterson & Whalen, 2001). However, memories for events that occurred before the age of 3 are not well remembered in adulthood. Accordingly, it is very unlikely that an adult will have access to original memories from that time frame (e.g., Rubin, 2000; West & Bauer, 1999); this is often referred to as *normal infantile amnesia*. If you try to remember aspects of your childhood before you were 3, you most likely will end up concluding that you are not 100% certain of the source of that memory, even if you are sure that an event occurred. Are you really sure you have a memory of falling down the stairs or have you been repeatedly told about it? Are you really sure you remember visiting that zoo, or have you just seen the picture many times? What is reported to be a source memory for an event before age 3 is often a reconstruction of the event that results from the person being repeatedly told about the event, seeing images of the event, or discussing the event with his or her parents (e.g., Loftus, 1993; Peterson, Sales, Rees, & Fivush, 2007). This is not to suggest that we should not believe what a child says to us; instead, it means that we must honestly recognize the limits of human memory both in children and in adults. Indeed, most memory, even in adulthood, is reconstructed in nature.

Where Was Attention Directed during the Event?

Attention itself directly affects what is encoded in memory (Chun & Turk-Browne, 2007). Much like an adjustable zoom lens on a camera, attention can be narrowed to very minute details (e.g., the song playing on the radio when the car accident occurred) or can be widened to take in an entire panorama (e.g., the position of the cars on the bridge in relation to where the injured are laying). Thus, an individual going through a traumatic event is most likely making adjustments to his or her attention. Furthermore, attention is inexorably linked to memory storage. If an individual is not paying attention to particular details, they will likely have less storage strength and will not be remembered as well. This phenomenon of where the focus of attention is drawn is well known to cognitive psychologists, often using the term "weapons focus" to illustrate how attention can be narrowed and how this narrowing influences memory (Loftus, 1979). The concept of weapons focus makes intuitive sense when you think about a robbery: when a criminal draws out a gun, the vast majority of others' attention is focused on the action surrounding the gun. All other details become peripheral; and sure enough, memory for the actions surrounding the weapon is often very good, whereas details outside of the lens of focus (e.g., your colleague screaming) are not as well remembered. Central details that are attended to are more likely to be remembered well, whereas peripheral details are not attended to, and thus not remembered as well (e.g., Christianson & Loftus, 1987, 1991; Clifford & Hollin, 1981; Kebeck & Lohaus, 1986). The selective nature of attention necessarily entails selective memory: one can't recall what was never attended to in the first place. This relationship suggests that at least some information that appears "missing" from memory may never have been been attended to.

Consistent with weapons focus, aspects of an event that are most related to severity or life threat are most likely to command attention and to be remembered well. Yet, the duration of the traumatic event may interact here as well. In a brief event (e.g., a car accident), attention is limited by both the time needed to orient to the event itself and the brief duration of the event. This often leads to the perception of the event happening before the person even knew what was going on, or even vagueness about what happened. Thus, because of the brevity of the event itself, what was attended to is limited, and what is remembered may be impaired. In contrast, during a long-drawn-out event (e.g., kidnapping over several days or weeks), a myriad of details are available to be attended to or not attended to. Again, just as in the case of weapons focus, salient events will most likely be attended to better than less salient ones, again, leading to some pieces of the event being remembered well and other pieces not as well.

With high levels of stress, the role of dissociation and its impact on attention may play a role in regard to storage strength. Specifically, *peritraumatic dissociation*, that is, dissociation during the traumatic event, is often implicated in impaired encoding. *Dissociation* refers to a subjective sense of numbing or detachment, reduced awareness of one's surroundings, derealization, depersonalization, or amnesia for important aspects of the event (Classen, Koopman, & Spiegel, 1993). Specifically, some theorists suggest that traumatic memories are often characterized by an "avoidant, dissociative" encoding style used as a defensive coping strategy in the face of extreme stress, enabling the traumatized individual to disengage attention from threatening stimuli and direct it elsewhere (e.g., Shilony & Grossman, 1993; Terr, 1994). For example, instead of paying attention to the rapist's face, a trauma survivor directs her attention out the window of the room and attends to the snow falling down quietly. Clinically, dissociative reactions are commonly reported in both chronic traumatic experiences such as childhood sexual abuse (e.g., Draijer & Langeland, 1999) and after single-episode trauma such as rape or assault (e.g., Dancu, Riggs, Hearst-Ikeda, Shoyer, & Foa, 1996). These reactions are often theoretically linked to inadequate encoding and processing of trauma, leading to both a disorganized, disintegrated trauma narrative and frequent, automatic memory intrusions (e.g., Brewin et al., 1996; Ehlers, Hackmann, & Michael, 2004; Foa & Hearst-Ikeda, 1996; Foa & Riggs, 1993). Accordingly, from this viewpoint, dissociation results in a trauma memory that is encoded in a fragmented or disorganized manner and this impaired encoding increases the likelihood of chronic PTSD.

It is unclear whether dissociation provides a unique encoding pathway separate from the more basic attentional mechanisms described above. Those whose attention has been shifted away from crucial aspects of the trauma memory (i.e., those who dissociate) ought to have more disorganized or fragmented memory traces than those who do not. However, it is nearly impossible to determine precisely where or how attention was directed during a traumatic event. Those who have more disorganized or fragmented encoding, for whatever reason, ought to be at greater risk for chronic PTSD. However, evidence for this is equivocal at best. Research instead suggests that PTSD is more strongly associated with perceived, rather than actual, memory fragmentation (Bedard-Gilligan & Zoellner, 2013). Moreover, improvements in trauma narrative organization during PTSD treatment are not consistently associated with improvements in PTSD symptoms (Zoellner & Bittinger, 2004). Thus, individuals with PTSD may feel like their memory for the traumatic event is incoherent and disorganized, potentially feeling like they ought to remember some aspect better than they do; however, the evidence for actual fragmentation being associated with PTSD is not as strong. Thus, at present, there are some holes in the argument that disrupted encoding via dissociation impairs trauma recovery.

In general, what does this mean regarding the role of attention? The role of attention is not something we can change; where attention was directed and what was encoded is determined at the time of the event. Thus, it is not something that can be modified to enhance recovery. Instead of improving encoding, however, it may be worthwhile to reduce the negative impact by preventing, minimizing, or erasing the initial encoding of the event. Initial research suggests that this might be accomplished through pharmacological agents such as beta-adrenergic blockers (e.g., propranolol) or protein synthesis inhibitors (Cohen et al., 2006; Pitman & Delahanty, 2005). Modulating early trauma memories in this manner raises both ethical (Glannon, 2006) and practical (Grillon, Cordova, Morgan, Charney,

& Davis, 2004) issues. Furthermore, possible "erasure" of the memory does nothing in regard to the potential negative impact of later reconstruction of the event by the individual (e.g., being told, reading newspaper, or watching video accounts of what happened). This reconstruction, to be discussed further below, is potentially as important as what was initially encoded.

Finally, the implications regarding the role of attention for traumatic memories are relatively simple. If anything, trauma survivors ought not be concerned when aspects of his or her memories feel like they are missing details or, quite the opposite, feel like their memory is really powerful and entrenched in memory. One's focus of attention is most likely a key, individual-specific mechanism that influences these perceptions. Thus, not all individuals are going to direct their attention in the same way and, as a consequence, remember in the same way.

Who Was Experiencing the Event?

We now turn to a final factor that has the potential to influence encoding and storage strength of the traumatic memory. Who you are and what you have experienced in the past most likely also influences the initial encoding of the event. In particular, one's pre-event experiences and cognitive abilities may impact what is stored in memory. Just like we think of attention as similar to a camera lens, our prior experiences also form a lens as to how we experience a traumatic event and what is initially encoded. Take, for example, a chess master and a chess novice being briefly shown a chessboard. If the board is unorganized both will remember information comparably; however, if the board is organized into a chess pattern, the master will have superior recall to the novice (Chase & Simon, 1973; Gobet & Simon, 1996a, 1996b). The master brings to the board a set of experiences that helps him or her organize and remember the information differently than the novice. What one person sees and what another person sees, even if presented identical stimuli and identical focus of attention, are not identical; prior experience matters. The most obvious, relevant extension of the role of prior experience is previous trauma exposure. Someone undergoing a similar event again (e.g., being raped, being hit by an improvised explosive device, experiencing a car accident) has a different experience than someone who has never been through a similar event before. This prior experience most likely not only strengthens and alters encoding of the subsequent event but also consistently has been associated with an increased likelihood of developing chronic PTSD (Brewin et al., 2000). Thus, prior experience shapes what is encoded and either directly or indirectly may be related to persistent trauma-related memory symptoms.

Cognitive ability may also impact storage strength. How well an individual generally encodes and remembers information likely affects how well he or she encodes and remembers a traumatic event. It is well documented that trauma-exposed individuals with PTSD are more likely to report problems with attention, memory, and lower general intellectual ability than those without PTSD (e.g., McNally & Shin, 1994; Vasterling et al., 2002). A number of human studies have shown lower hippocampal volume, a key brain region implicated in memory functioning and accompanying cognitive-processing deficits in individuals with PTSD (e.g., Bremner et al., 1995; Villarreal et al., 2002). Yet it is unclear is these deficits existed before or were a consequence of trauma exposure and PTSD. A growing number of studies point to the former hypothesis (Gilbertson et al., 2002, 2007), namely that pretrauma differences in cognitive ability may act as a risk factors for developing PTSD. In a particularly important series of studies, Gilbertson and colleagues ingeniously evaluated hippocampal volume and cognitive performance in monozygotic twin pairs (twins who share identical genetic material) but who were discordant for combat exposure (one was exposed to combat and the other was not). Pairs were grouped according to whether the combat-exposed brother developed PTSD or not. The *combat-unexposed cotwins* of combat veterans with PTSD largely displayed similar reduced hippocampal volume and cognitive impairment as their brothers, both of which were lower than that of non-PTSD combat veterans and their brothers. The brain and brain functioning of the brother who did not go into combat was associated with combat-related PTSD symptoms in the other brother. Thus, lower hippocampal volume and cognitive impairments were largely due to shared genetic factors and not to trauma exposure, arguing instead that these factors may serve as premorbid risk factors in PTSD. A logical extension of this is that pretrauma factors such as reduced hippocampal volume and impaired ability to integrate information during encoding may increase one's likelihood to develop PTSD.

Conclusions: What, Then, Is Initially Encoded in Memory?

This answer to this question is simple. We simply do not know. So many factors contribute to determining what gets encoded and what doesn't that it becomes very difficult to answer the question of what should or shouldn't be remembered. Yet, both individuals working with trauma survivors and trauma survivors themselves often wish for their memory of the event to be different. Either longing for details that may never have been there or trying to uncover details that may never have been there may be fruitless. Instead, it probably makes most sense to accept what was initially encoded. Lastly, key aspects of the trauma memory are most likely very well encoded, having high storage strength, and as we will see below, this storage strength is something that persists over time. Thus, the nature of trauma memories is powerful and persistent. We now turn away from storage strength and to the role of retrieval.

RETRIEVAL OF THE TRAUMATIC MEMORY

The perceived importance of initial encoding has led our field to empha-size storage strength and, potentially inappropriately, minimize the role of subsequent retrieval on recovery following trauma exposure. Although what was initially encoded in memory forms the basis for what eventually will be recalled about the traumatic event, the subsequent retrieval of the traumatic memory may be just as important, *if not more important*, in determining who will recover and who will have persistent memory-related problems such as cued and uncued reexperiencing of the event, flashbacks, and trauma-related nightmares. As we will see, memory is dynamic, our recall of our past experiences is reconstructed through various filters, and, importantly, *the very act of our remembering has the ability to change the representation of that past experience in memory.* Thus, memories, even traumatic ones, are dynamic. To understand this flux, we must further understand the relative role of storage and retrieval strength.

If we think of memories, including traumatic ones, in terms of Bjork and Bjork's (1992) new theory of disuse, a representation in memory is a function of both its storage strength and its retrieval strength. This dis-tinction between storage and retrieval and the importance of retrieval is not new and draws heavily on past strong theoretical and empirical work, with similiar constructs seen historically in the work of both Hull (1943) and Estes (1955). Storage strength for memory traces reflects how well learned or interassociated something is, reflecting not only original learn-ing but also the accumulated total learning history of the event. In trauma exposure, it is strong for key memory traces. Retrieval strength, on the other hand, reflects how readily accessible the traces of the memory are for retrieval. In trauma exposure, retrieval strength is also strong for key memory traces. Of particular note, the probability that something will be recalled is completely determined by its retrieval strength (Bjork & Bjork, 2006). Thus, retrieval strength modulates our experience of our memories.

What can and cannot be retrieved at any point in time is extremely dependent on the cues that are available (Koriat, 2000). This process is highly adaptive and is thought to underlie everyday remembering and adaptive forgetting. For example, old, out-of-date information (e.g., the old address of a friend) becomes nonretrievable and does not interfere with the recall of new and more relevant information (e.g., the current address of a friend). This old information is not "forgotten" in the absolute sense of the word: should circumstances change, making the old information relevant again, it can be recalled or relearned rapidly as retrieval strength is again strengthened (e.g., if you went back to the old neighborhood where your friend lived, you may then be able to easily recall his or her address).

The Importance of Retrieval Strength

Based on what we discussed earlier in regard to encoding, the initial storage strength for particular memory traces associated with a traumatic event is most likely very strong. According to Bjork and Bjork's (1992) model, storage strength does not decrease over time; that is, if it is initially strong, it will always stay strong. Storage strength can grow, though, as a function of subsequent retrieval. Because decreasing storage strength is not possible, what we care about, then, is retrieval strength, as retrieval strength can both increase and decrease; and, most importantly, as mentioned above, retrieval strength directly impacts what is actually remembered.

The very act of retrieving modifies the human memory system. According to Bjork and Bjork (1992), two key principles are worth noting. First, for a trace to be recalled in response to a given cue, its representation must be discriminated from other representations in memory associated with that cue and be reconstructed from its representation. Second, retrieval strength of any particular trace decreases when other traces are subsequently experienced or retrieved. This means that retrieving one piece of information actually hurts retrieval of other pieces of information. More importantly, competition for retrieval strength happens at the level of retrieval cues. These retrieval cues are things that have been associated with a given item in the past, such as real or imagined aspects of the environment, interpersonal contexts, emotions, or physical states (Bjork & Bjork, 2006). We will discuss each of these principles in more depth as they have relevance to how we understand the act of remembering.

The first principle focuses on how retrieval is highly "cue-dependent" (Tulving, 1983; Tulving & Pearlstone, 1966). As mentioned earlier, cues can take many forms, real or imagined. If the original environmental or situational cues are present that are associated with a certain memory, a normally inaccessible memory becomes accessible. As suggested earlier, if we return to an old neighborhood where we grew up or to a school we once attended, access to those cues allows us to be able to retrieve information that without those cues would be inaccessible (Bjork & Bjork, 1992). The importance of cues in retrieval of certain memories also helps explain why reexperiencing symptoms are so common; encountering a cue has the ability to easily trigger related memories. Although one possible implication for trauma survivors would be to try to minimize the presence of cues, this is not entirely possible; cues are not just external situations but also can be more internal thoughts, feelings, and images. Furthermore, avoidance of nondangerous, trauma-related cues limits the range of activities a trauma survivor is willing to engage in and ends up limiting his or her daily life functioning. If it is not adaptive to try to eliminate these cues, then we need to think of how to use or modify these retrieval events in a more adaptive manner.

This second principle is referred to as "retrieval-induced forgetting," reflecting how recall of some items impairs recall of other related items (e.g., Anderson, 2003; Anderson, Bjork, & Bjork, 1994; Bjork, 1989; Geisleman, Bjork, & Fishman, 1983). As seen immediately after a traumatic event, the vast majority of individuals experience cued or uncued retrieval of aspects of the traumatic memory (e.g., intrusive memories, flashbacks, nightmares; e.g., Rothbaum, Foa, Riggs, Murdock, & Walsh, 1992). It should not be assumed that these reexperiencing events are benign in nature, as they are retrieval events and accordingly further *enhance* retrieval strength and storage strength for whatever aspects of the traumatic memory are being reexperienced and *impair* retrieval strength of other aspects. To be more concrete, when Carol, the driver of the vehicle in the accident discussed above, sees a vehicle that resembles the one involved in the accident (cue) and then reexperiences the image of the truck driving erratically (cued memory trace), it enhances the likelihood of this memory trace being subsequently retrieved. However, it also simultaneously impairs retrieval for other materials associated with that cue, that is, it becomes more difficult to subsequently retrieve that she repeatedly honked her horn to warn the other driver (uncued memory trace). Thus, retrieval strength for this uncued memory trace will actually decrease. Furthermore, highly memorable and fear-inducing pieces of the trauma memory are likely to result in distress and hence may be terminated quickly or actively suppressed, resulting in repeated differential retrieval of portions of the trauma memory. The cumulative result, then, would be increased retrieval strength of these worst parts, or "hot spots" of trauma memory with an experience of unavailability of other pieces of memory or hypomnesia for pieces of the trauma memory. Thus, the presence of intrusions, to some extent, may make future similar intrusions more likely, and may actually reduce the likelihood of retrieval of other important aspects of the traumatic event that may be important for trauma recovery.

The Key Role of Retrieval Practice

If we follow Bjork and Bjork's theory and line of research further, active retrieval of an item increases storage strength and retrieval strength more than does passively experiencing that item (e.g., Anderson, Bjork, & Bjork, 2000; Ciranni & Shimamura, 1999; Roediger & Karpicke, 2006). This retrieval practice phenomenon is now commonly used in enhancing teaching. For example, having a student explain to another student the principles of how to solve a particular problem is a powerful learning experience for the "explainer." Furthermore, the benefits of successful retrieval are larger the more difficult or involved the act of retrieval (e.g., Green & Kittur, 2006). Taking this teaching example further, having the "explainee" then attempt to solve the problem, on his or her own, even when it is difficult, rather than watching the explainer solve the problem for them, is a powerful learning experience for the "explainee." Thus, the practice of effortful, purposeful retrieval more dramatically improves subsequent remembering than simple reexperiencing of an item. This raises the possibility that the effects of reexperiencing on the traumatic memory can potentially be mitigated through active, effortful retrieval.

Taking a step backward, in some respects, the logical conclusions of this research may seem counterintuitive. When trying to "forget" the traumatic event, why would we be talking about the importance of subsequent retrieval? Subsequent retrieval enhances memory rather than helps in this forgetting process. Yet, as suggested earlier, when dealing with a traumatic event, forgetting probably is not possible. Instead, it is more realistic to work toward better controlling what is remembered and when it is remembered. While a horrific event such as a horrible car accident is always going to be an awful event, what we are instead suggesting is shifting or enhancing the retrieval of other important and related memory traces. These other trauma-related memory traces, similar to those traces that are being reexperienced, have good storage strength but not necessarily good retrieval strength; consequently, through repeated retrieval of those other memory traces, their retrieval strength should be able to be increased. This then actually changes what someone remembers when they are confronted with a trauma-related memory cue. Coming back to our earlier example, by repeatedly retrieving the memory of how hard she tried to prevent the accident (e.g., by honking, trying to evade the other driver, avoiding crashing into the streambed), when confronted with a vehicle that resembles the one that crashed into her, Carol may be more able to easily recall how hard she tried to prevent the accident, rather than the fear and distress she experienced at that time. The goal then isn't forgetting (e.g., escaping/avoiding), but changing or reconstructing the trauma memory in a more effective manner. It is important to note here that we are not talking about adding new or false information to the trauma memory. Instead, the goal is to alter the retrieval strength of what is being recalled and what is not from the traumatic event in order to reduce trauma memory–related distress and impairment. This focus on the role of cue competition is also reminiscent of extinction learning and context ambiguity theory (e.g., Bouton, 1994, 2000; Bouton & Swartzentruber, 1991) discussed in Chapter 11.

What does effortful retrieval practice look like? For one thing, passive reexperiencing symptoms, such as having an intrusive image of the trauma, may inadvertently strengthen some memory traces without shifting competition for retrieval strength that happens at the level of retrieval cues. What ought one do when he or she experience a reexperiencing symptom? A common response is to distract one's attention or think of something else, effectively truncating or avoiding the cued memory (e.g., when reexperiencing the fear and helplessness of the car accident while at her home,

Carol may turn her TV on very loudly while going through her grocery list in her head). Instead, however, one should use reexperiencing symptoms as a cue to deliberately think about related, but potentially more adaptive, aspects of the traumatic event (e.g., how she yelled for everyone to "hold on" and tried very hard to stay on the road). With practice, this deliberate thinking should eventually introduce more competition and help alter relative retrieval strengths. Similarly, activities such as writing about or purposely recalling details about the trauma memory ought to be more powerful at shifting retrieval strength than more passive activities such as reading about one's trauma memory or listening to one's trauma memory. Similarly, just remembering vaguely (e.g., "I think about it all the time."), without expending concerted retrieval effort, would also not be as powerful a form of retrieval. This is particularly important for trauma survivors who question why more deliberate remembering would be different from their everyday remembering. Remember, the more the individual has to work to retrieve details, the more likely both retrieval strength and storage strength will be enhanced. A final related application is in the area of trauma "hot spots," those traces of the memory that are most distressing. Hot spots are probably key targets for this type of effortful retrieval practice, where again the importance is in retrieval of more adaptive memory traces. But what type of hot spot content should one be the focus of effortful retrieval? What is likely to promote more adaptive recovery and what might detract from it? One possible answer is the role of meaning.

The Role of Meaning

Up to this point, we have been focusing on memory traces, but these effects can be more broadly understood within a network model of memory. Often we think of trauma memories as fitting into some overarching schema, or packet of information that we associate with a concept (Bartlett, 1932). These associations affect our memory, providing filters that affect our retrieval (see Norman, Newman, & Detre, 2007, for a neural network model of retrieval-induced forgetting). Specifically, the more that we meaningfully relate pieces of information to one another during retrieval practice, termed *elaborative processing*, the better we can retrieve that information (e.g., Craik & Tulving, 1975). Consistent with elaborative processing, subjective organization, or a person's perception of organization, grouping things together in larger units based on meaningful relationships has been shown to be helpful as well (e.g., Tulving, 1962, 1968). Thus, elaborative processing yields the strongest memory performance.

What would adaptive, elaborative, meaning-based processing at the time of retrieval practice look like for trauma survivors? Of particular relevance to trauma survivors may be the role of self in retrieval (e.g., Barclay & DeCooke, 1988). Key candidates for shifting and elaborating the meaning of the traumatic event regarding the self may be in regard to negative beliefs about one's self, others, and the world (e.g., Ehlers & Clark, 2000; Epstein, 1991; Foa & Rothbaum, 1998; Janoff-Bulman, 1985, 1992; McCann & Pearlman, 1990; Resick & Schnicke, 1992). For example, Epstein (1991) emphasized key positive beliefs that may be impacted as a result of trauma exposure; specifically that the self is worthy, others are trustworthy, the world is benign, and the world is meaningful. Indeed, these beliefs often discriminate between trauma-exposed individuals with and without PTSD (Ali, Dunmore, Clark, & Ehlers, 2001; Foa, Ehlers, Clark, Tolin, & Orsillo, 1999; Mechanic & Resick, 1993). More generally, these beliefs may contribute to a sense of ongoing danger that contributes to the development of PTSD (e.g., Dunmore, Clark, & Ehlers, 1999).

Thus, in order to achieve more elaborative, meaning-based retrieval practice, linking of the retrieval to a larger sense of meaning that is particularly relevant for the trauma survivor should significantly enhance later retrieval strength. It is important to note that the focus is on linking cues and memory traces in an adaptive manner, not further reifying unadaptive beliefs (e.g., that the world is dangerous). Taken together, effortful retrieval practice ought to include elaboration of meaning, particularly regarding meaning for one's self. In some respect, this harkens back to Barlett's (1932) concept of "effort after meaning," where providing an overarching meaning to an incomprehensible situation aids in future remembering. The focus, then, is finding meaning as part of the effortful retrieval as a means to shaping future retrieval. If we return to the example of Carol, whose cued reexperiencing has her consistently remembering the image of the car swerving into her vehicle and reduced remembering of how she fought to avoid an accident, through retrieval practice, she then builds the retrieval strength of the memory of how she did try to prevent the collision and also makes a conceptual shift in meaning such that she no longer believes that she just let the accident happen. This elaborative retrieval practice not only increases the likelihood of this being recalled in the future, but also decreases the likelihood of recall of the image of the car swerving into her. Thus, future retrieval ought to be altered in a more adaptive manner; that is, reexperiencing symptoms may not be as distressing and may not be as frequent.

The Role of Repetition and Overlearning

One final note on retrieval bears discussion. To increase retrieval strength, retrieval practice needs to happen not just once but repeatedly. Furthermore, even after retrieval strength results in near perfect performance (e.g., reexperiencing symptoms no longer are as distressing or as frequent), additional overlearning should help maintain this performance. Overlearning, here, simply refers to continuing to do retrieval practice. Specifically, in response to repetition and overlearning, while retrieval strength eventually hits an asymptote of perfect performance, storage strength can continue to be accumulated. This increased storage strength then helps to slow the loss of retrieval strength (e.g., continuing to no longer have distressing reexperiencing symptoms). This means that the best results of effortful retrieval practice come with lots of practice. Indeed, there is a growing literature in regard to how to make this practice most optimal (see Bjork & Bjork, 2006; Lang, Craske, & Bjork, 1999); but suffice it to say, more practice is better.

Conclusion: A Reconstructive View of Traumatic Memory

What we are proposing here is that we, as a field, shift away from a predominant focus on the encoding of the traumatic event and instead adopt a reconstructed view of traumatic memory, emphasizing the role of retrieval in shaping the experience of the trauma survivor and the development of chronic PTSD. Taking a view of memory as dynamic and reconstructive, as opposed to passive or reactive, not only is in line with current cognitive thought (e.g., Brown & Craik, 2000) but also provides a more comprehensive and practical understanding of the role of posttrauma processes in recovery.

Taking a reconstructive view of trauma memory also has implications for understanding the veracity of memory. As discussed above, retrieval processes are highly cue-dependent, but they are also erratic and fallible (Bjork & Bjork, 1992), sometimes having undesirable consequences. Specifically, errors in the memory (e.g., false memories or source-monitoring failures) do occur particularly at later retrieval (e.g., Loftus, 1997; Roediger & McDermott, 1999), but also possibly at initial encoding of the event (e.g., Loftus, 1997). These types of errors are also present in individuals with PTSD (Bremner, 2000; Zoellner, Foa, Bridigi, & Przeworski, 2000). Thus, errors happen and individuals with PTSD are not immune to them. Thus, within a reconstructive view of memory, it is assumed that there are going to be occasional inaccuracies.

A reconstructive view of memory also argues against a traditional file cabinet view of memory. In this view, pieces of information are stored in different files and organized in a certain way. Once pieces of information are stored in the cabinet all you have to do is go back into that file cabinet, retrieve the correct file, and access the piece of information you are looking for. When you put it back, it remains there unchanged. Instead, in a reconstructive view of memory, the very act of retrieving information from that file cabinet changes representations in the memory system; it changes what you have access to and what you do not have access to in the future in that file cabinet. Thus, the contents of the file cabinet are constantly in flux, depending on previous accessing of the cabinet, changing positions in terms of their retrieval strength. You can't always find what you want and sometimes get things you don't want. Accordingly, we are not passive recorders of our experiences but are active participants in our memory. We have the ability to shape what we remember, to better control the retrieval of memories of a particular event, no matter how well stored in memory. This has significant implications for understanding both natural and therapeutic recovery following traumatic events.

Potential Implications

Notably, some current work suggests that sleep, particularly rapid eye movement (REM) sleep seen during dreaming, is an important consolidator of extinction learning (Pace-Schott et al., 2009, 2011; Spoormaker et al., 2010). The very act of retrieving a memory is thought to make it temporarily more malleable. This is a hypothesized process, known as memory reconsolidation, that allows the memory to be updated with new information for a brief period (approximately 6–24 hours) after it is retrieved. Indeed, mere exposure to safety information within this window after recalling an aversive memory was sufficient to reduce the fear in response to the memory even 1 year later (Schiller et al., 2010). This fear reduction on subsequent retrieval is thought to arise because the original fear memory itself has been altered through the incorporation of safety information during the critical reconsolidation window. Although this interpretation is still under debate and has not consistently been replicated in humans (e.g., Kindt & Soeter, 2013), the demonstrated effects of retrieval on the nature of response to the memory reinforce our previous point that deliberate retrieval practice, and enhancing attention to the nonthreatening aspects of a memory, can reduce fear during subsequent retrieval. The logical extension of this work is that repeated, effortful retrieval of the trauma memory in a way that promotes fear reduction (i.e., extinction) followed by adequate sleep may consolidate a memory in such a way as to promote resilience. Alternatively, retrieval that does not promote fear reduction followed by adequate sleep may consolidate a memory in a way that hinders recovery. The research to address these questions is currently being conducted.

Interventions designed to aid traumatic recovery must be especially careful of the impact that they can have on how memories are processed. An example of this is group debriefing interventions designed to aid post-trauma stress management by having individuals discuss the event and make emotional interpretations about its meaning and impact while cognitively processing the implications of the event in a group format (Everly & Michell, 2001; Hammond & Brooks, 2001). Though well intentioned, these interventions have been a source of much controversy due to empirical findings that argue against immediate and compulsory trauma-focused treatment (Litz, Gray, Bryant, & Adler, 2002). Criticial incident stress debriefing (CISD), for example, may interfere with natural recovery from traumatic experiences and may inadvertently lead to false or other information being encoded as a personally experienced fact (see McNally, Bryant, & Ehlers, 2003, for a review). Experimental studies have found that misinformation provided by a confederate during a typical debriefing intervention frequently leads to that false information being recalled as a source memory (Devilly et al., 2007). Furthermore, this incorrect information appears to be stable over time, suggesting that once it is incorporated into the individual's memory, his or her confidence in its validity persists (Devilly et al., 2007; Gerrie, Belcher, & Garry, 2006). This may be exacerbated by ongoing stress, loss, and grief that may make an individual particularly vulnerable to these effects. Furthermore, immediate debriefing in the wake of traumatic events has been shown to have either inert or iatrogenic effects in terms of trauma recovery. Individuals who have been debriefed consistently have higher rates of PTSD than nondebriefed individuals, and debriefing is assocated with greater psychiatric symptoms including anxiety and functional impairment (Bisson & Deahl, 1994; Carlier, Lamberts, Van Uchelen, & Gersons, 1998; Mayou, Ehler, & Hobbs, 2000). As a result, a Cochrane review of the literature regarding psychological debriefing concluded that the compulsory use of this technique should be stopped because of this lack of support (Rose, Bisson, Churchill, & Wessely, 2009).

However, given what is known about aspects of memory retrieval that promote trauma recovery, several specific ideas can be further incorporated into existing interventions for chronic PTSD. Psychoeducation about the nature of memory retrieval and memory change may be beneficial for many patients. It can be both reassuring and empowering to learn that some of the more unpleasant aspects of trauma memories are malleable and sensitive to changes that patients can make in the way they retrieve them. It also encourages a shift in perspective from attributing symptoms to a stable, global, personal defect (e.g., "I'm experiencing X and can't get over it, so there must be something wrong with me") to one that allows for the identification of specific memory characteristics that the patient can change with repeated practice (e.g., "How does thinking about my trauma this way affect how I experience the memory of it, and what can I do to improve this?"). Importantly, this provides a rationale that can enhance motivation to engage in other memory-oriented procedures designed to enhance recovery. Patients can also be encouraged to voluntarily approach the memory of their trauma repeatedly and in great detail. This is a fundamental aspect of some existing inteventions for PTSD, including prolonged exposure therapy and trauma-focused cognitive-behavioral therapy (CBT), and it has strong empirical support (e.g., Bradley, Greene, Russ, Dutra, & Westen, 2005; Institute of Medicine, 2007).

OTHER RELATED CONSEQUENCES
OF TRAUMA EXPOSURE AND PTSD

Before we leave the topic of attention and memory, two additional memory-related phenomena seen in individuals with PTSD are worthwhile to note. These are selective attention to threat-related material and problems with retrieving specific autobiographical memories, particularly for positive ones. Although the research has not been conducted to adequately determine whether or not these are pretrauma vulnerability factors, these phenomena are more theoretically linked with the consequence of trauma exposure and PTSD.

Attention to Threat

Using our example of Carol, who survived a horrific motor vehichle accident, whenever she is anywhere near other vehicles she is vigilant and scans her environment to look for any clues regarding potential danger. These clues could be any sound, any shadow, any unexpected movement. She is primed to look for threat, both to a greater degree and in more situations than people without PTSD. Once she perceives even mild potential threat, she mentally dwells on it for a long time and has difficulty paying attention to anything else. All of this occurs so automatically that it is difficult for her to control. This is exactly what selective attention to threat-relevant information is about. Selective attention to threat-related material is a common information-processing phenomenon found across the anxiety disorders (see Bar-Haim, Lamy, Pergamin, Bakermans-Kranenburg, & van IJzendoorn, 2007, for a review). Basically, individuals with anxiety-based disorders tend to orient toward threat-relevant information much more so than individuals without an anxiety-based disorder. Again, this is the camera lens of attention searching out the environment for cues that might signal danger or potential future threat. This selective attention to threat can also extend to making threat-related interpretation errors regarding ambiguous stimuli (e.g., Mathews & Mackintosh, 2000; White, Suway, Pine, Bar-Haim, & Fox, 2011). Thus, for example, for a motor vehicle accident survivor like Carol, any movement from the periphery of her visual field is perceived to be an out-of-control driver about to crash into her, rather than some mundane event such as a well-controlled car backing out of a driveway. The interpretation of vague information is directed toward keeping the individual safe; it is like a car alarm set to detect threat, but one that goes off with the most innocuous stimuli.

What does this mean for individuals with PTSD? Their daily life is spent orienting to innocuous stimuli in the environment that are nevertheless perceived as potentially threatening. For many, this constant, uncontrollable orienting toward, and difficulty disengaging from, potential threat makes them feel like they are going crazy. Simply knowing that this is a natural and automatic reaction that is designed to protect them from future danger, albeit more primed than necessary, may help mitigate some of these perceptions. See Mobini and Grant (2007) for an extended discussion of clinical implications of an attentional bias to threat. Recently, novel computerized interventions that retrain these threat-oriented biases in attention (see Hakamata et al., 2010, for a review) and interpretation have been showing some promise in anxiety (e.g., Mackintosh, Mathews, Yiend, Ridgeway, & Cook, 2006).

Difficulty in Remembering Specific Positive, Past Memories

When asked to remember autobiographical memories from key words like "happy," trauma survivors with PTSD often have greater difficulty than trauma survivors without PTSD retrieving memories of specific instances. Instead of saying "that day on the beach last summer when the sun was glistening off the water as it set," they would say "a day at the beach," exemplifying broad, general categories of events rather than a particular instance, even with repeated prompting. Although this may not seem like a big difference on the surface, being able to retrieve specific positive autobiographical memories differentiates individuals with and without PTSD (e.g., McNally et al., 1994) and individuals who are depressed and those who are not (e.g., Williams et al., 1996).

Why might this be the case? There are a variety of theories put forth (e.g., Philippot, Schaefer, & Herbette, 2003; Watkins & Teasdale, 2001, 2004; Williams et al., 1996), but most of them incorporate some idea of helping individuals regulate distressing emotions. Intense emotion can hamper specificity and interfere with the emotion regulation that is necessary for the effortful retrieval of specific memories. Put simply, this means that to the extent that it is difficult to deal with positive or negative emotions, it will be harder to retrieve specific emotional memories. That is, sometimes thinking about positive things (e.g., specific positive memories can also be emotionally intense, not because they elicit positive emotions but because they too elicit strong negative emotions—highlighting the belief that things are not the same anymore) is just as difficult as thinking about negative things, and retrieving a more general memory helps protect the individual from these intense emotions. If we then think about this difficulty in general, more effort is going to be required to elicit detailed specific memories. This effort may be on the part of the person retrieving the memory, having to use more cognitive resources or manage his or her emotions more carefully, or may be on the part of the listener, having to give more examples and cues to get specific details from the individual. Accordingly, avoidance of specific memories may serve a general purpose of helping the individual function on a daily basis, though in the long term, this negatively reinforced habit maintains reliance on avoidance to regulate emotion.

SUMMARY AND CLINICAL RECOMMENDATIONS

By way of summary, let's return to our example of the car accident that Carol and her friends were involved in. Who of the four friends in the car is going to have more initial reexperiencing symptoms? Who is going on to develop chronic PTSD? The honest answer, if we integrate what we have been discussing, is that we do not yet know. The answer potentially lies in retrieval strength, and, based on our example, we know nothing about the aftermath of the car accident, where retrieval processes become key. Clearly, prior-to-the-accident experiences of those in the car and their experience during the accident itself shape initial storage strength of the memory. This itself can account for some, but not all, of the variability in who is likely to develop chronic reexperiencing of the event. But the retrieval strength of various memory traces for these individuals has yet to be determined. All is not written at the time of the traumatic event, and what happens afterward in terms of retrieval may actually be more important for recovery than what happened during the event.

To summarize key points:

1. Initial encoding of the traumatic event creates strong storage strength. Thus, the traumatic memory will generally be powerful and easily cued for the trauma survivor. This strong storage most likely cannot be decreased.
2. The traumatic event itself, past experiences, and attention all influence what is initially encoded regarding the traumatic event. Yet, these factors are very hard to identify retrospectively, making it difficult to say what should and shouldn't be stored in memory.
3. Reexperiencing symptoms are passive forms of retrieval that enhance retrieval strength, thus *increasing* the likelihood of future reexperiencing symptoms *and* actually *impairing* retrieval of other potentially more adaptive aspects of the trauma memory.
4. Effortful retrieval practice of the trauma memory, accessing important information not normally accessed, and focusing on elaborative meaning processing has the potential to alter the subsequent experience of the trauma memory, in an adaptive manner.
5. Repeated effortful retrieval practice helps solidify this learning.

So, if all of the individuals in the car accident experience some degree of reexperiencing and avoidance of trauma-related cues after the car accident, how might natural and therapeutic recovery look for these four individuals? To facilitate this recovery, the old adage of "guarding your heart and your mind" seems most relevant. This means actively paying attention to and modifying what a trauma survivor is feeling and thinking about. This would potentially entail being purposeful when thinking of the event, not trying to get rid of distressing images and thoughts when confronted with them, and effortfully thinking of other related adaptive details and thoughts. This would potentially also entail elaborative, deliberate, and repeated retrieval of the memory of the accident, not at times of reexperiencing. What might this look like? It might be as simple as talking with friends and family about what happened, or it might be repeatedly thinking or writing about the accident deliberatively and purposely, being sure to include details and meaning elements that would lead to more adaptive functioning. How much effortful retrieval is necessary may depend on how much difficulty an individual is having with the trauma memory; that said, repeated retrieval and overlearning are generally good things. These details and meaning might even be as simple as thinking thoughts such as "I did all I could do to avoid the accident [and reviewing details to know that it is true]. Accidents happen, but they don't happen every time I drive. There was nothing more that I could do." Whether or not this effortful retrieval is accomplished during natural and therapeutic recovery, the person is actively working to shift what information he or she retrieves about the traumatic event. This isn't the power of positive thinking. Bad things happened, and often they could happen again. Finding meaning after trauma exposure means finding a truth that the survivor can live with about what happened and moving forward with this truth in hand.

ACKNOWLEDGMENTS

Preparation of this chapter was supported in part by a grant to Lori A. Zoellner (No. R01MH66347, Lori Zoellner, Principal Investigator). We would like to thank Hillary Smith for her careful read of and reference help on this chapter.

REFERENCES

Ali, T., Dunmore, E., Clark, D., & Ehlers, A. (2002). The role of negative beliefs in posttraumatic stress disorder: A comparison of assault victims and non victims. *Behavioural and Cognitive Psychotherapy, 30*(3), 249–257.

Anderson, M. C. (2003). Rethinking interference theory: Executive control and the mechanisms of forgetting. *Journal of Memory and Language, 49*, 415–445.

Anderson, M. C., Bjork, R. A., & Bjork, E. L. (1994). Remembering can cause forgetting: Retrieval dynamics in long-term memory. *Journal of Experimental Psychology: Learning, Memory, and Cognition, 20*(5), 1063–1087.

Anderson, M. C., Bjork, E. L., & Bjork, R. A. (2000). Retrieval-induced forgetting:

Evidence for a recall-specific mechanism. *Psychonomic Bulletin and Review*, 7, 522–530.

Bar-Haim, Y., Lamy, D., Pergamin, L., Bakermans-Kranenburg, M. J., & van IJzendoorn, M. H. (2007). Threat-related attentional bias in anxious and nonanxious individuals: A meta-analytic study. *Psychological Bulletin*, 133, 1–24.

Barclay, C. R., & DeCooke, P . A. (1988). Ordinary everyday memories: Some of the things of which selves are made. In U. Neisser & E. Winograd (Eds.), *Remembering reconsidered: Ecological and traditional approaches to the study of memory* (pp. 91–125). New York: Cambridge University Press.

Bartlett, F. C. (1932). *Remembering*. Oxford, UK: Oxford University Press.

Bedard-Gilligan, M., & Zoellner, L. A. (2013). Dissociation and memory fragmentation in posttraumatic stress disorder: An evaluation of the dissociative encoding hypothesis. *Memory, 20*, 277–299.

Bisson, J. I., & Deahl, M. P. (1994). Psychological debriefing and prevention of post-traumatic stress: More research is needed. *British Journal of Psychiatry*, 165(6), 717–720.

Bjork, R. A. (1989). Retrieval inhibition as an adaptive mechanism in human memory. In H. L. Roediger & F. I. M. Craik (Eds.), *Varieties of memory and consciousness: Essays in honor of Endel Tulving* (pp. 309–330). Hillsdale, NJ: Erlbaum.

Bjork, R. A., & Bjork, E. L. (1992). A new theory of disuse and an old theory of stimulus fluctuation. In A. Healy, S. Kosslyn, & R. Shiffrin (Eds.), *From learning processes to cognitive processes: Essays in honor of William K. Estes* (Vol. 2, pp. 35–67). Hillsdale, NJ: Erlbaum.

Bjork, R. A., & Bjork, E. L. (2006). Optimizing treatment and instruction: Implications of a new theory of disuse. In L.-G. Nilsson & N. Ohta (Eds.), *Memory and society: Psychological perspectives* (pp. 109–133). New York: Psychology Press.

Blanchard, E. B., Hickling, E. J., Galovski, T., & Veazey, C. (2002). Emergency room vital signs and PTSD in a treatment seeking sample of motor vehicle accident survivors. *Journal of Traumatic Stress*, 15(3), 199–204.

Bouton, M. E. (1994). Context, ambiguity, and classical conditioning. *Current Directions in Psychological Science, 3*, 49–53.

Bouton, M. E. (2000). A learning theory perspective on lapse, relapse, and the maintenance of behavior change. *Health Psychology, 19*, 57–63.

Bouton, M. E., & Swartzentruber, D. (1991). Sources of relapse after extinction in Pavlovian and instrumental learning. *Clinical Psychology Review, 11*, 123–140.

Bradley, R., Greene, J., Russ, E., Dutra, L., & Westen, D. (2005). A multidimesnional meta-analysis of psychotherapy for PTSD. *American Journal of Psychiatry, 162*, 214–227.

Brewin, C. R., Andrews, B., & Valentine, J. D. (2000). Meta-analysis of risk factors for posttraumatic stress disorder in trauma-exposed adults. *Journal of Consulting and Clinical Psychology*, 68(5), 748–766.

Brewin, C. R. (2001). Cognitive and emotional reactions to traumatic events: Implications for short-term intervention. *Advances in Mind–Body Medicine, 17*, 163–168.

Brewin, C. R., Dalgleish, T., & Joseph, S. (1996). A dual representation theory of posttraumatic stress disorder. *Psychological Review, 103*, 670–686.

Bremner, J. D. (2000). A biological model for delayed recall of childhood abuse. *Journal of Aggression Maltreatment and Trauma, 4*(2), 165–183.

Bremner, J. D., Randall, P., Scott, T. M., Bronen, R. A., Delaney, R. C., Seibyl, J. P., et al. (1995). MRI-based measurement of hippocampal volume in patients with combat-related posttraumatic stress disorder. *American Journal of Psychiatry, 152*, 973–981.

Brown, S. C., & Craik, F. I. M. (2000). Encoding and retrieval of information. In E. Tulving & F. I. M. Craik (Eds.), *The Oxford handbook of memory* (pp. 93–107). New York: Oxford University Press.

Bryant, R. A., Harvey, A. G., Guthrie, R. M., & Moulds, M. L. (2000). A prospective study of psychophysiological arousal, acute stress disorder, and posttraumatic stress disorder. *Journal of Abnormal Psychology, 109*, 341–344.

Carlier, I. V. E., Lamberts, R. D., Van Uchelen, A. J., & Gersons, B. P. R. (1998). Disaster-related post-traumatic stress in police officers: A field study of the impact of debriefing. *Stress Medicine, 14*(3), 143–148.

Chase, W. G., & Simon, H. A. (1973). Perception in chess. *Cognitive Psychology, 4*, 55–81.

Christianson, S.-Å. (1992). Emotional stress and eyewitness memory: A critical review. *Psychological Bulletin, 112*(2), 284–309.

Christianson, S.-Å, & Loftus, E. F. (1987). Memory for traumatic events. *Applied Cognitive Psychology, 1*(4), 225–239.

Christianson, S.-Å., & Loftus, E. F. (1991). Remembering emotional events: The fate of detailed information. *Cognition and Emotion, 5*, 81–108.

Chun, M. M., & Turk-Browne, N. B. (2007). Interactions between attention and memory. *Current Opinion in Neurobiology, 17*, 177–184.

Ciranni, M. A., & Shimamura, A. P. (1999). Retrieval-induced forgetting in episodic memory. *Journal of Experimental Psychology: Learning, Memory, and Cognition, 25*, 1403–1414.

Classen, C., Koopman, C., & Spiegel, D. (1993). Trauma and dissociation. *Bulletin of the Menninger Clinic, 57*(2), 178–194.

Clifford, B. R., & Hollin, C. R. (1981). Effects of the type of incident and the number of perpetrators on eyewitness memory. *Journal of Applied Psychology, 66*(3), 364–370.

Cohen, H., Kaplan, Z., Matar, M. A., Loewenthal, U., Kozlovsky, N., & Zohar, J. (2006). Anisomycin, a protein synthesis inhibitor, disrupts traumatic memory consolidation and attenuates posttraumatic stress response in rats. *Biological Psychiatry, 60*(7), 767–776.

Craik, F. I. M., & Tulving, E. (1975). Depth of processing and the retention of words in episodic memory. *Journal of Experimental Psychology: General, 104*(3), 268–294.

Dancu, C. V., Riggs, D. S., Hearst-Ikeda, D., Shoyer, B. G., & Foa, E. B. (1996). Dissociative experiences and posttraumatic stress disorder among female victims of criminal assault and rape. *Journal of Traumatic Stress, 9*, 253–267.

Devilly, G. J., Ciorciari, J., Piesse, A., Sherwell, S., Zammit, S., Cook, F., et al. (2007). Dissociative tendencies and memory performance on directed-forgetting tasks. *Psychological Science, 18*(3), 212–217.

Draijer, N., & Langeland, W. (1999). Childhood trauma and perceived parental dysfunction in the etiology of dissociative symptoms in psychiatric inpatients. *American Journal of Psychiatry, 156*(3), 379–385.

Dunmore, E. C., Clark, D. M., & Ehlers, A. (1999). Cognitive factors involved in the onset and maintenance of posttraumatic stress disorder (PTSD) after physical or sexual assault. *Behaviour Research and Therapy, 37,* 809–829.

Ehlers, A., & Clark, D. M. (2000). A cognitive model of persistent posttraumatic stress disorder. *Behaviour Research and Therapy, 38,* 319–345.

Ehlers, A., Hackmann, A., & Michael, T. (2004). Intrusive re-experiencing in posttraumatic stress disorder: Phenomenology, theory, and therapy. *Memory, 12*(4), 403–415.

Epstein, S. (1991). Impulse control and self-destructive behaviour. In L. P. Lipsitt & L. L. Mitick (Eds.), *Self-regulatory behaviour and risk-taking: Causes and consequences* (pp. 273–284). Norwood, NJ: Ablex.

Estes, W. K. (1955). Statistical theory of spontaneous recovery and regression. *Psychological Review, 62*(3), 145–154.

Everly, G. S., & Mitchell, J. T. (2001). America under attack: The "10 commandments" of responding to mass terrorist attacks. *International Journal of Emergency Mental Health, 3*(3), 133–135.

Foa, E. B., Ehlers, A., Clark, D. M., Tolin, D. F., & Orsillo, S. M. (1999). The Posttraumatic Cognitions Inventory (PTCI): Development and validation. *Psychological Assessment, 11*(3), 303–314.

Foa, E. B., & Hearst-Ikeda, D. (1996). Emotional dissociation in response to trauma: An information-processing approach. In L. K. Michelson & W. J. Ray (Eds.), *Handbook of dissociation: Theoretical, empirical, and clinical perspectives* (pp. 207–224). New York: Plenum Press.

Foa, E. B., & Riggs, D. S. (1993). Post-traumatic stress disorder in rape victims. In J. Oldham, M. B. Riba, & A. Tasman (Eds.), *American Psychiatric Press review of psychiatry* (Vol. 12, pp. 273–303). Washington, DC: American Psychiatric Press.

Foa, E. B., & Rothbaum, B. O. (1998). *Treating the trauma of rape: Cognitivebehavioral therapy for PTSD.* New York: Guilford Press.

Geiselman, R. E., Bjork, R. A., & Fishman, D. L. (1983). Disrupted retrieval in directed forgetting: A link with posthypnotic amnesia. *Journal of Experimental Psychology: General, 112*(1), 58–72.

Gerrie, M. P., Belcher, L. E., & Garry, M. (2006). "Mind the gap": False memories for missing aspects of an event. *Applied Cognitive Psychology, 20*(5), 689–696.

Gilbertson, M. W., Shenton, M. E., Ciszewski, A., Kasai, K., Lasko, N. B., Orr, S. P., et al. (2002). Smaller hippocampal volume predicts pathologic vulnerability to psychological trauma. *Nature Neuroscience, 5*(11), 1242–1247.

Gilbertson, M. W., Williston, S. K., Paulus, L. A., Lasko, N. B., Gurvits, T. V., Shenton, M. E., et al. (2007). Configural cue performance in identical twins discordant for posttraumatic stress disorder: Theoretical implications for the role of hippocampal function. *Biological Psychiatry, 62*(5), 513–520.

Glannon, W. (2006). Neuroethics. *Bioethics, 20*(1), 37–52.

Gobet, F., & Simon, H.A. (1996a). The roles of recognition processes and look-ahead search in time-constrained expert problem solving: Evidence from grand-master-level chess. *Psychological Science, 7*(1), 52–55.

Gobet, F., & Simon, H. A. (1996b). Templates in chess memory: A mechanism for recalling several boards. *Cognitive Psychology, 31,* 1–40.

Green, C., & Kittur, A. (2006). Retrieval-induced forgetting in a multiple-trace memory model. *Proceedings of the Twenty-Eighth Annual Meeting of the Cognitive Science Society,* Vancouver, Canada.

Grillon, C., Cordova, J., Morgan, C. A., Charney, D. S., & Davis, M. (2004). Effects of the beta-blocker propranolol on cued and contextual fear conditioning in humans. *Psychopharmacology (Berlin), 175*(3), 342–352.

Hakamata, Y., Lissek, S., Bar-Haim, Y., Britton, J. C., Fox, N. A., Leibenluft, E., et al. (2010). Attention bias modification treatment: A meta-analysis toward the establishment of novel treatment for anxiety. *Biological Psychiatry, 68,* 982–990.

Hammond, J., & Brooks, J. (2001). The World Trade Center attack. Helping the helpers: The role of critical incident stress management. *Critical Care, 5,* 315–317.

Institute of Medicine. (2007). *PTSD compensation and military service.* Washington, DC: National Academies Press.

Janoff-Bulman, R. (1985). The aftermath of victimization: Rebuilding shattered assumptions. In C. R. Figley (Ed.), *Trauma and its wake: Vol. 1. The study and treatment of post-traumatic stress disorder.* New York: Brunner/Mazel.

Kebeck, G., & Lohaus, A. (1986). Effect of emotional arousal on free recall of complex material. *Perceptual and Motor Skills, 63*(2, Pt.1), 461–462.

Kindt, M., & Soeter, M. (2011). Reconsolidation in a human fear conditioning study: A test of extinction as updating mechanism. *Biological Psychology, 92*(1), 43–50.

Koriat, A. (2000). The feeling of knowing: Some metatheoretical implications for consciousness and control. *Consciousness and Cognition, 9*(2), 149–171.

Kroll, N. E. (1972). The von Restorff effect as a function of method of isolation. *Psychonomic Science, 26,* 333–334.

Lang, A. J., Craske, M. G., & Bjork, R. A. (1999). Implications of a new theory of disuse for the treatment of emotional disorders. *Clinical Psychology: Science and Practice, 6*(1), 80–94.

Litz, B. T., Gray, M. J., Bryant, R. A., & Adler, A. B. (2002). Early intervention for trauma: Current status and future directions. *Clinical Psychology: Science and Practice, 9,* 112–134.

Loftus, E. F. (1979). Reactions to blatantly contradictory information. *Memory and Cognition, 7*(5), 368–374.

Loftus, E. F. (1993). The reality of repressed memories. *American Psychologist, 48*(5), 518–537.

Loftus, E. I. (1997). Memories for a past that never was. *Current Directions in Psychological Science, 6,* 60–65.

Lynn, S. J., Knox, J. A., Fassler, O., Lilienfeld, S. O., & Loftus, E. F. (2004). Memory, trauma, and dissociation. In G. M. Rosen & S. J. Lynn (Eds.), *Post traumatic stress disorder: Issues and controversies* (pp. 163–186). West Sussex, UK: Wiley.

Mackintosh, B., Mathews, A., Yiend, J., Ridgeway, V., & Cook, E. (2006). Induced biases in emotional interpretation influence stress vulnerability and endure despite changes in context. *Behavior Therapy, 37*(3), 209–222.

Mathews, A., & Mackintosh, B. (2000). Induced emotional interpretation bias and anxiety. *Journal of Abnormal Psychology, 109*(4), 602–615.

Mayou, R. A., Ehlers, A., & Hobbs, M. (2000). Psychological debriefing for road traffic accident victims. *British Journal of Psychiatry, 176*(6), 589–593.

McCann, I. L., & Pearlman, L. A. (1990). *Psychological trauma and the adult survivor: Theory, therapy, and transformation.* New York: Brunner/Mazel.

McGaugh, J. L. (2000). Memory—a century of consolidation. *Science, 287,* 248–251.

McNally, R. J. (2003). Progress and controversy in the study of posttraumatic stress disorder. *Annual Review of Psychology, 54,* 229–252.

McNally, R. J. (2003). *Remembering trauma.* Cambridge, MA: Belknap Press of Harvard.

McNally, R. J. (2004). Conceptual problems with the DSM-IV criteria for posttraumatic stress disorder. *International Journal on the Biology of Stress, 63*(10), 1–14.

McNally, R. J., Bryant, R. A., & Ehlers, A. (2003). Does early psychological intervention promote recovery from posttraumatic stress? *Psychological Science in the Public Interest, 4*(2), 45–79.

McNally, R. J., & Shin, L. M. (1994). Association of intelligence with severity of posttraumatic stress disorder symptoms in Vietnam combat veterans. *American Journal of Psychiatry, 152,* 936–938.

Mechanic, M. B., & Resick, P. A. (1993, October). *The Personal Beliefs and Reactions Scale: Assessing rape-related cognitive schemata.* Paper presented at the annual meeting of the International Society for Traumatic Stress Studies, San Antonio, TX.

Mobini, S., & Grant, A. (2007). Clinical implications of attentional bias in anxiety disorders: An integrative literature review. *Psychotherapy: Theory, Research, Practice, Training, 44*(4), 450–462.

Moscovitch, M., & Craik, F. I. M. (1976). Depth of processing, retrieval cues, and uniqueness of encoding as factors in recall. *Journal of Verbal Learning and Verbal Behavior, 15*(4), 447–458.

Nelson, C. A. (1995). The ontogeny of human memory: A cognitive neuroscience perspective. *Developmental Psychology, 31,* 723–738.

Norman, K. A., Newman, E. L., & Detre, G. (2007). A neural network model of retrieval-induced forgetting. *Psychological Review, 114*(4), 887–953.

Ozer, E. J., Best, S. R., Lipsey, T. L., & Weiss, D. S. (2003). Predictors of posttraumatic stress disorder and symptoms in adults: A meta-analysis. *Psychological Bulletin, 129*(1), 52–73.

Pace-Schott, E. F., Milad, M. R., Orr, S. P., Rauch, S. L., Stickgold, R., & Pitman, R. K. (2009). Sleep promotes generalization of extinction of conditioned fear. *Sleep, 32*(1), 19–26.

Pace-Schott, E. F., Shepherd, E., Spencer, R. M., Marcello, M., Tucker, M., Propper, R. E., et al. (2011). Napping promotes inter-session habituation to emotional stimuli. *Neurobiology of Learning and Memory, 95*(1), 24–36.

Peterson, C., & Bell, M. (1996). Children's memory for traumatic injury. *Child Development, 67*(6), 3045–3070.

Peterson, C., Sales, J. M., Rees, M., & Fivush, R. (2007). Parent–child talk and children's memory for stressful events. *Applied Cognitive Psychology, 21*(8), 1057–1075.

Peterson, C., & Whalen, N. (2001). Five years later: Children's memory for medical emergencies. *Applied Cognitive Psychology, 15*(7), S7–S24.

Peterson, M. A. (1999). What's in a stage name? *Journal of Experimental Psychology: Human Perception and Performance,25,* 276–286.

Philippot, P., Schaefer, A., & Herbette, G. (2003). Consequences of specific processing of emotional information: Impact of general versus specific autobiographical memory priming on emotion elicitation. *Emotion, 3*(3), 270–283.

Pitman, R. K. (1988). Post-traumatic stress disorder, conditioning, and network theory. *Psychiatric Annals, 18*(3), 182–189.

Pitman, R. K., & Delahanty, D. L. (2005). Conceptually driven pharmacological approaches to acute trauma. *CNS Spectrums, 10*(2), 99–106.

Pitts, M. W., & Takahashi, L. K. (2011). The central amygdala nucleus via corticotropin-releasing factor is necessary for time-limited consolidation processing but not storage of contextual fear memory. *Neurobiology of Learning and Memory, 95*(1), 86–91.

Resick, P. A., & Schnicke, M. K. (1992). Cognitive processing therapy for sexual assault victims. *Journal of Consulting and Clinical Psychology, 60,* 748–756.

Roediger, H. L., & Karpicke, J. D. (2006). Test-enhanced learning. *Psychological Science, 17*(3), 249–255.

Roediger, H. L., & McDermott, K. B. (1999). False alarms and false memories. *Psychological Review, 106,* 406–410.

Rose, S., Bisson, J., Churchill, R., & Wessely, S. (2009). Psychological debriefing for preventing post traumatic stress disorder (PTSD). *Cochrane Database of Systematic Reviews,* Issue 2 (Article No. CD000560), DOI: 10.1002/14651858. CD000560.

Rothbaum, B. O., Foa, E. B., Riggs, D. S., Murdock, T., & Walsh, W. (1992). A prospective examination of post-traumatic stress disorder in rape victims. *Journal of Traumatic Stress, 5*(3), 455–475.

Rubin, D. C. (2000). The distribution of early childhood memories. *Memory, 8*(5), 265–269.

Schacter, D. L., Norman, K. A., & Koutsaal, W. (1997). The recovered memory debate: A cognitive neuroscience perspective. In M. A. Conway (Ed.), *Recovered memories and false memories* (pp. 63–99). Oxford, UK: Oxford University Press.

Schiller, D., Monfils, M., Raio, C. M., Johnson, D., LeDoux, J. E., & Phelps, E. A. (2010). Blocking the return of fear in humans using reconsolidation update mechanisms. *Nature, 463,* 49–53.

Shalev, R. Y., Sahar, T., Freedman, S., Peri, T., Glick, N., Brandes, D., et al. (1998). A prospective study of heart rate response following trauma and subsequent development of posttraumatic stress disorder. *Archives of General Psychiatry, 55,* 553–559.

Shilony, E., & Grossman, F. K. (1993). Depersonalization as a defense mechanism in survivors of trauma. *Journal of Traumatic Stress, 6,* 119–128.

Shobe, K. K., & Kihlstrom, J. F. (1997). Is traumatic memory special? *Current Directions in Psychological Science, 6*(3), 70–74.

Spoormaker, V. I., Schröter, M. S., Gleiser, P. M., Andrade, K. C., Dresler, M., Wehrle, R., et al. (2010). Development of a large-scale functional brain network during human non-rapid eye movement sleep. *Journal of Neuroscience, 30*(34), 11379–11387.

Squire, L. R., & Alvarez, P. (1995). Retrograde amnesia and memory consolidation: A neurobiological perspective. *Current Opinion in Neurobiology, 5,* 169–177.

Terr, L. (1994). *Unchained memories.* New York: Basic Books.

Titus, T. G., & Robinson, J. A. (1973). Pseudo-primacy effects in free recall. *Perceptual and Motor Skills, 37,* 891–899.

Tulving, E. (1962). The effect of alphabetical subjective organization on memorizing unrelated words. *Canadian Journal of Psychology/Revue Canadienne de Psychologie, 16*(3), 185–191.

Tulving, E. (1968). When is recall higher than recognition? *Psychonomic Science, 10,* 53–54.

Tulving, E. (1983). *Elements of episodic memory* (Vol. 2). Oxford, UK: Clarendon Press.

Tulving, E., & Pearlstone, Z. (1966). Availability versus accessibility of information in memory for words. *Journal of Verbal Learning and Verbal Behavior, 5*(4), 381–391.

van der Kolk, B. A. (1996). The complexity of adaptation to trauma: Self-regulation, stimulus discrimination, and characterological development. In B. A. van der Kolk, A. C. McFarlane, & L. Weisaeth (Eds.), *Traumatic stress: The effects of overwhelming experience on mind, body, and society* (pp. 182–213). New York: Guilford Press.

van der Kolk, B. A., Burbridge, J. A., & Suzuki, J. (1997). The psychobiology of traumatic memory: Clinical implications of neuroimaging studies. *Annals of the New York Academy of Sciences, 821,* 99–113.

van der Kolk, B. A., & Fisler, R. (1994). Childhood abuse and neglect and loss of self-regulation. *Bulletin of Menninger Clinic, 58,* 145–168.

van der Kolk, B. A., & Kadish, W. (1987). Amnesia, dissociation, and the return of the repressed. In B. A. van der Kolk (Ed.), *Psychological trauma* (pp. 173–190). Washington, DC: American Psychiatric Press.

Vasterling, J. J., Duke, L. M., Brailey, K., Constans, J. I., Allain, A. N., & Sutker, P. B. (2002). Attention, learning, and memory performances and intellectual resources in Vietnam veterans: PTSD and no disorder comparisons. *Neuropsychology, 16*(1), 5–14.

Villarreal, G., Hamilton, D. A., Petropoulos, H., Driscoll, I., Rowland, L. M., Griego, J. A., et al. (2002). Reduced hippocampal volume and total white matter volume in posttraumatic stress disorder. *Biological Psychiatry, 52*(2), 119–125.

Watkins, E., & Teasdale, J. D. (2001). Rumination and overgeneral memory in depression: Effects of self-focus and analytic thinking. *Journal of Abnormal Psychology, 110*(2), 353–357.

Watkins, E., & Teasdale, J. D. (2004). Adaptive and maladaptive self-focus in depression. *Journal of Affective Disorders, 82*(1), 1–8.

Weaver, T. L., & Clum, G. A. (1995). Psychological distress associated with interpersonal violence: A meta-analysis. *Clinical Psychology Review, 15*(2), 115–140.

West T. A., & Bauer P. J. (1999). Assumptions of infantile amnesia: Are there differences between early and later memories? *Memory, 7*(3), 257–278.

White, L. K., Suway, J. G., Bar-Haim, Y., Pine, D., & Fox, N. A. (2011). Cascading effects: The influence of attention bias to threat on the interpretation of ambiguous information. *Behavior Research and Therapy, 49*(4), 244–251.

Williams, J. M. G., Ellis, N. C., Tyers, C., Healy, H., Rose, G., & Macleod, A. K. (1996). The specificity of autobiographical memory and imageability of the future. *Memory and Cognition, 24*(1), 116–125.

Zoellner, L. A., & Bittinger, J. (2004). On the uniqueness of trauma memories in PTSD. In G. Rosen (Ed.), *Posttraumatic stress disorder: Issues and controversies* (pp. 147–162). New York: Wiley.

Zoellner, L. A., Foa, E. B., Brigidi, B. D., & Przeworski, A. (2000). Are trauma victims susceptible to "false memories"? *Journal of Abnormal Psychology, 109*, 517–524.

Chapter 8

Understanding Posttrauma Cognitions and Beliefs

J. Gayle Beck, Jason Jacobs-Lentz, Judiann McNiff Jones,
Shira A. Olsen, *and* Joshua D. Clapp

Ashley is a 23-year-old African American woman. When she was in her junior year of college, Ashley began dating Rodney, a handsome and charming man who was employed in the school's information technologies (IT) department. Rodney was kind and generous to Ashley when they first met, frequently walking her from one class to the other and making sure that she got to her car safely when she was on campus at night. As the relationship proceeded, Rodney became controlling, needing to know where Ashley was at all times, accusing her of infidelity, and wanting to limit her time with friends and family. Just as Ashley was considering breaking up with Rodney, she learned that she was pregnant. Raised with traditional values, Ashley felt that it was her duty to marry Rodney to provide a stable home for the baby. Within the first year of marriage, Rodney became verbally abusive, telling Ashley that she was fat and stupid and that no one else could love her. By the baby's first birthday, Rodney's abuse had spiraled into hitting, kicking, and threatening Ashley with a gun. At this point, Ashley packed herself and the baby and fled to her mother's home, three states away.

When Ashley sought mental health assistance, her primary complaint was posttraumatic stress disorder (PTSD) symptoms, including intrusive thoughts about the abuse, flashbacks, avoidance of abuse-related cues, emotional numbing, difficulty concentrating, and a heightened startle response. In describing the intimate partner violence (IPV) that she had endured, her description was peppered with statements such as "I should have known better than to take up with him" and "Maybe the abuse occurred because of the way I acted." Moreover, Ashley noted "Men are not what they seem. I don't think I will ever trust again." Ashley understood that the PTSD symptoms were a result of IPV exposure but felt that they signified weakness and indicated that her life was destroyed.[1]

Ashley's case exemplifies many of the cognitions and beliefs that characterize PTSD following the experience of a trauma. Trauma can change people in many ways, including an impact on thoughts and beliefs that pervade the survivor's consciousness. In this chapter, we begin with a brief review of current theoretical models of trauma and PTSD, with an eye toward examining how specific types of cognitions and beliefs may be associated with posttrauma recovery and its converse, the development of PTSD. Recognizing the key role that thoughts and beliefs play in the aftermath of a trauma, this chapter discusses different forms of cognitions about the self and the world, with particular attention to how these thoughts influence emotion and behavior. Importantly, cognitions can be targeted with our current psychosocial treatments, as is discussed. As we illustrate in this chapter, the field has made considerable progress in understanding the significant role that cognitions and beliefs play in the aftermath of trauma and progress in this domain has been facilitated by well-crafted theories. As noted in the next section, these theories arrive at a surprising degree of consensus regarding posttrauma thoughts and beliefs.

THEORETICAL PERSPECTIVES
ON TRAUMA-RELATED COGNITIONS AND BELIEFS

Even before the introduction of PTSD into the third edition of the *Diagnostic and Statistical Manual of Mental Disorders* (DSM-III; American Psychiatric Association, 1980), negative thoughts and beliefs had been discussed in theoretical models of trauma response. As noted in this section, the negative cognitions and beliefs associated with trauma center around a handful of themes, representing an element of commonality across theories. In

---

[1]This case represents a mixture of various clients whom we have seen in our clinical work with women who have experienced intimate partner violence. Any resemblance to a specific individual is purely coincidental.

this section, a collection of influential trauma models are briefly reviewed, highlighting shared cognitive processes in these accounts.

Schema-Based Theories

Early stress response models focused primarily on changes in schematic knowledge or belief structures. Within this literature, schemas pertain to cognitive structures whose purpose is to organize knowledge and beliefs regarding some aspect of the self or the world. Information consistent with preexisting schemas is easily incorporated; processing of information that is incongruent with part of existing schemas is believed to be more effortful.

Horowitz's (1986) stress–response model is a prototype for schema models of trauma. He proposed that exposure to stressful events is marked by an initial emotional response, followed by a period of active processing in which the individual attempts to resolve discrepancies between the trauma experience and preexisting beliefs. Horowitz proposes that active processing of traumatic events is marked by alternating phases of intrusion and denial. Intrusions are characterized by unproductive rumination about the event and generalization of the consequences of the experience to more broad life domains. Ashley's perception that her PTSD symptoms signaled weakness is an example of this generalization. In response to intrusive symptoms, the stress–response model proposes a corresponding denial phase, characterized by emotional numbing, withdrawal, and behavioral constriction. Horowitz's stress–response model predicts that alternating intrusion and denial phases will continue until the realities of the trauma experience and schematic structures are congruent. Resolution of these discrepancies is believed to be gradual, as it requires incorporation of new information with preexisting beliefs and thoughts. Individuals with particularly rigid pretrauma beliefs are postulated to need more time for this incorporation process. Horowitz acknowledges that traumatic experiences may not necessarily be incongruent with preexisting schemas for some people. In particular, individuals may report preexisting negative thoughts that map onto those that typically follow a traumatic experience; in this instance, Horowitz suggests that these preexisting thoughts serve as a resiliency factor. More often, however, negative preexisting schemas are expected to impede adaptive completion and set the stage for the development of PTSD.

Other schema-based models have expanded stress–response theory by specifying specific belief structures impacted by trauma and elaborating on processes involved in the reconciliation of traumatic experiences and these preexisting beliefs (Epstein, 1991; Janoff-Bulman, 1992; McCann & Pearlman, 1990). One of the more influential authors in this literature, Janoff-Bulman (1992) proposes that trauma violates fundamental beliefs about the benevolence and justness of the world, the meaningfulness of life, and the worthiness of one's self. An example of this might include a rape victim who states, "I thought that my college campus was safe" or a victim of a traumatic crime who asks, "Why me? What have I done to deserve this?" Survivors are forced to assimilate trauma-related information with previously held just-world beliefs and may arrive at a dysfunctional conclusion such as "I was to blame for this event." Ashley's sense that she was somehow responsible for Rodney's abuse exemplifies this type of conclusion. Alternatively, the previously held schema can be modified to incorporate new experiences in a more adaptive fashion (e.g., "Sometimes bad things happen to good people"). McCann and Pearlman (1990) elaborated on this theory by extending the scope of themes that are affected by a trauma to include disruptions in beliefs about trust, power, safety, esteem, and intimacy. Elaborating on outcomes specified by these other schema models, Resick and Schnicke (1992) postulate that some individuals may experience overaccommodation following trauma exposure. Overaccommodation is unique to trauma survivors in that it involves a radical change in belief structures. In particular, beliefs stemming from the trauma are generalized from specific events (e.g., "Rodney can't be trusted") to broad situations (e.g., "Nobody can be trusted").

Emotional Processing Theory

Emotional processing theory (Foa, Steketee, & Rothbaum, 1989) attributes posttrauma symptoms to pervasive fear structures that develop following trauma. For PTSD, this network is composed of information about the feared stimuli; information about the verbal, physiological, and behavioral responses to these stimuli; and interpretive information regarding the meaning of these stimuli and responses. The magnitude of trauma exposure is related to the intensity of responding and the accessibility of this fear structure. Meaning elements within the fear structure may pertain to beliefs involving the probability of future danger ("It could happen again") and negative expectations regarding the consequences of encountering the feared stimuli ("Returning to the location will be awful" or "My anxiety will become overwhelming").

Consistent with schema-based theories, Foa and colleagues (Foa & Riggs, 1993; Foa & Rothbaum, 1998) propose that violations of basic assumptions of safety contribute to the pervasiveness of the fear structure. Schematic representations of the self as entirely incompetent and the world as completely dangerous are proposed to maintain associations within the fear network and perpetuate PTSD symptomatology. For example, Ashley felt that men in general were untrustworthy and she must protect herself against ever being hurt again by an intimate partner. Like Horowitz's model, emotional processing theory suggests that individuals with more rigid pretrauma beliefs (e.g., "Bad things only happen to bad people") may be at increased risk for developing PTSD when these beliefs are violated. Additionally, interpretation of posttrauma symptoms as evidence of weakness may contribute to or reinforce representations of the self as incompetent. Perceptions of others as blaming or unhelpful also are proposed to contribute to global beliefs of the world as dangerous and hostile within emotional processing theory.

Dual Representation Theory

Using cognitive and neuroscience models, Brewin, Dalgleish, and Joseph (1996) proposed the dual representation theory (DRT), which postulates that memories of the traumatic event are represented in two neurocognitive systems. The first representation involves the conscious experience of the trauma (termed *verbally accessible memory* [VAM]), which contains autobiographical information about sensory features of the situation, the individual's emotional and physiological reactions, and his or her interpretations of the event. Information contained within the VAM is readily accessible and can be deliberately accessed and edited. The situationally accessible memory (SAM) system, by contrast, contains information restricted to sensory, physiological, and motor aspects of the trauma, which are triggered automatically when an individual encounters a situation with sensory elements consistent with the traumatic event.

Much like schema-based theories, DRT proposes that trauma violates basic assumptions resulting in perceptions of the world as uncontrollable and unpredictable. Memories of the event as well as attributions regarding the cause and meaning of the traumatic experience are represented within the VAM. By contrast, conditioned emotional reactions and associated stimulus–response elements proposed by emotional processing theory are believed to be represented in the SAM. DRT proposes that successful resolution of trauma exposure requires modification of elements contained in both the VAM and the SAM. Much like other theories, DRT postulates that this cognitive processing can be prolonged for some people, particularly in cases where there is a large discrepancy between preexisting beliefs and the trauma experience. DRT also proposes that avoidance, a hallmark symptom of PTSD, can result in premature inhibition of processing. This theory postulates that premature inhibition is characterized by impaired memory for the trauma, anxious avoidance of trauma cues, and somatization.

Cognitive Theory

Within cognitive theory, negative cognitions play a central role in the development and maintenance of posttrauma symptomatology. For example,

Ehlers and Clark (2000) speculate that individuals who develop PTSD experience a pervasive sense of current threat relative to those who experience a successful resolution of trauma. Similar to previous models, the locus of threat can be external (e.g., "The world is full of dangerous people") or internal (e.g., "I am not good at taking care of myself"). Negative appraisals of the traumatic event and its aftermath are one mechanism proposed to contribute to ongoing perceptions of threat.

Specific cognitive appraisals occurring throughout the course of the traumatic experience and recovery are specified as potential contributors to PTSD symptoms. Negative appraisals of the traumatic event may be overgeneralized, contributing to inflated perceptions of danger across a range of life domains, as previously exemplified by Ashley's perceptions of men. Similar to previous work by Foa and colleagues (1989), negative appraisals also are believed to reinforce beliefs that the world is a dangerous place, that the probability of future victimization is high, and that the individual is incapable of handling the implications of the event. Ehlers and Clark (2000) also emphasize that negative appraisals regarding how one felt or responded during the event may result in generalized negative beliefs about the self (e.g., "I didn't try to escape, which means I wanted it to happen").

Like other models reviewed in this section, cognitive models posit that negative appraisals of the consequences of trauma may contribute to the maintenance of psychopathology. Normative reactions to trauma (e.g., nightmares, intrusive memories, exaggerated startle) may be interpreted as evidence that one is going crazy or permanently damaged, perpetuating symptomatology by producing negative emotions and promoting dysfunctional coping strategies. Additionally, appraisals of others as unresponsive or rejecting reinforce beliefs of the world as hostile. Withdrawal from support networks as a consequence of these appraisals may prevent the individual from utilizing others to assist in processing of the event. Finally, appraisal of functional consequences of the trauma (e.g., changes in health, finances, employment) as evidence of permanent change or ruin, contributes directly to distress and pathology. Ashley's belief that her life had been destroyed by the IPV is an example of this type of thinking.

Ehlers and Clark (2000) also postulate that specific appraisals are associated with specific emotion states: perceptions of danger contribute to fear, perceptions of responsibility contribute to guilt, and perceptions of loss contribute to sadness. The negative emotions that these appraisals produce perpetuate additional negative appraisals by biasing memory and interpretation of events. In this way, maladaptive beliefs and emotions form a self-sustaining, feed-forward cycle that perpetuates perceptions of threat, negative emotion, and PTSD symptomatology.

Ehlers and Clark's (2000) model also introduces a novel construct hypothesized to contribute to negative beliefs. "Mental defeat" refers to the perceived loss of autonomy and control during the traumatic experience and has been associated with chronic PTSD and poor treatment response. Ehlers and Clark propose that individuals who experience mental defeat are more likely to experience negative beliefs about the self and to view themselves as permanently damaged, as exemplified by the case of Ashley.

Summary

As noted in this brief review, although each type of theory highlights distinct psychological processes in its account of the etiology and maintenance of PTSD, there are commonalities across these accounts. In particular, theoretical models of PTSD identify the following thoughts and beliefs as relevant:

1. Negative thoughts about the self, which can include perceptions of incompetence or self-blame.
2. Negative thoughts about the world, which can include perceptions that danger lurks everywhere and that situations previously believed to be benign are unjust and threatening.
3. Negative beliefs about the meaning of posttrauma symptoms, including perceptions that one has "gone crazy" or been permanently changed.
4. Perceptions of loss of control and autonomy during the trauma can set the stage for more generalized perceptions of helplessness.

As is reviewed in the next section, these thoughts can take a variety of forms, which has important implications for understanding and treating individuals with PTSD.

UNDERSTANDING THE NATURE OF NEGATIVE THOUGHTS AND BELIEFS

Although general categories of negative thoughts and beliefs have been highlighted by various theories of PTSD, it is notable that these have been specified further as the field has developed. In this section, we examine the specific nature of negative thoughts and beliefs, anchored by specific assessment devices. Discussion of instruments for the measurement of dysfunctional cognitions and beliefs is intended to facilitate empirically supported clinical practice. We also examine the links between negative thoughts, negative emotions, and behaviors, as illustrated by the case of Ashley.

When working with a trauma survivor, it is important to get a detailed sense of his or her negative thoughts about him- or herself. This information can help you as a therapist to understand the daily presence of trauma symptoms in your patient's life, as well as individualize intervention. As well, some forms of cognitive therapy, such as cognitive processing therapy (e.g., Resick & Schnicke, 1992) require a careful understanding of the patient's dysfunctional cognitions, so a thorough pretreatment assessment is necessary. However, it is important to recognize that trauma survivors typically may be hesitant to articulate these thoughts. In Ashley's case, she was reluctant to acknowledge that she felt weak and useless, particularly as this message echoed Rodney's verbal abuse. Somehow, by articulating these negative thoughts, Ashley felt that it meant that Rodney's assessment of her was true. The use of self-report scales can ease the discomfort that some trauma patients experience when asked directly about their negative thoughts about themselves.

Negative Thoughts about the Self: Incompetence and Lack of Control

Negative cognitions about one's incompetency and lack of self-control have played a salient role in examination of posttrauma functioning. Items reflecting negative thoughts about the self have been included in several self-report scales, including the Posttraumatic Cognitions Inventory (PTCI; Foa, Ehlers, Clark, Tolin, & Orsillo, 1999) and the World Assumption Scale (WAS; Janoff-Bulman, 1996). Items on the PTCI that assess negative thoughts about the self include "I am a weak person" and "If I think about the trauma, I will not be able to handle it." These thoughts are correlated with PTSD, anxiety, and depression, suggesting that this particular type of negative cognition is associated with a range of negative emotions (Beck et al., 2004). The WAS also assesses negative thoughts about the self, focusing on low self-worth, including items such as "I have a low opinion of myself" and "I have reason to be ashamed of my personal character" (Janoff-Bulman, 1996). Although not utilized as heavily in research, the content of these items seem to overlap with measures of low self-esteem and may be particularly useful to include during therapy with trauma patients who are struggling with generalized perceptions of incompetence.

A related aspect of negative cognitions involves mental defeat, which Ehlers and Clark (2000) suggest is a significant predictor of poor posttrauma functioning. Assessment efforts in this domain are not quite as developed, although this research team has developed a 29-item questionnaire that captures mental defeat (e.g., Dunmore, Clark, & Ehlers, 2001) and includes items such as "I mentally gave up." Clinically, this arena seems more difficult to assess than specific cognitive content (e.g., specific negative thoughts about one's incompetence), particularly in patients who lack insight or psychological sophistication. Given the potentially salient role of mental defeat (see section titled "Links with PTSD"), it would be helpful to have clinically informed assessment instruments of this cognitive process.

When considering thoughts of incompetence and lack of control, it is notable that in our clinical experience these thoughts can contribute in other ways to the radiating impact of trauma, as the survivor may not feel capable of accomplishing the many tasks involved in recovering from a traumatic experience. In Ashley's case, these tasks included locating adequate housing, securing a restraining order against Rodney, deciding whether to begin divorce proceedings, negotiating child custody, gaining employment, and reestablishing herself socially within her new environment. Thoughts about incompetence and lack of control were a clear impediment to Ashley when she considered these tasks. Therapeutically, these thoughts stood in the way of formulating concrete plans for each task, as well as implementing these plans. Irrespective of the intervention selected to use with a given patient, addressing the motivational consequences of a steady stream of negative thoughts of incompetence and lack of control is a primary clinical task.

Negative Thoughts about the Self: Self-Blame

Negative thoughts about the self can extend to perceptions of responsibility and self-blame. Importantly, this cognitive content is assessed by many scales in this domain. The PTCI, for example, has a self-blame scale, which includes items such as "The event happened because of the way I acted." A related scale that assesses self-blame is the Personal Beliefs and Reactions Scale (PBRS; Resick, Schnicke, & Markway, 1991), which was developed to examine distorted perceptions of responsibility among women who have experienced sexual assault. The PBRS correlates significantly and in the anticipated direction with coping measures (e.g., Mechanic & Resick, 1993). As expected, the self-blame subscale of the PBRS correlates significantly with PTSD severity (e.g., Owens & Chard, 2001) and the scale is able to differentiate women with PTSD from those without it (Mechanic & Resick, 1993).

Working definitions of self-blame are conceptually somewhat murky in the larger domain of psychological assessment (e.g., Tangney & Dearing, 2002). Within the trauma arena, however, self-blame and guilt have been conceptualized as sharing overlapping features, as discussed cogently by Kubany and colleagues (1996). For example, the Trauma-Related Guilt Inventory (TRGI; Kubany et al., 1996) includes a guilt cognitions subscale. This assesses hindsight bias (the belief that one should have known what would happen, as exemplified by Ashley's belief that "I should have known better than to take up with him"), wrongdoing (a violation of personal standards), and lack of justification for actions taken or not taken. Within Kubany and colleagues' conceptualization, guilt is clearly associated with perceptions of responsibility and self-blame, as indexed by items such as "I was responsible for causing what happened." Clinically, these cognitions often echo a distorted sense of responsibility. For example, Ashley felt that by not separating from Rodney when he first became controlling and domineering, she was responsible for the abuse. While this belief is not rational, it clearly illustrates self-blame within an individual with PTSD.

Distorted perceptions of responsibility could seemingly drive different emotions and behaviors, relative to other types of negative cognitions and beliefs. In addition to feelings of guilt, one could speculate that self-blame would be associated with depression, reduced self-esteem, social anxiety, and perhaps feelings of shame. Data from Vietnam-era combat veterans and women who had experienced IPV supports these associations (Kubany et al., 1996). It is important to note that conceptualization and assessment of some of the "moral" emotions (shame, guilt, pride) has been critiqued for construct overlap (e.g., Rizvi, 2010). From a clinical perspective, it remains to be determined if these emotions show differential associations with specific dysfunctional cognitions in trauma survivors. Given work on other types of negative thoughts reviewed above, it seems wise to not expect a tight one-to-one correspondence between dysfunctional thoughts and specific emotions, contrary to predictions from cognitive theory.

In considering thoughts of self-blame, Ashley clearly believed that she was responsible for the abuse and violence she endured. In particular, she believed that the abuse happened because of something that she had done or said. Paradoxically, these cognitions may have influenced her perceptions of the nature and severity of the spousal abuse and kept her romantically involved with Rodney. As with thoughts about incompetence and lack of control, specific forms of cognitive therapy can be helpful in addressing this type of cognitive distortion.

Negative Thoughts about the World: Danger

As noted in the review of theoretical perspectives, posttrauma thoughts and beliefs can be focused externally and include perceptions and beliefs about the dangerousness of the world. These thoughts can be evaluated using the PTCI, which contains a subscale assessing negative thoughts about the world (e.g., "The world is a dangerous place" and "You can never know who will harm you"). These thoughts also have been shown to correlate with PTSD, anxiety, and depression (Beck et al., 2004), which suggests that they are not unique to any specific negative emotion. Clinically, it seems intuitive that a generalized sense of threat and danger could be associated with a number of negative emotions (e.g., fear, anger, depression) and negative coping behaviors (e.g., social withdrawal, insistence on carrying a weapon when one leaves home). Ashley carried negative beliefs about the dangerousness of the world, particularly focused on men. She believed that all men were inherently untrustworthy and capable of violence. These beliefs had generalized to some extent and extended to most strangers (irrespective of sex). Guided by these beliefs, Ashley avoided contact with people she did not know. Our clinical conceptualization of this case suggested that negative beliefs about danger and threat motivated Ashley's avoidance behavior, which then functioned as a maintaining factor for PTSD symptomatology.

Another facet of negative thoughts about dangerousness can be found on the WAS. One dimension of this scale focuses on the benevolence of the world and contains items such as "People are basically kind and helpful." Within the WAS, endorsement of beliefs about benevolence of the world is negatively associated with endorsement of beliefs about poor self-control in the prevention of bad events. This suggests an important link between negative thoughts about the world and negative thoughts about the self, as those individuals who acknowledge that the world is potentially harmful are more likely to also acknowledge that they have little or no control over whether harmful things happen. Our clinical experience suggests that when these two types of cognitive distortions occur together, patients with PTSD may be characterized by helplessness, another issue that would appear to be a primary clinical task.

Negative Thoughts about the World: An Unjust World

Following trauma exposure, negative thoughts about the world can extend beyond thoughts of threat and danger and include thoughts about unjustness. The WAS is the measure that most directly assesses perceptions of justness. Items in this domain include "Generally, people deserve what they get in this world" and "People will experience good fortune if they themselves are good." Some authors have discussed how expressions of hostility and antagonism may serve as basic survival skills for individuals who view the world as unjust (Chemtob, Novaco, Hamada, Gross, & Smith, 1997). In particular, when faced with a world that seems unfair and somewhat random, Chemtob and colleagues (1997) examined how hostility and anger are justified by individuals with PTSD as appropriate forms of self-protection. Clinically, it is notable that excessive irritability can be the most notable emotion expressed by an individual with PTSD; if this occurs, it would be worthwhile to explore the patient's perceptions of whether the world is just. Importantly, perceptions of unjustness do not always show significant associations with posttrauma symptomatology (e.g., Owens & Chard, 2001), suggesting that they may not be a unique signifier of the disorder.

In considering the clinical presentation of these types of negative thoughts, Ashley endorsed beliefs in a just world that had been violated by her experience with Rodney. She vacillated between feeling that she had experienced IPV because she was not a good person and feeling angry about what Rodney had done to her, stating "He was so unfair to me." From a clinical perspective, Ashley's feelings of being wronged by Rodney seemed to motivate adaptive coping. As an example, these thoughts appeared to help her take specific positive actions, such as obtaining a restraining order and deciding to file for divorce. In contrast, her thoughts about being a bad person were associated with depression, inactivity, and related negative thoughts about her own incompetence and responsibility for the abuse.

In sum, negative thoughts and beliefs can take many forms following the experience of trauma. As noted in this review, these thoughts and beliefs do not necessarily map onto specific negative emotions in a one-to-one fashion. Contrary to theoretical predictions, these cognitions seem to be associated with a variety of negative emotions (anxiety, depression, anger, shame, guilt). Importantly, dysfunctional cognitions seemingly can motivate both adaptive and maladaptive behaviors, such as behavioral activation or social withdrawal. As clinicians, we should seek to understand the functional relationship between thoughts, emotions, and behaviors. For example, Ashley felt like she had somehow caused the abuse. This belief was associated with feelings of both shame and guilt, which contributed to her social withdrawal. Related literature has documented that social withdrawal is associated with increased depressed mood, which further compounded Ashley's sense of responsibility for the abuse. Assessment of dysfunctional cognitions can be difficult, but fortunately the field has developed sound measures that allow us clinically to capture posttrauma cognitions and beliefs in a more systematic and standard fashion. In addition to their clinical assets, these measures have greatly facilitated research on risk and resiliency following trauma, as reviewed in the next section of this chapter.

HOW DO NEGATIVE BELIEFS AND COGNITIONS INFLUENCE RISK AND RESILIENCY AFTER TRAUMA?

Although negative beliefs and cognitions have been well documented among individuals with PTSD, we are beginning to understand more clearly how these thought processes influence risk and resiliency following trauma. This section examines the predictive power of negative cognitions in longitudinal studies and explores factors that influence this trajectory, with discussion of clinical implications for prevention and intervention. Because cognitions are modifiable, this domain represents a prime target for our efforts, in an effort to reduce risk or heighten resiliency in the immediate aftermath of trauma.

Links with PTSD

Recognition of the importance of negative thoughts has motivated a collection of prospective longitudinal studies. In these studies, survivors are assessed in the initial days or weeks following trauma and then reassessed 6–12 months later, to determine which variables predict the development of PTSD. As summarized by Ehlers and Clark (2006), negative beliefs about the self and the world shortly after the trauma have been shown to correlate significantly with PTSD severity often assessed 6–12 months later, such that higher levels of negative beliefs at time 1 are associated with higher levels of PTSD symptomatology at time 2. Importantly, these associations remain significant when controlling statistically for other risk factors (Dunmore et al., 2001). These studies strongly suggest that negative thoughts and beliefs play an important role in maintaining PTSD and exert their influence separately from other risk factors. As noted in Ashley's case, negative thoughts and beliefs do not fade in their influence over time and may seem clinically interwoven with PTSD symptoms.

Moreover, other aspects of negative cognitions have been examined within this literature. For example, negative interpretations of immediate posttrauma PTSD symptoms at time 1 (e.g., "These intrusions mean that I really am losing my mind") showed large and significant correlations with PTSD status at time 2 (Ehlers & Clark, 2006). As well, negative interpretations of others' responses after trauma and perceptions that one has been permanently changed by trauma have both been shown to be significantly associated with PTSD severity. These studies have involved adult survivors of assault and serious motor vehicle accidents (MVAs), demonstrating that these findings are not unique to any one type of extreme event. Ashley's negative cognitions illustrate the long-lasting nature of these thoughts, as she had been separated from Rodney for approximately 6 months at the time she sought help. Clinically, it is somewhat baffling to understand how a patient can maintain irrational beliefs (e.g., "Maybe the abuse occurred because of the way I acted") after he or she is removed from a traumatic relationship. The reader is reminded that trauma also shapes a person's attention and memory (e.g., Ehlers, Ehring, & Kleim, 2012), such that he or she may process information in a fashion that maintains negative thoughts and beliefs.

In considering risk and resiliency, risk factors for the development of PTSD appear to differ somewhat from risk factors for the maintenance of PTSD (Vogt, King, & King, 2007). This also holds true for cognitions and beliefs. Early efforts to differentiate etiological versus maintaining factors tended to compare variables that predict PTSD symptomatology in the immediate aftermath of the trauma with those that predict symptoms months later. For example, Dunmore and colleagues (2001) reported that specific cognitions during trauma exposure (e.g., "I am completely overwhelmed" [mental defeat]) appear to predict PTSD symptoms in the immediate aftermath of a trauma. In contrast, negative appraisals of initial symptoms and negative perceptions of others' reactions contributed to the maintenance of PTSD symptoms at 9 months in this sample of assault victims. This pattern is reflected in the case of Ashley, who continued to focus on distorted perceptions of responsibility and self-blame in the months after she fled from Rodney. This is an important finding, as it suggests that interventions that are designed to be used immediately after a trauma need to target mental defeat while treatments for individuals diagnosed with PTSD need to consider a broader spectrum of negative thoughts about the self and the world, in order to address cognitive factors that maintain the disorder.

Links with Anxiety and Quality of Life

The focus on negative beliefs and thoughts in the trauma literature has included study of their role in anxiety and reduced quality of life. For example, Grills-Taquechel, Littleton, and Axsom (2011) examined women who had been exposed to the Virginia Tech campus shootings. High self-worth beliefs measured pretrauma (using the WAS) served as a protective factor against anxiety and reductions in quality of life following the trauma. In contrast, pretrauma beliefs that one had no control over outcomes and that life events are random appeared to be risk factors in that high self-controllability scores (pretrauma) interacted with high levels of trauma exposure to predict anxiety. Likewise, strong beliefs in the randomness of events (pretrauma) interacted with high levels of trauma exposure to predict anxiety. Taken together, these data indicate that negative thoughts, especially thoughts about one's lack of control and the randomness of life, are risk factors for anxiety and reductions in life quality following trauma.

Links with Comorbidity

Because comorbid disorders are normative among individuals with PTSD (e.g., Brady, Killeen, Brewerton, & Lucerini, 2000), it is important to determine if negative beliefs and cognitions are specific to PTSD. Moreover, because the preceding section suggests that negative thoughts can influence the development of anxiety after trauma, it is important to examine how specific these thoughts are with respect to their emotional consequences. For example, dysfunctional cognitions could be reflective of general distress and predict many different psychiatric conditions (e.g., depression, PTSD). Ehring, Ehlers, and Glucksman (2008) examined this question in a study of MVA survivors, who were assessed in the emergency room following their accident, as well as four times in the 6 months afterward. These authors were interested in whether specific negative cognitions predicted PTSD, depression, and travel phobia, or instead whether negative cognitions were not disorder-specific. Analyses indicated that specific cognitive variables predicted the severity of subsequent PTSD, in particular negative thoughts about the self, rumination about the trauma, and efforts to suppress thoughts about the trauma. Specific cognitive variables also predicted depression, particularly self-devaluation and depressive ruminations. Cognitive variables were less unique in the prediction of travel phobia. It is important to note that most predictors were disorder-specific, as this suggests that specific kinds of negative thoughts and beliefs predict two different forms of psychopathology that are common in the aftermath of a trauma (PTSD and depression). Clearly, if we are to design early intervention programs to be delivered in the immediate aftermath of a trauma, it seems important to target the specific negative thoughts that set the stage for PTSD and depression.

Links with Coping Strategies

Although understanding the predictive role of negative beliefs and cognitions following trauma is important, it is equally important to consider how these processes effect coping strategies. Ehlers and Steil (1995) and Steil and Ehlers (2000) have hypothesized several propositions linking negative cognitions with dysfunctional coping strategies, each of which can heighten the risk for developing chronic PTSD. Ehlers and Steil proposed that negative idiosyncratic interpretations of intrusion symptoms maintained PTSD through two pathways. First, these dysfunctional interpretations are distressing and this contributes to heightened physiological arousal. Second, these interpretations motivate both cognitive and behavioral avoidance, which block efforts to emotionally process the traumatic event and prevent reduction in distress to trauma-related cues. Steil and Ehlers subsequently elaborated this model, highlighting how thought suppression, rumination, and distraction are likely to serve as cognitive avoidance strategies and act in concert with behavioral avoidance. In two cross-sectional studies with MVA survivors, these authors examined this model, particularly the dysfunctional meaning that participants ascribed to their intrusions, the amount of distress produced by the intrusions, the degree of avoidance to reminders of the accident that was reported, and how often rumination, thought suppression, and distraction were used to manage posttrauma intrusions. Consistent with prediction, if intrusions were interpreted to indicate mental illness, incompetence, a permanent negative personality change, or a sign of impending threat, greater distress was reported. These types of negative beliefs and thoughts were associated with dysfunctional coping strategies, in particular thought suppression, rumination, distraction, and behavioral avoidance of trauma cues. Ironically, at least one of these coping strategies (thought suppression) can increase the actual occurrence of intrusive thoughts (e.g., Shipherd & Beck, 1999). Not surprisingly, increased use of avoidance strategies was associated with increased PTSD severity. These studies document that negative thoughts act in concert with negative coping strategies in determining an individual's psychological state following trauma. Although intuitive, the functional link between negative thoughts and dysfunctional coping is important, particularly in considering interventions for trauma survivors.

Of equal importance are coping strategies that buffer an individual from symptomatology. Bennett, Beck, and Clapp (2009) explored a range of thought control strategies, including distraction, worry, self-punishment, social control (e.g., talking to a friend about one's intrusive thoughts), and reappraisal (e.g., reevaluating the meaning of the thought). This study examined whether thought control strategies intermediated the relationship between PTSD and dysfunctional cognitions in MVA survivors. Increased levels of PTSD were associated with greater use of worry and self-punishment as a means to control negative thoughts. In turn, higher levels of worry and self-punishment were associated with greater severity of dysfunctional thoughts. Distraction and social control emerged as positive cognitive coping strategies; higher levels of these thought control strategies were associated with lower levels of PTSD and lower levels of dysfunctional thoughts. Reappraisal failed to show a significant intermediary association between PTSD and dysfunctional cognitions. In considering these findings, it is notable that distraction has been reported by other authors to be a negative approach to coping (e.g., Steil & Ehlers, 2000). Collectively, these studies suggest that thought suppression, rumination, worry, avoidance, and self-punishment serve as dysfunctional methods for coping with negative thoughts. In contrast, positive social contact appears to serve as a positive method, much as discussed in Chapter 13 (this volume). As noted, many preventative interventions incorporate psychoeducation about the potential effects of these coping strategies, in an effort to reduce the likelihood of ongoing distress and the development of PTSD in the early days following a trauma. Clinicians working with individuals diagnosed with PTSD can assess the presence of negative thoughts and how individuals are currently coping with these cognitions. Prior to beginning exposure or other forms of therapy, it may be useful to ask the patient to seek greater social support and to try to cease active thought suppression, rumination, worry, and self-punishment.

Links with Interpersonal Functioning

In considering other possible influences to trauma outcomes, social support typically emerges as an important predictor (e.g., Brewin, Andrews, & Valentine, 2000; Ozer, Best, Lipsey, & Weiss, 2003). Ashley's case illustrates how the lack of social support can contribute to increased risk following trauma. Because Rodney isolated her from friends and family, Ashley was left without support from others. As noted in the previous section, positive social support appears to play an adaptive role in reducing negative thoughts about the self and the world. Likewise, negative support easily can be postulated to strengthen negative beliefs about oneself and the world. To date, one investigation has focused on the role of dysfunctional cognitions in understanding the association between functioning within one's romantic relationship and the maintenance of PTSD symptoms (Robinaugh et al., 2011). The sample included individuals who had experienced a serious MVA that involved physical injury. Dysfunctional cognitions (about the self, the world, and self-blame) significantly accounted for the association between perceived support from a romantic partner 4 weeks following the MVA and the persistence of PTSD symptoms 3 months later. Although actual observation of the partner's behavior was missing from this study, it is salient to note that negative thoughts appear to influence a person's perception of the extent and quality of support offered by their significant other.

Summary: Risk and Resilience

In general, the studies in this section illustrate the radiating impact that dysfunctional cognitions exert in the aftermath of trauma exposure. In particular, negative thoughts and beliefs are associated with the development of PTSD symptoms, anxiety, and comorbid disorders; reductions in perceived quality of life; and perceptions of one's romantic partner. Importantly, how people cope with negative thoughts and beliefs can alter the effect of these thoughts. Although we are not yet able to determine empirically if negative thoughts are cause or corollary to these outcomes, it is salient to note that negative thoughts represent a potential target for psychoeducation in the early days following a trauma, in an effort to target individuals who are at risk for negative mental health outcomes.

One might also ask how negative cognitions interact with other risk factors that have been empirically identified, particularly pretrauma variables (e.g., Brewin et al., 2000; Ozer et al., 2003). Although we, as a field, have considerable evidence to support the role of factors such as female gender, minority race, low socioeconomic status, and previous exposure to trauma or adversity as risk factors for the development of PTSD, we have yet to examine how these more static factors interact with negative thoughts to enhance risk for PTSD. One could speculate, for example, that exposure to previous traumatic events could prime the beliefs that "The world is a dangerous place" or "I am not able to take care of myself." Subsequent trauma conceivably could confirm and strengthen these beliefs. To date, these kinds of speculations have not been examined, although empirical work of this sort would be very useful in developing interventions for at-risk individuals. It is only when we have a deeper understanding of the operative processes behind pretrauma variables that prevention and early intervention efforts can advance efficiently (Kazdin & Blase, 2011). In this context, it would seem useful to consider outcomes other than PTSD, including posttraumatic growth (Calhoun & Tedeschi, 2006) and resilience (Bonanno, 2004).

IMPLICATIONS FOR CHANGE EFFORTS

Negative cognitions and beliefs have been clearly linked with poor mental health outcomes following a trauma, in particular PTSD. At present, research suggests that these thoughts can serve as a target for change efforts, in particular within prevention efforts for individuals who have been recently exposed to a trauma and within treatment for individuals with diagnosed PTSD. This section will briefly discuss the implications of our current knowledge about negative thoughts and beliefs for these change efforts.

Prevention and Early Intervention

As reviewed by Au, Silva, Delaney, and Litz (2012), a number of prevention and early intervention programs have been designed and evaluated, including various approaches to psychological debriefing (PD), psychological first aid, psychoeducation, and various applications of cognitive-behavioral therapy (CBT). Although a detailed review of these programs is beyond the scope of the current chapter, it is important to recognize that many of these programs, with the exception of some forms of PD, include provision of information on psychological and physiological stress reactions, healthy ways of coping, and maladaptive coping responses to avoid or monitor. Discussion of negative thoughts and beliefs are a core component of this information, which is particularly important in light of research concerning the saliency of mental defeat in the etiology of PTSD and the more pernicious role of negative thoughts about the self and the world in the maintenance of the disorder.

To date, one report has examined the role of negative cognitions in response to early intervention programs (Zoellner, Feeny, Eftekhari, & Foa, 2011). This study examined if negative thoughts responded to early intervention programs. Women who had recently experienced sexual assault were given 4 weeks of either brief CBT, supportive counseling, or assessment-only, with measurement of dysfunctional thoughts before and afterward (using the WAS and the PBRS). Negative beliefs about the self and the world improved across all interventions, with somewhat less positive change noted following supportive counseling. Because PTSD symptoms and negative posttrauma thoughts and beliefs show a natural recovery trajectory following a trauma for most individuals (e.g., Gilboa-Schechtman & Foa, 2001), it is important for future work to strive to develop early intervention programs that can change negative cognitions and PTSD symptoms above and beyond the passage of time. Additionally, future work is needed to explore if individual characteristics that appear to heighten the risk for PTSD (such as notable endorsement of mental defeat) might predict a particularly good response to early interventions following trauma.

Treatment

Considerably greater effort has been devoted to developing and testing treatments for individuals with PTSD. At present, there are several empirically supported treatments for PTSD, including cognitive processing therapy (CPT; Resick & Schnicke, 1992). CPT is postulated to work directly to correct distorted thinking by helping patients with PTSD learn to question the factual basis of their dysfunctional thoughts. Moreover, patients are taught to replace their faulty assumptions with more balanced statements that will be associated with healthier emotional responses. Owens, Pike, and Chard (2001) reported that improvements were noted on the PBRS and the WAS following CPT. Importantly, these cognitive changes were maintained at 1-year follow-up, suggesting that CPT produces lasting changes in how individuals with PTSD think about themselves and the world. Other forms of treatment, such as prolonged exposure therapy, have also been shown to produce reductions in dysfunctional guilt-related cognitions in patients with PTSD, although the reduction noted in this study was smaller than that noted in CPT (Resick et al., 2002). Interestingly, although the addition of cognitive restructuring did not enhance prolonged exposure, Foa and Rauch (2004) noted that reductions in negative thoughts as indexed by the PTCI were significantly associated with reductions in PTSD for both exposure-alone and exposure plus cognitive restructuring. Greater understanding of how various treatments for PTSD impact negative thoughts and beliefs would be useful for clinical practice, particularly for patients with high levels of dysfunctional thoughts.

SUMMARY AND CLINICAL RECOMMENDATIONS

Pulling this chapter together, it is fitting to spell out specific clinical recommendations, particularly given the role that negative thoughts play in posttrauma adaptation. As has been reviewed in this chapter, negative thoughts and beliefs can exert a powerful influence following a trauma. In particular, mental defeat, as well as negative thoughts about the self and the world, have been shown to be salient in the etiology and maintenance of PTSD. Research has shown that negative thoughts are associated with reduced quality of life and diagnostic comorbidity, and they also effect one's perception of one's romantic partner. Current efforts at prevention address negative thoughts via the provision of information, although it is unknown if this is effective at reducing dysfunctional cognitions and beliefs per se. Among the established treatments, CPT has been shown to reduce negative thoughts and these gains appear to last after treatment is over. Other treatments that do not explicitly target negative thoughts, such as exposure therapy, also produce reductions in negative thoughts, although these reductions may be smaller than those obtained with CPT.

From a clinical standpoint, some specific recommendations emerge from this literature:

1. When working with people shortly after a trauma, provide accurate information about anticipated trauma-related symptoms, including specific forms of negative thoughts that may become pervasive. Remembering that most people emerge from a trauma without PTSD, it is salient to help the survivor understand that negative thoughts and beliefs are a natural sequelae of the trauma experience and not reflective of "reality." This is particularly important when addressing perceptions of mental defeat in the early aftermath of a trauma.

2. Help the trauma survivor to anticipate negative thoughts about the self and the world. In our clinical experience, it is particularly important to be aware of distortions in perceptions of responsibility, generalization of negative beliefs stemming from the trauma, and perceptions of the self as incompetent, as these attributions may be particularly difficult for the trauma survivor to objectively assess.

3. The use of standardized measures can assist in assessing the patient with PTSD, especially given individual sensitivities in discussing negative thoughts. These measures can be helpful in assuring both thorough and objective appraisals of the nature and severity of these beliefs.

4. Strive to understand the functional connection between negative thoughts and specific coping strategies. Although the literature has focused on thought suppression, worry, rumination, avoidance, and seeking social support, there are a number of other strategies to consider (e.g., excessive alcohol use, excessive sleeping). Like Ashley, there may be times when negative thoughts serve to keep a trauma survivor exposed to negative events (in this case, abuse from Rodney). Because avoidance is a cardinal component of PTSD, be certain to assess efforts to cognitively avoid negative thoughts.

5. Encourage the patient with PTSD to learn to be their own scientist when addressing dysfunctional thoughts in therapy. Although CPT explicitly incorporates training patients in the observation of their own thoughts and behavior, this approach can be incorporated within most other approaches to the treatment of PTSD. Gaining

dispassionate awareness of dysfunctional thoughts can assist the patient with PTSD in learning to step away from these cognitions, which can increase motivation for treatment as well as help the patient be able to observe his or her own positive change.

In sum, the field has made considerable progress in understanding the salient role that negative thoughts play in poor mental health following a trauma. It would seem fitting that we begin to explore thoughts and beliefs that are associated with positive outcomes, particularly since these have not been examined empirically to the same extent. Negative thoughts can color posttrauma adaptation through influencing emotions and behaviors. As noted, we have learned a considerable amount about these cognitive processes. Additional work in this arena will certainly continue to enhance our prevention and treatment efforts for survivors of trauma.

ACKNOWLEDGMENTS

Support for this work is provided in part by the Lillian and Morrie Moss Chair of Excellence position (to J. Gayle Beck) and National Institute of Mental Health Award No. F31 MH083385 (to Joshua D. Clapp).

REFERENCES

American Psychiatric Association. (1980). *Diagnostic and statistical manual of mental disorders* (3rd ed.). Washington, DC: Author.

Au, T. M., Silva, C., Delaney, E. M., & Litz, B. T. (2012). Individual approaches to prevention and early intervention. In J. G. Beck & D. M. Sloan (Eds.), *Handbook of traumatic stress disorders* (pp. 363–380). New York: Oxford University Press.

Beck, J. G., Coffey, S. F., Palyo, S. A., Gudmundsdottir, B., Miller, L. M., & Colder, C. R. (2004). Psychometric properties of the Posttraumatic Cognitions Inventory (PTCI): A replication with motor vehicle accident survivors. *Psychological Assessment, 16,* 289–298.

Bennett, S. A., Beck, J. G., & Clapp, J. D. (2009). Understanding the relationship between posttraumatic stress disorder and trauma cognitions: The impact of thought control strategies. *Behaviour Research and Therapy, 47,* 1018–1023.

Bonanno, G. A. (2004). Loss, trauma, and human resilience: Have we underestimated the human capacity to thrive after extremely aversive events? *American Psychologist, 59,* 20–28.

Brady, K. T., Killeen, T. K., Brewerton, T., & Lucerini, S. (2000). Co-morbidity of psychiatric disorders and posttraumatic stress disorder. *Journal of Clinical Psychiatry, 61,* 22–32.

Brewin, C. R., Andrews, B., & Valentine, J. D. (2000). Meta-analysis of risk factors for posttraumatic stress disorder in trauma-exposed adults. *Journal of Consulting and Clinical Psychology, 68,* 748–766.

Brewin, C. R., Dalgleish, T., & Joseph, S. (1996). A dual representation theory of posttraumatic stress disorder. *Psychological Review, 103,* 670–686.

Calhoun, L. G., & Tedeschi, R. G. (2006). The foundations of posttraumatic growth. In L. G. Calhoun & R. G. Tedeschi (Eds.), *Handbook of posttraumatic growth* (pp. 1–23). Mahwah, NJ: Erlbaum.

Chemtob, C. M., Novaco, R. W., Hamada, R. S., Gross, D. M., & Smith, G. (1997). Anger regulation deficits in combat-related posttraumatic stress disorder. *Journal of Traumatic Stress, 10,* 17–36.

Dunmore, E., Clark, D. M., & Ehlers, A. (2001). A prospective investigation of the role of cognitive factors in persistent posttraumatic stress disorder (PTSD) after physical or sexual assault. *Behaviour Research and Therapy, 39,* 1063–1084.

Ehlers, A., & Clark, D. M. (2000). A cognitive model of posttraumatic stress disorder. *Behaviour Research and Therapy, 38,* 319–345.

Ehlers, A., & Clark, D. M. (2006). Predictors of chronic posttraumatic stress disorder: Traumatic memories and appraisals. In B. O. Rothbaum (Ed.), *Pathological anxiety: Emotional processing in etiology and treatment* (pp. 39–55). New York: Guilford Press.

Ehlers, A., Ehring, T., & Kleim, B. (2012). Information processing in posttraumatic stress disorder. In J. G. Beck & D. M. Sloan (Eds.), *Handbook of traumatic stress disorders* (pp. 191–218). New York: Oxford University Press.

Ehlers, A., & Steil, R. (1995). Maintenance of intrusive memories in posttraumatic stress disorder: A cognitive approach. *Behavioural and Cognitive Psychotherapy, 23,* 217–249.

Ehring, T., Ehlers, A., & Glucksman, E. (2008). Do cognitive models help in predicting the severity of posttraumatic stress disorder, phobia, and depression after motor vehicle accidents?: A prospective longitudinal study. *Journal of Consulting and Clinical Psychology, 76,* 219–230.

Epstein, S. (1991). The self-concept, the traumatic neurosis, and the structure of personality. In D. J. Ozer, J. M. Healy Jr., & A. J. Stewart (Eds.), *Perspectives on personality* (Vol. 3, pp. 63–98). London: Jessica Kingsley.

Foa, E. B., Ehlers, A., Clark, D. M., Tolin, D. F., & Orsillo, S. M. (1999). The Posttraumatic Cognitions Inventory (PTCI): Development and validation. *Psychological Assessment, 11,* 303–314.

Foa, E. B., & Rauch, S. A. M. (2004). Cognitive changes during prolonged exposure versus prolonged exposure plus cognitive restructuring in female assault survivors with posttraumatic stress disorder. *Journal of Consulting and Clinical Psychology, 72,* 879–884.

Foa, E. B., & Riggs, D. S. (1993). Post-traumatic stress disorder in rape victims. In J. Oldham, M. B. Riba, & A. Tasman (Eds.), *Review of psychiatry* (Vol. 12, pp. 273–303). Washington, DC: American Psychiatric Association.

Foa, E. B., & Rothbaum, B. O. (1998). *Treating the trauma of rape: Cognitive behavioral therapy for PTSD.* New York: Guilford Press.

Foa, E. B., Steketee, G., & Rothbaum, B. O. (1989). Behavioral/cognitive conceptualization of posttraumatic stress disorder. *Behavior Therapy, 20,* 155–176.

Gilboa-Schechtman, E., & Foa, E. B. (2001). Patterns of recovery from trauma: The use of intraindividual analyses. *Journal of Abnormal Psychology, 110,* 392–400.

Grills-Taquechel, A. E., Littleton, H. L., & Axsom, D. (2011). Social support, world assumptions, and exposure as predictors of anxiety and quality of life following a mass trauma. *Journal of Anxiety Disorders, 25,* 498–506.

Horowitz, M. J. (1986). Stress–response syndromes: A review of posttraumatic and adjustment disorders. *Hospital and Community Psychiatry, 37,* 241–249.

Janoff-Bulman, R. (1992). *Shattered assumptions: Towards a new psychology of trauma.* New York: Free Press.

Janoff-Bulman, R. (1996). Psychometric review of the World Assumptions Scale. In B. H. Stamm (Ed.), *Measurement of stress, trauma, and adaptation* (pp. 440–442). Lutherville, MD: Sidran Press.

Kazdin, A. E., & Blase, S. L. (2011). Rebooting psychotherapy research and practice to reduce the burden of mental illness. *Perspectives in Psychological Science, 6,* 21–37.

Kubany, E. S., Haynes, S. N., Abueg, F. R., Manke, F. P., Brennan, J. M., & Stahura, C. (1996). Development and validation of the Trauma-Related Guilt Inventory (TRGI). *Psychological Assessment, 8,* 428–444.

McCann, I. L., & Pearlman, L. A. (1990). *Psychological trauma and the adult survivor: Theory, therapy, and transformation.* New York: Brunner/Mazel.

Mechanic, M., & Resick, P. A. (1993, October). *The Personal Beliefs and Reactions Scale: Assessing rape-related cognitive schemata.* Paper presented at the 8th annual meeting of the International Society for Traumatic Stress Studies, San Antonio, TX.

Owens, G. P., & Chard, K. M. (2001). Cognitive distortions among women reporting childhood sexual abuse. *Journal of Interpersonal Violence, 16,* 178–191.

Owens, G. P., Pike, J. L., & Chard, K. M. (2001). Treatment effects of cognitive processing therapy on cognitive distortions of female child sexual abuse survivors. *Behavior Therapy, 32,* 413–424.

Ozer, E. J., Best, S. R., Lipsey, T. L., & Weiss, D. S. (2003). Predictors of posttraumatic stress disorder and symptoms in adults: A meta-analysis. *Psychological Bulletin, 129,* 52–73.

Resick, P. A., Nishith, P., Weaver, T. L., Astin, M. C., & Feuer, C. A. (2002). A comparison of cognitive processing therapy, prolonged exposure and a waiting condition for the treatment of posttraumatic stress disorder in female rape victims. *Journal of Consulting and Clinical Psychology, 70,* 867–879.

Resick, P. A., & Schnicke, M. K. (1992). Cognitive processing therapy for sexual assault victims. *Journal of Consulting and Clinical Psychology, 60,* 748–756.

Resick, P. A., Schnicke, M. K., & Markway, B. G. (1991, November). *Personal Beliefs and Reactions Scale: The relation between cognitive content and posttraumatic stress disorder.* Paper presented at the 25th annual convention of the Association for the Advancement of Behavior Therapy, New York.

Rizvi, S. (2010). Development and preliminary validation of a new measure to assess shame: The Shame Inventory. *Journal of Psychopathology and Behavioral Assessment, 32,* 438–447.

Robinaugh, D. J., Marques, L., Traeger, L. N., Marks, E. H., Sung, S. C., Beck, J. G., et al. (2011). Understanding the relationship of perceived social support to posttrauma cognitions and posttraumatic stress disorder. *Journal of Anxiety Disorders, 25,* 1072–1078.

Shipherd, J. C., & Beck, J. G. (1999). The effects of suppressing traumarelated thoughts in women with PTSD. *Behaviour Research and Therapy, 37*, 99112.

Steil, R., & Ehlers, A. (2000). Dysfunctional meaning of posttraumatic intrusions in chronic PTSD. *Behaviour Research and Therapy, 38*, 537–558.

Tangney, J. P., & Dearing, R. L. (2002). *Shame and guilt.* New York: Guilford Press.

Vogt, D. S., King, D. W., & King, L. A. (2007). Risk pathways for PTSD: Making sense of the literature. In M. J. Friedman, T. M. Keane, & P. A. Resick (Eds.), *Handbook of PTSD: Science and practice* (pp. 99–115). New York: Guilford Press.

Zoellner, L. A., Feeny, N. C., Eftekhari, A., & Foa, E. B. (2011). Changes in negative beliefs following three brief programs for facilitating recovery after assault. *Depression and Anxiety, 28*, 532–540.

Chapter 9

Disclosure of Traumatic Events

Denise M. Sloan *and* Blair E. Wisco

Joe always felt a heightened sense of responsibility for other people, whether it be the soldiers who were under his command or his wife and children. During his combat deployment, Joe experienced one particular event that troubled him for many years. One day a group of children approached a soldier in Joe's troop and gave this other soldier a gift box. Given Joe's nature to protect others, Joe carefully watched the interaction between the soldier and children. As the children ran off, a bomb exploded, killing the soldier. Joe watched horrified as the soldier fell to the ground. He felt a surge of anger toward the children who he was certain knew they were handing the soldier a bomb. As Joe aimed his rifle at the children running from the scene, he heard his commanding officer order him to drop his rifle. Joe did not obey the command so the rifle was kicked out of his hands. Joe was ordered to immediately leave the scene. Although he was very angry, Joe followed the command. As he walked away, he felt angry and confused. Joe couldn't understand why his commanding officer stopped him. He was sure that that commanding officer saw what happened. Joe started to doubt his action and his anger toward the children he viewed as a threat. He also felt guilt because he had children of his own. He wondered how he could have aimed his rifle at children and what this meant about the kind of person he was. Because Joe felt intense guilt and shame regarding his actions, he never discussed the incident with anyone for more than 40 years. The incident haunted Joe. He had recurring nightmares and intrusive thoughts of the soldier who was killed, as well as intrusive thoughts about his action toward the children. He feared what others would think of him if they knew about the incident. Over 40 years later, Joe was able to describe the incident in detail to his therapist.

During his disclosure, he recalled that he did not view the children as children during the incident. Instead, he viewed them as enemy threats that could kill the soldiers under his command. He also realized that his action of aiming his rifle was an instinct to protect his soldiers. These were all new insights that Joe was able to have because he, for the first time, was able to discuss the event with someone else. He had previously tried to avoid thinking about the incident; and when he would have thoughts about the event, he would try to push the thoughts away. Joe commented that the disclosure allowed him the opportunity to think about the event from a different standpoint, and it also allowed him to remember important details of the event. Following his disclosure, Joe no longer felt guilty about his actions during the event and he also no longer experienced nightmares and intrusive thoughts about the event. Joe was also surprised and relieved that the therapist did not view Joe as a "bad person" for his actions. Because the disclosure to the therapist was so positive, Joe felt able to discuss the incident with his wife and several friends. Joe was pleasantly surprised to find that everyone he disclosed the event to had similar reactions; they understood why he aimed the rifle at the children and they did not believe his actions reflected poorly upon him.[1]

Disclosure is thought to be critical in promoting recovery from exposure to a traumatic experience. However, when to disclose, to whom to disclosure, and how much to disclose are critical determinants of the extent to which one benefits from the disclosure. In this chapter, we provide a definition for disclosure and describe the characteristics that influence whether or not benefits from disclosure are derived. We then present theories of why trauma disclosure is beneficial, and review the empirical evidence that supports each of these theories. We conclude with a description of the clinical implications of trauma disclosure.

DEFINITION OF DISCLOSURE

Broadly defined, *disclosure* refers to the communication of personally relevant information, thoughts and feelings. Disclosure can be verbal or

---

[1]This case represents a mixture of various clients whom we have seen in our clinical work who have experienced posttraumatic stress disorder. Any resemblance to a specific individual is purely coincidental.

written (letter, e-mail), and beneficial effects have been observed with both formats (see Frattaroli, 2006, for a review).

IMPORTANT CHARACTERISTICS OF DISCLOSURE

Although a wealth of research demonstrates the various benefits resulting from trauma disclosure (Frattaroli, 2006), there are circumstances in which disclosure can be detrimental. Within social relationships, several factors determine whether or not disclosure will yield beneficial outcome, including the degree to which we disclose, to whom we disclose, and the context of the disclosure. Who is most likely to benefit from disclosure is another important consideration. In general, few individual difference variables reliably moderate the effects of disclosure, which seems to be generally beneficial across a wide variety of samples (Frattaroli, 2006).

Depth of Disclosure

Disclosure can vary along a dimension of depth (Derlega, Metts, Petronio, & Margulis, 1993). An example of minimal depth disclosure would be a trauma survivor disclosing that he or she was in a car accident. An example of disclosure of greater depth would be a person disclosing the details of the car accident, their thoughts and feelings surrounding the accident, as well as how they believe the accident changed their outlook and the meaning of life. The first example involves disclosure of superficial information, whereas the second example involves emotional information about the self and details about the trauma event. The more details that are provided regarding a traumatic experience, the more likely the person will describe his or her emotional response to the traumatic event. However, a person can provide details of a traumatic experience without describing his or her thoughts and feelings in response to the event. For instance, Joe would frequently disclose that he served in a combat zone, which is superficial disclosure because the disclosure does not provide details of specific combat experiences that affected Joe. If Joe disclosed that he was in combat, witnessed a soldier killed, and described his actions during the incident he would be providing a detailed disclosure but he would be omitting important information regarding his thoughts and feelings surrounding the incident. The emotional information is critical for promoting resilience and recovery from a traumatic event (e.g., Sloan & Marx, 2004b). In the case of Joe, the emotional information involves his feelings of fear for the safety of the soldiers during the incident and his feelings of guilt that he aimed his rifle at children. The additional disclosure of Joe wondering if his actions meant that he was as "bad person" is also important. By disclosing this emotional information regarding his thoughts and feelings, Joe had the opportunity to gain a different perspective on his actions during the incident, which reduced his feelings of guilt.

Context of Disclosure

Disclosures to individuals with whom we have an ongoing relationship can increase psychological well-being and can strengthen our relationship with that person (Reis & Shaver, 1988). However, disclosures to a relative stranger can be viewed as odd or inappropriate; and, as a result, the stranger may be unlikely to respond in a positive manner, ultimately leaving the discloser feeling unsupported (Reis & Shaver, 1988). Of course, there are exceptions. For instance, if the stranger is a new therapist, then the disclosure would be viewed as appropriate and therefore potentially beneficially. Also, if an ongoing relationship is unsupportive, then the trauma survivor may not benefit from the disclosure.

Research also indicates that, in some situations, it is best to suppress or inhibit self-disclosures. In a longitudinal investigation of adjustment to the death of a spouse, Bonanno and colleagues (2002) found that greater disclosure of distress was related to greater reports of grief several months later. Paradoxically, bereaved adults who displayed initial suppression of emotional disclosures (in terms of their feelings of grief surrounding the death of their spouse), reported less grief several months later and improved self-reported physical health. These findings suggest that suppression of disclosure can be adaptive in certain situations. An important methodological aspect of this study is that the disclosure of grief was to a stranger (i.e., an experimenter). As noted earlier, disclosure to a relative stranger may differ from disclosure to someone with whom one has a close, ongoing relationship. Taken together, these findings indicate that choosing the appropriate time to disclose and the appropriate people to disclose to (e.g., close friends) is important in whether or not the disclosure will lead to successful recovery from a traumatic event.

Whether a trauma survivor discloses to another person, rather than a personal journal, also influences whether or not benefits are derived. Radcliffe, Lumley, Kendall, Stevenson, and Beltran (2007) examined the importance of an audience for disclosure. These investigators randomly assigned participants to one of four conditions. Participants were assigned to either a disclosure condition in which they shared their written disclosure narratives (i.e., submitted to an experimenter), to a disclosure condition in which they did not share their written disclosure narratives (i.e., not submitted), or to one of two nondisclosure control groups. Participants assigned to one of the disclosure conditions were informed prior to the writing sessions whether or not they would be required to submit their disclosure narratives. Although both disclosure groups showed greater improvements than did the control groups, individuals who shared their disclosure narrative displayed a broader range of psychological and physical health benefits than did the individuals who did not share their disclosure narrative. This finding suggests that, regardless of whether or not there is an audience, people do benefit from disclosure. However, those who share their disclosures with others reap the greatest benefits. Returning to our case example, Joe disclosed his trauma to a therapist, a trained professional. After having a positive experience with this disclosure, he opened up to his wife and close friends. Disclosing to several people may have helped Joe gather more evidence that others would not judge him harshly for his actions or reject him because of his trauma history. It's unlikely that Joe would have derived the same benefits from simply writing about the trauma event without discussing it with others.

Timing of Disclosure

Disclosure that happens soon after a traumatic event appears to be important for recovery or resilience. For instance, all of the available early interventions for trauma survivors involve disclosure. Psychological debriefing, an example of an early trauma intervention, has a primary goal of promoting the expression of thoughts and feelings about the trauma event. Although there are a variety of psychological debriefing approaches, the most common form is critical incident stress debriefing (CISD), which is a single-session, individual- or small group–based discussion of the traumatic event. CISD has the goals of alleviating acute distress and preventing long-term psychiatric morbidity in trauma survivors (see Gray & Litz, 2005, for a review). CISD is delivered shortly after traumatic exposure and provides a venue for individuals to engage in disclosure by discussing their emotional reactions to the traumatic event (Everly, Flannery, & Mitchell, 2000). This discussion is led by a CISD facilitator who asks survivors to discuss what happened during the traumatic event and then to share what they thought and felt as it was occurring (Mitchell & Everly, 1996). Group members then identify and discuss any posttraumatic symptoms they may have experienced since the event (Mitchell & Everly, 1996). CISD also provides psychoeducation on common reactions to trauma and adaptive coping strategies (Mitchell & Everly, 1996). Despite the intuitive appeal of CISD, research has not found CISD to be more effective than no treatment control conditions, and in some cases CISD has been found to be detrimental (see Gray & Litz, 2005). There are a number of possibilities for why CISD has not been found effective, including the possibility that CISD prompts individuals to disclose their traumatic event but does not incorporate sufficient repetition to habituate them to trauma-related cues (McNally, Bryant, & Ehlers, 2003). Supporting this speculation, a dismantling study found that disclosure increased PTSD symptoms among trauma survivors with high initial hyperarousal symptoms (e.g., increased heart rate), compared to those who received psychoeducation debriefing or no treatment (Sijbrandij, Olff, Reitsma, Carlier, & Gersons, 2006). These findings suggest that a single session of trauma disclosure can prolong or even escalate psychological and physiological arousal in survivors who have increased reactivity immediately after a traumatic event (Sijbrandij et al., 2006). Indeed, as is described later in this chapter, trauma disclosure that happens repeatedly is more beneficial than disclosure that occurs only once. For Joe, he waited over 40 years to disclose the trauma event, and this delay in disclosing resulted in years of intrusive thoughts, nightmares, and feelings of guilt. Had he disclosed the event soon after it occurred, he would have likely been spared years of suffering. To summarize, the available evidence indicates that disclosure that occurs soon after the trauma event is important for recovery; however, the disclosure should occur on multiple occasions to facilitate recovery.

Individual Differences in Disclosure

There has also been great interest in identifying who benefits the most from disclosure. A meta-analysis of written disclosure found that studies including participants with histories of trauma had larger effect sizes compared to studies that did not select for trauma exposure (Frattaroli, 2006). This meta-analysis also found that participants with higher stress levels and worse physical health derived more benefit from disclosure. These effects may be due to ceiling effects for healthier individuals, who have less room to improve. Few demographic variables have been found to reliably moderate the effects of disclosure (Frattaroli, 2006). Several studies have found that written trauma disclosure is equally beneficial for males and females (Epstein, Sloan, & Marx, 2005; Sheese, Brown, & Graziano, 2004). However, women are more likely to self-disclose than men (see Dindia & Allen, 1992, for a review) and consequently may derive more benefits from trauma disclosure. Nevertheless, when men do disclose, they experience benefits that are comparable to those experienced by women. In the case of Joe, he was reluctant to disclose his trauma history at first, but benefited from disclosure when he did finally choose to discuss his trauma. The high level of distress Joe experienced in response to the trauma event was a clear indicator of his need to disclose the event, and the likely benefits he would derive from such disclosure.

THEORETICAL MODELS OF TRAUMA DISCLOSURE

There is no consensus on how disclosure confers its benefits. Several theoretical models of disclosure have been proposed (for reviews, see Frattaroli, 2006; Sloan & Marx, 2004b), but some are more relevant to trauma disclosure. Two of these models parallel the theoretical bases for cognitive-behavioral treatment for PTSD: exposure and cognitive processing/assimilation. A third model, emotional inhibition, proposes that disclosure is beneficial because it allows an individual to express the emotions and thoughts surrounding a traumatic experience rather than suppressing these reactions (Pennebaker, 1989). Finally, the social support model suggests that trauma disclosure is beneficial because it deepens or enhances the trauma survivors' existing social relationships, thereby strengthening their social support system (Pennebaker, 1997).

Exposure Model

The exposure model is based on behavioral and information processing theories of PTSD and other anxiety disorders. Most behavioral theories of anxiety disorders posit that avoidance serves to maintain anxiety symptoms (e.g., Mowrer, 1960). Individuals are motivated to avoid stimuli associated with anxiety (e.g., heights, spiders) because avoiding these stimuli offers an immediate reduction in distress. However, avoidance of feared stimuli maintains anxiety in the long term because individuals do not have the opportunity for their heightened anxiety response to habituate and to learn that feared stimuli are not dangerous. The importance of avoidance in the maintenance of PTSD has been recognized for many years (e.g., Keane, Zimering, & Caddell, 1985), and avoiding talking or thinking about a trauma event is a diagnostic criterion for PTSD (American Psychiatric Association, 2013). In trauma survivors, feared stimuli can include the trauma memory itself, stimuli that remind the individual of the trauma memory (e.g., Vietnamese individuals in the case of a Vietnam veteran, highways in the case of motor vehicle accident survivor), or stimuli eliciting emotional reactions associated with the trauma memory (e.g., a hot and rainy day that is similar to weather in Vietnam). According to emotional processing theory of PTSD (Foa & Kozak, 1986; Rachman, 1980), these stimuli are represented in memory as a pathological fear structure. Fear structures in general allow for quick responses to threatening situations but become pathological when they involve excessive response elements, are resistant to modification, and the associations among the different elements do not accurately represent reality. According to emotional processing theory, exposure to the trauma memory allows for correction of the pathological fear structure because new information (i.e., that the trauma memory is not dangerous) is learned. In the case of Joe, he avoided memories of the trauma events and places that might remind him of the event (e.g., any place in which he thought he might see or have to interact with Vietnamese individuals, such as Asian-themed restaurants). Joe's view of Chinese restaurants as dangerous was inaccurate, and his avoidance of such restaurants prevented him from correcting this erroneous belief.

Exposure is a therapeutic technique developed to counter avoidance. In the treatment of PTSD, exposure allows the individual to repeatedly confront his or her trauma memory and trauma reminders, which promotes reduction of pathological fear/anxiety. Trauma disclosure can be considered a form of exposure, as the individual is confronting his or her trauma memory by recounting the event. According to the exposure model (Foa & Kozak, 1986), repeated trauma disclosure should be more effective than a single disclosure. Repeated disclosure represents the willingness to confront the trauma memory and provides greater opportunity for learning that the trauma memory is not dangerous, as well as the opportunity to correct previously held irrational beliefs regarding the trauma event (e.g., "I should have been able to stop the event from happening"). In order for disclosure to be effective, the trauma survivor must recount the event in details and describe the emotions and thoughts he or she experienced during the event. By recounting the trauma event in this way, the survivor is able to more accurately identify erroneous beliefs about the event and replace these incorrect beliefs with correct information.

In the case of Joe, disclosing the trauma event to his therapist allowed Joe to recall important aspects of the event, such as how he viewed the children during the event (i.e., as the enemy, not as children). He also remembered that several of soldiers who witnessed the incident later relayed to him that they would have done the same thing that he did if they had witnessed the exchange between the children and the solider, and they had a rifle near them. Joe had not previously remembered any of these important details because he was unwilling to remember the event, thereby not allowing himself the opportunity to remember fully important details of the incident.

Several lines of work demonstrate that trauma disclosure initially elicits high negative affect followed by significant reduction of negative affect with repeated disclosure. One line of work comes from the written disclosure experimental procedure developed by Pennebaker and Beall (1986; also referred to as expressive writing) in which individuals write about traumatic or stressful life events, typically for 20 minutes on three separate occasions. Individuals are instructed to write about their deepest emotions surrounding the event as well as to provide details of the event. Sloan and colleagues (Sloan & Marx, 2004a; Sloan, Marx, & Epstein, 2005; Sloan, Max, Epstein, & Lexington, 2007) have found that individuals assigned to write about (or disclose) traumatic events display initially high levels of negative affect and arousal, which significantly decreases by the last disclosure session. In addition, Sloan and her colleagues have found that both the initial activation of negative affect and arousal as well as the reduction of negative affect and arousal is significantly associated with reductions in PTSD symptom severity. Sloan and colleagues (2005) also found that repeatedly writing about the same traumatic event leads to significantly better outcome than writing about different trauma events at each disclosure session, consistent with the exposure model.

Research from imaginal exposure therapy also supports the contention that exposure underlies the benefits of trauma disclosure. In exposure treatment, trauma survivors repeatedly recount (disclose) the trauma experience to a therapist by providing details of the trauma event as well as thoughts and feelings they experienced while the trauma occurred. Jaycox, Foa, and Morral (1998) examined female rape survivors with PTSD who engaged in nine sessions of either prolonged exposure alone or prolonged exposure plus stress inoculation training. Prolonged exposure treatment involved both imaginal exposure that took place during the sessions and *in vivo* exposures that occurred outside of the therapy sessions. Jaycox and colleagues found that rape survivors who reported high initial distress and across-session reduction of distress had greater treatment gains than participants who did not display this pattern of response. Thus, although all of the women disclosed their trauma, and derived benefit from the disclosure, the women who most fully engaged in the treatment (as evidenced by initially high distress ratings) gained the greatest benefits. This finding indicates that disclosure alone is not sufficient to activate the fear structure. A trauma survivor must fully disclose both the details of the trauma event and the emotions surrounding the event. Similar findings were reported by Sloan and colleagues (2007) who found that trauma survivors participating in written disclosure had significantly greater reductions in PTSD symptoms when instructed to disclose their deepest emotions, rather than just their thoughts surrounding the trauma event.

Several other studies of exposure-based treatment for PTSD provide support for the exposure model. Pitman, Orr, Altman, and Longpre (1996) found a trend for reduction of heart rate during imaginal exposure sessions and overall improvement in PTSD symptom severity. van Minnen and Hagenaars (2002) found that mean and peak distress ratings during the first session of imaginal exposure did not differ between PTSD treatment responders and nonresponders; however, treatment responders had greater reduction of self-reported distress from the first to the second session relative to nonresponders. Similarly, Rauch, Foa, Furr, and Filip (2004) found that peak distress rating during the first session of imaginal exposure was not associated with PTSD outcome, but between-session reduction of self-reported distress did predict greater reductions in PTSD symptom severity. Taken together, although there are some exceptions (see Rauch et al., 2004; van Minnen & Hagenaars, 2002), studies have found that initially high negative affect or distress leads to reductions in PTSD symptom severity. More consistent findings have been obtained with between-session reduction of negative affect, such that greater reduction of negative affect or distress is associated with beneficial outcome. These findings support the premise that, at least in part, exposure accounts for the beneficial outcome observed with trauma disclosure. Indeed, exposure is regarded as a central component of evidence-based treatments for PTSD (e.g., Institute of Medicine, 2007).

These findings also underscore the importance of trauma survivors feeling distress when initially disclosing their trauma experience. If the trauma survivor discloses his or her thoughts and feelings (emotional disclosure) in relation to the event, he or she is more likely to experience distress during the disclosure. The distress should be viewed as a good sign that he or she is disclosing in a way that will be beneficial to him or her. The findings for exposure theory also underscore the importance for repeated disclosure which should be accompanied by decreasing distress levels with successive disclosures. For Joe, he reported very high initial distress when he first disclosed the trauma event. However, by the last time he recounted the event to the therapist, he reported feeling minimal distress. Indeed, Joe stated that he had a sense of relief that he had finally disclosed the event.

Cognitive Processing/Assimilation Model

Several different cognitive models of PTSD exist, but most share the common feature of maladaptive schemas, or core beliefs, that are either confirmed or challenged by experiencing a trauma (e.g., Ehlers & Clark, 2000). When a traumatic event occurs, one's conceptualization of the trauma must be modified to fit into existing beliefs (assimilation) or existing beliefs must be modified to accommodate the traumatic event (overaccommodation; Chard, Schuster, & Resick, 2012). For example, people commonly hold the belief that the world is a safe place before experiencing a traumatic event. After the trauma, a person might respond by blaming him- or herself for not preventing the event from occurring (assimilation) or change his or her belief to now judge the world as a dangerous place (overaccomodation). Several maladaptive schemas associated with trauma have been identified (Ehlers & Clark, 2000), and common themes have emerged, such as concerns related to safety, trust, power/control, esteem, and intimacy (Chard et al., 2012).

Foa and Riggs (1993) speculated that the recovery process of trauma involves organizing and streamlining the traumatic memory and that trauma survivors with disorganized memories exhibit PTSD symptoms. The process of trauma disclosure offers the opportunity for trauma memories to become more organized and less fragmented, thereby promoting recovery. As with the exposure model, repeated disclosure is important as the trauma memory is likely to become more organized with repeated disclosures. When disclosing to others, one might also receive feedback that challenges maladaptive schemas (e.g., "It wasn't your fault," "There wasn't anything you could have done to prevent it"). However, disclosure to others could be detrimental if feedback serves to reinforce the maladaptive schemas (e.g., "You should have known better than to be out late at night").

For Joe, his trauma disclosure allowed him the opportunity to realize that he wasn't viewing the children as children during the incident. He also was able to correct the belief that he was a bad person because he aimed the rifle at the children. Rather, he was a good person who was doing the best that he could in a bad situation. Gaining this insight allowed Joe to no longer feel guilty about the event and to change his interpretation of his actions during the incident, which he came to view as reasonable and understandable given the circumstances.

The empirical literature generally supports the cognitive processing/assimilation model. Drawing from the written disclosure literature, several investigators have found that the percentage of cognitive insight words increases as individuals write repeatedly about a stressful event. The increase in cognitive insight is also related to beneficial outcome (e.g., Pennebaker & Francis, 1996). These findings are consistent with the notion that repeated disclosure allows for the opportunity to correct irrational thoughts and integrate the trauma event into a new or a revised schema. Although these findings support cognitive processing as an important component of successful recovery from a trauma event, several written disclosure studies have not found evidence that increases in cognitive insight are related to beneficial outcome (e.g., Park & Blumberg, 2002).

Sloan and colleagues (2012) also found support for the cognitive processing theory of trauma disclosure. These investigators found that trauma survivors who were randomly assigned to disclose (through writing) their trauma experience over the course of several sessions reported a significant decrease in trauma-related cognitions (e.g., negative worldviews, negative self views, and self-blame) compared with the trauma-related cognitions prior to the disclosure sessions, as well as compared to trauma survivors who were assigned to a wait-list condition.

Supporting Foa and Riggs's (1993) contention that trauma memories that are disorganized are associated with greater PTSD symptoms, several studies have documented that more disorganized trauma memories are associated with increased PTSD symptom severity (e.g., Amir, Stafford, Freshman, & Foa, 1998; Foa, Molnar, & Cashman, 1995; Zoellner, Alvarez-Conrad, & Foa, 2002). Moreover, Foa and colleagues (1995) found that women who engaged in imaginal exposure displayed an increase in the organization of their trauma narrative from the first to the last treatment session, and the increased organization was related to a reduction in depression symptoms. Moreover, a decrease of fragmentation of the trauma narrative was related to the reduction in PTSD symptom severity. van Minnen and colleagues (2002) attempted to replicate these findings with a group of treatment responders and nonresponders. These investigators found that treatment responders, relative to nonresponders, showed a greater decrease in disorganized thought during the course of imaginal exposure therapy. In contrast, Moulds and Bryant (2005) found no differences in organization of trauma narratives written before and after cognitive-behavioral treatment among a sample of 15 individuals diagnosed with acute stress disorder. However, Moulds and Bryant did find that narratives that increased in organization after treatment contained fewer references to dissociative symptoms. Taken together, these findings generally support the cognitive processing theory by demonstrating that repeated trauma disclosure may lead to an increase in the coherence and organization of the trauma memory, which facilitates recovery from a traumatic event.

Overall, findings generally support cognitive processing theory to underlie beneficial outcome associated with trauma disclosure. However, there are some studies that have not found support for this model (see Zoellner & Bittinger, 2003). One reason for the mixed findings may be the different methods that have been used to measure cognitive processing and the difficulty in quantifying cognitive processes. It should also be noted that Foa and Kozak (1986) argued that maladaptive cognitions are corrected through the process of exposure, and there is some evidence to support this contention (e.g., Rauch & Foa, 2006).

Emotional Inhibition Model

Pennebaker (1989, 1997) proposed that emotional inhibition underlies the beneficial outcome associated with written disclosure of stressful life experiences, including trauma. Inhibition is conceptualized as not thinking or talking about stressful experiences. Inhibition can also comprise suppressing emotional expression by controlling one's language and behaviors, including facial expressions and body language (Pennebaker & Beall, 1986). Inhibition-based theories of psychological well-being have been influential since Freud's original writing on the benefits of catharsis, or releasing anxiety by talking about previously suppressed memories (e.g., Freud, 1961). Inhibition is thought to create a stressful physiological and cognitive burden that takes a toll on physical and psychological health over time. Disclosure through either talking or writing about a stressful life event is thought to relieve the stress associated with inhibition, leading to physical and psychological health benefits (Pennebaker, 1997).

In the case example, Joe inhibited talking about the trauma event for over 40 years. The suppression of this event caused considerable distress for Joe. He frequently worried what other people might think of him if they knew about the event, he ruminated about what his actions on that day meant about the kind of person he was, and he felt guilty that the soldier was killed because he believed there might have been something he could have done to prevent it. Being able to disclose the event to his therapist and later to his wife and friends resulted in Joe being able to discuss his thoughts and feelings with others. Joe stated that he felt like a "weight had been lifted" after disclosing the trauma event to others.

Although the emotional inhibition theory has long been thought to underlie the beneficial effects of disclosure (Freud, 1961), the evidence to support this theory is scant. There is evidence that writing about traumatic experiences leads to improved immune functioning (Pennebaker, Kiecolt-Glaser, & Glaser, 1988; Petrie, Booth, Pennebaker, Davison, & Thomas, 1995), which peripherally supports the model that trauma disclosure provides the opportunity to release stress on the system caused by emotional inhibition. However, other data do not support the emotional inhibition theory. For example, trauma survivors who have previously disclosed their trauma experience are just as likely to reap benefits from trauma disclosure as those who have not previously disclosed their trauma experience (e.g., Greenberg & Stone, 1992). This finding may be related to the need to disclose repeatedly and/or to disclose in a more detailed manner in order to achieve benefits associated with disclosure.

Emotional inhibition could also be conceptualized as a form of avoidance, consistent with the exposure model described previously (Mowrer, 1960). That is, the trauma survivor avoids disclosure due to fear of the trauma memory.

Social Support Model

More recently, Pennebaker and Graybeal (2001) proposed that disclosure is beneficial by promoting what they termed "social integration." More specifically, disclosing to others about one's stressful or traumatic experiences promotes a feeling of closeness and informs others about one's inner state. Conversely, when keeping traumatic events secret, one remains socially isolated and potentially less able to cope with negative thoughts and feelings associated with the event. Such personal disclosures serve to strengthen the social relationship (Reis & Shaver, 1988). The increased strength of social relationships is thought to account for recovery from a stressful or traumatic event.

Pennebaker (1997) has speculated that the emotional inhibition theory accounts for the initial beneficial effects associated with disclosure; however, these beneficial effects are maintained for months afterward because the written disclosure increases the likelihood that the individual will disclose the event to individuals with whom he or she has an existing social relationship. Such personal disclosures serve to strengthen the social relationship (Reis & Shaver, 1988). The increased strength of social relationships is thought to account for recovery from a stressful or traumatic event.

After disclosing the trauma event to his wife, Joe noticed that he and his wife were closer than they had been in many years. His wife felt closer to Joe because she now understood what he had experienced and what he had been dealing with for so many years. She also felt closer to Joe because he clearly trusted her enough to share his traumatic experience with her. Joe felt closer to his wife because he no longer feared that she might discover the "secret" he had been keeping from her and others for so many years. He experienced her comfort once he disclosed the event and that she didn't judge him the way he had feared she might.

The social support model has received less attention in the research literature to date; nevertheless, there are a number of findings that support this model. Participants assigned to disclose trauma or stressful life events are more likely than control participants to talk about their experience in the weeks or months following the disclosure (e.g., Kovacs & Range, 2000) and are more likely to report having received socially supportive behaviors from friends and family following their disclosure (Heffner-Johnson, 2002). In addition, individuals who disclose their traumatic or stressful life events are more likely to make small changes in their friendship networks and even laugh more than control participants in the days and weeks following disclosure (Pennebaker & Graybeal, 2001). Sheese and colleagues (2004) found that individuals who have greater social supports prior to their disclosure are more likely to show reductions in depression and physical health symptoms after disclosure relative to people with limited social support. Overall, the available evidence indicates a clear connection between disclosure and improved social relationships. However, the exact nature of this association, and how one affects the other, is unknown.

SUMMARY AND CLINICAL RECOMMENDATIONS

There are a number of factors that appear important in determining whether or not one reaps benefits from trauma disclosure.

Depth of Disclosure

Providing only broad or scant details of the trauma event is not beneficial for recovery. Instead, the disclosure should contain a detailed account of the trauma event, including the emotions and thoughts the person experienced during the event. Providing greater details will also allow the person to organize the trauma memory and better recognize misattributions relating to the event, such as inaccurate beliefs that he or she could have prevented the event from occurring. By providing greater details and describing emotions and thoughts that occurred during the event, the person is better able to engage in the disclosure. Greater engagement in the trauma disclosure appears important to experiencing initially high levels of negative affect and arousal, which has been shown to be an important predictor of trauma recovery. Greater depth of disclosure can be encouraged by prompting the trauma survivor for additional details if they are initially describing the experience with scant information. Asking questions should be balanced by allowing the trauma survivor to fully describe the event and his or her thoughts and feelings of the event, rather than interrupting the person.

Repeated Disclosure

The available research indicates that disclosing the trauma on a single occasion may not be sufficient for trauma recovery. Repeated disclosure appears to facilitate the organizing and streamlining of the trauma memory; both are important to trauma recovery. Also, repeated disclosure is important in terms of providing the opportunity for the trauma survivors to experience fear reduction of initially high levels of negative affect and arousal. Reduction of negative affect and arousal has also been shown to be critical to successful trauma recovery. Trauma survivors should be encouraged to repeatedly describe the trauma experience. For instance, if the survivor states that he or she wants to put the event behind him or her, he or she should be encouraged to first describe the event several times in order to successfully "put the event" behind him or her. Friends and family members should make sure that the trauma survivor is discussing his or her experience while at the same time not forcing the person to disclose the event when he or she is not ready to do so. Gentle encouragement is best.

Form of Disclosure

Trauma disclosure can take different forms. One can write about the trauma event or talk about it with another person. Given the associated social benefits and additional benefits to viewing the trauma from another perspective, it would seem best to disclose to another person. This would be particularly helpful in the case of a person with whom one has a close, ongoing relationship. However, if a trauma survivor is uncomfortable or unable to disclose to another person, benefits can be obtained from disclosure through writing. If the trauma survivor cannot identify anyone he or she feels close with, the person may be best served by writing about the trauma event rather than disclosing the event with someone who is an acquaintance more than a friend. Similarly, if the trauma survivor has had prior experiences of friends and/or relatives being judgmental, it may be best to write about the event rather than disclose to someone who might question the survivor's role or actions in the trauma event.

Timing of Disclosure

The available research indicates that disclosure that takes place soon after the trauma event plays a critical role in resilience/recovery from the experience. Thus, trauma survivors should be encouraged to discuss the event in the days or weeks following the experience in order to facilitate recovery. But even when a person discloses the event many years following the trauma, similar benefits are observed. Whenever disclosure occurs, the trauma survivor will have the opportunity to describe his or her thoughts and feelings surrounding the event, his or her reactions to the event, and to correct any erroneous beliefs regarding the event. As previously described, the disclosure should occur multiple times and should provide detailed information in order to reap the greatest benefits.

Disclosure has long been recognized as important for developing and sustaining social relationships. Research conducted over the last two decades has uncovered the importance of disclosure in recovery from traumatic events. Indeed, trauma disclosure is a core component of early interventions for trauma survivors. By disclosing a trauma event, the survivor has the opportunity to organize the trauma memory and correct irrational beliefs he or she may hold surrounding the event. The survivor also has the opportunity to learn that the trauma memory itself is not dangerous and that he or she is able to tolerate the negative emotions elicited by the trauma memory. Trauma disclosure may also strengthen existing social relationships. The strengthening of social relationships further facilitates recovery from a traumatic experience. Taken together, disclosure represents a cornerstone for successful recovery from a traumatic event.

REFERENCES

American Psychiatric Association. (2013). *Diagnostic and statistical manual of mental disorders* (5th ed.). Arlington, VA: Author.

Amir, N., Stafford, J., Freshman, M. S., & Foa, E. B. (1998). Relationship between trauma narratives and trauma pathology. *Journal of Traumatic Stress, 11,* 385–392.

Bonanno, G. A., Wortman, C. B., Lehman, D. R., Tweed, R. G., Haring, M., Sonnega, J., et al. (2002). Resilience to loss and chronic grief: A prospective study from pre-loss to 18 months post-loss. *Journal of Personality and Social Psychology, 83,* 1150–1164.

Chard, K. M., Schuster, J. L., & Resick, P. A. (2012). Empirically supported psychological treatments: Cognitive processing therapy. In J. G. Beck & D. M. Sloan (Eds.), *Handbook of traumatic stress disorders* (pp. 439–448). New York: Oxford University Press.

Derlega, V. J., Metts, S., Petronio, S., & Margulis, S. T. (1993). *Self-disclosure.* Newbury Park, CA: Sage.

Dindia, K., & Allen, M. (1992). Sex differences in self-disclosure. A meta-analysis. *Psychological Bulletin, 112,* 106–124.

Elhers, A., & Clark, D. M. (2000). A cognitive model of posttraumatic stress disorder. *Behavior Research and Therapy, 38,* 319–345.

Epstein, E. M., Sloan, D. M., & Marx, B. P. (2005). Getting to the heart of the matter: Written disclosure, gender, and heart rate. *Psychosomatic Medicine, 67*, 413–419.

Everly, G. S., Flannery, R. B., & Mitchell, J. T. (2000). Critical incident stress management (CISM): A review of the literature. *Aggression and Violent Behavior, 5*, 23–40.

Foa, E. B., & Kozak, M. J. (1986). Emotional processing of fear: Exposure to corrective information. *Psychological Bulletin, 99*, 20–35.

Foa, E. B., Molnar, C., & Cashman, L. (1995). Change in rape narratives during exposure therapy for posttraumatic stress disorder. *Journal of Traumatic Stress, 8*, 675–690.

Foa, E. B., & Riggs, D. S. (1993). Posttraumatic stress disorder in rape victims. In J. Oldham, M. B. Riba, & A. Tasman (Eds.), *American Psychiatric Press review of psychiatry* (pp. 273–303). Washington, DC: American Psychiatric Press.

Frattaroli, J. (2006). Experimental disclosure and its moderators: A meta-analysis. *Psychological Bulletin, 132*, 823–865.

Freud, S. (1961). *The ego and the id.* In J. Strachey (Ed. & Trans.), *The standard edition of the complete psychological works of Sigmund Freud* (Vol. 19, pp. 3–66). London: Hogarth Press. (Original work published 1923)

Gray, M. J., & Litz, B. T. (2005). Behavioral interventions for recent trauma: Empirically informed practice guidelines. *Behavior Modification, 29*, 189–215.

Greenberg, M. A., & Stone, A. A. (1992). Emotional disclosure about traumas and its relation to health: Effects of previous disclosure and trauma severity. *Journal of Personality and Social Psychology, 63*, 75–84.

Heffner-Johnson, K. L. (2002). *A biosocial approach to the study of trauma disclosure and health.* Doctoral dissertation, University of Nevada, Reno. *Dissertation Abstracts International, 62*(8), 3848B.

Institute of Medicine. (2007). *Treatment of posttraumatic stress disorder: An assessment of the evidence.* Washington, DC: National Academies Press.

Jaycox, L. H., Foa, E. B., & Morrel, A. R. (1998). Influence of emotional engagement and habituation on exposure therapy for PTSD. *Journal of Consulting and Clinical Psychology, 66*, 185–192.

Keane, T. M., Zimering, R. T., & Caddell, J. M. (1985). A behavioral formulation of posttraumatic stress disorder in Vietnam veterans. *Behavior Therapist, 8*, 9–12.

Kovacs, S. H., & Range, L. M. (2000). Writing projects: Lessening undergraduates' unique suicidal bereavement. *Suicide and Life-Threatening Behavior, 30*, 50–60.

McNally, R. J., Bryant, R. A., & Ehlers, A. (2003). Does early psychological intervention promote recovery from posttraumatic stress? *Psychological Science in the Public Interest, 4*, 45–79.

Mitchell, J. T., & Everly, G. S. Jr. (1996). *Critical incident stress debriefing: An operations manual for the prevention of traumatic stress among emergency services and disaster workers* (2nd ed.). Ellicott City, MD: Chevron.

Moulds, M. L., & Bryant, R. A. (2005). Traumatic memories in acute stress disorder: An analysis of narratives before and after treatment. *Clinical Psychologist, 9*, 10–14.

Mowrer, O. H. (1960). *Learning theory and behavior.* New York: Wiley.

Park, C. L., & Blumberg, C. J. (2002). Disclosing trauma through writing: Testing the meaning-making hypothesis. *Cognitive Therapy and Research, 26,* 597–616.

Pennebaker, J. W. (1989). Confession, inhibition, and disease. In L. Berkowitz (Ed.), *Advances in experimental social psychology* (pp. 211–244). New York: Academic Press.

Pennebaker, J. W. (1997). Writing about emotional experiences as a therapeutic process. *Psychological Science, 8,* 162–166.

Pennebaker, J. W., & Beall, S. K. (1986). Confronting a traumatic event: Toward an understanding of inhibition and disease. *Journal of Abnormal Psychology, 95,* 274–281.

Pennebaker, J. W., & Francis, M. (1996). Cognitive, emotional, and language processes in disclosure. *Cognition and Emotion, 10,* 601–626.

Pennebaker, J. W., & Graybeal, A. (2001). Patterns of natural language use: Disclosure, personality, and social integration. *Current Directions in Psychological Science, 10,* 90–93.

Pennebaker, J. W., Kiecolt-Glaser, J., & Glaser, R. (1988). Disclosure of traumas and immune functioning: Health implications for psychotherapy. *Journal of Consulting and Clinical Psychology, 56,* 239–245.

Pennebaker, J. W., Mayne, T. J., & Francis, M. E. (1997). Linguistic predictors of adaptive bereavement. *Journal of Personality and Social Psychology, 72,* 863–871.

Petrie, K. J., Booth, R. J., Pennebaker, J. W., Davison, K. P., & Thomas, M. G. (1995). Disclosure of trauma and immune response to a hepatitis B vaccination program. *Journal of Consulting and Clinical Psychology, 63,* 787–792.

Pitman, R. K., Orr, S. P., Altman, B., & Longpre, R. E. (1996). Emotional processing and outcome of imaginal flooding therapy in Vietnam veterans with chronic post-traumatic stress disorder. *Comprehensive Psychiatry, 37,* 409–418.

Rachman, S. (1980). Emotional processing. *Behaviour Research and Therapy, 18,* 51–60.

Radcliffe, A. M., Lumley, M. A., Kendall, J., Stevenson, J. K., & Beltran, J. (2007). Written emotional disclosure: Testing whether social disclosure matters. *Journal of Social and Clinical Psychology, 26,* 362–384.

Rauch, S. A. M., & Foa, E. B. (2006). Emotional processing theory and exposure therapy for PTSD. *Journal of Contemporary Psychotherapy, 36,* 61–65.

Rauch, S. A. M., Foa, E. B., Furr, J. M., & Filip, J. C. (2004). Imagery vividness and perceived anxious arousal in prolonged exposure treatment for PTSD. *Journal of Traumatic Stress, 17,* 461–465.

Reis, H. T., & Shaver, P. (1988). Intimacy as an interpersonal process. In S. Duck (Ed.), *Handbook of personal relationships* (pp. 367–389). Chichester, UK: Wiley.

Sheese, B. E., Brown, E. L., & Graziano, W.G., (2004). Emotional expression in cyberspace: Searching for moderators of the Pennebaker disclosure effect via e-mail. *Health Psychology, 23,* 457–464.

Sijbrandij, M., Olff, M., Reitsma, J. B., Carlier, I. V., & Gersons, B. P. (2006). Emotional or educational debriefing after psychological trauma: Randomised controlled trial. *British Journal of Psychiatry, 189,* 150–155.

Sloan, D. M., & Marx, B. P. (2004a). A closer examination of the structured written disclosure procedure. *Journal of Consulting and Clinical Psychology, 72,* 165–175.

Sloan, D. M., & Marx, B. P. (2004b). Taking pen to hand: Evaluating possible theories underlying written disclosure paradigm. *Clinical Psychology: Science and Practice, 11,* 121–137.

Sloan, D. M., Marx, B. P., Bovin, M. J., Feinstein, B. A., & Gallagher, M. W. (2012). Written exposure therapy as an intervention for PTSD: A randomized clinical trial. *Behaviour Research and Therapy, 50,* 627–635.

Sloan, D. M., Marx, B. P., & Epstein, E. M. (2005). Further examination of the exposure model underlying written emotional disclosure. *Journal of Consulting and Clinical Psychology, 73,* 549–554.

Sloan, D. M., Marx, B. P., Epstein, E. M., & Lexington, J. (2007). Does altering the instructional set affect written disclosure outcome? *Behavior Therapy, 38,* 155–168.

van Minnen, A., & Hagenaars, M. (2002). Fear activation and habituation patterns as early process predictors of response to prolonged exposure treatment in PTSD. *Journal of Traumatic Stress, 15,* 359–367.

van Minnen, A., Wessel, I., Dijkstra, T., & Roelofs, K. (2002). Changes in PTSD patients' narratives during prolonged exposure therapy: A replication and extension. *Journal of Traumatic Stress, 15,* 255–258.

Zoellner, L. A., & Bittinger, J. N. (2003). On the uniqueness of trauma memories in PTSD. In G. M. Rosen (Ed.), *Posttraumatic stress disorder: Issues and controversies* (pp. 147–162). West Sussex, UK: Wiley.

Zoellner, L. A., Alvarez-Conrad, J., & Foa, E. B. (2002). Peritraumatic dissociative experiences, trauma narratives, and trauma pathology. *Journal of Traumatic Stress, 15,* 49–57.

Chapter 10

Dissociation during and after Trauma

Agnes van Minnen, Rianne de Kleine,
and Muriel Hagenaars

Linda was 8 years old when her mother married her stepfather. Linda and her stepfather were close, he was very funny, and she loved playing games with him. Also, Linda had a very vivid imagination, and her stepfather made up his own bedtime stories based on her prompts. However, after some months his goodnight kisses became more and more intimate, and he progressively started to touch her sexually. Linda did not resist because it felt as if she was frozen and could not move; it was like she could not feel anything, emotionally or physically, not even the pain he caused her by penetrating her. During the sexual assaults she created another world for herself and sometimes did not even register how much time he spent in her bed. In this other world, it seemed like it was not her but someone else's body that was being abused. Afterward, she sometimes wondered whether it had really happened or whether she had dreamt it and often could not recall any details of that particular night. When Linda was 14, her mother divorced her stepfather and the sexual abuse stopped. However, in the years after the abuse had ended, Linda continued to feel numb and was incapable of enjoying happy moments, even her birthday. She did not sleep well and postponed going to bed because she was afraid of the recurrent nightmares and because her bedroom reminded her too vividly of the abuse. In the mornings, when she had to go to school, she felt as if she was not really in this world and felt like a robot. Also, when she was reminded of her sexual abuse, by a television program, for instance, it felt as if it was all happening again, and she froze up. Linda also felt hypervigilant most of the time and unable to cope with these feelings; she started to drink. Although the alcohol helped her to relax a little, it also numbed her feelings even more. At the age of 19, Linda sought treatment for her problems and was diagnosed with posttraumatic stress disorder (PTSD).[1]

What are the consequences of experiencing dissociative symptoms during a traumatic event and subsequent, persistent dissociative symptoms with respect to the development of PTSD? Is dissociation necessarily a bad thing and should we try to prevent it? In Linda's case, the dissociation during the sexual abuse seemed to have helped her to get through these traumatic events and may even have had a positive effect. However, she continued to dissociate after the abuse had stopped, which may have hampered her recovery. This leads us to the question: When is dissociation in relation to trauma functional and when does it become dysfunctional?

Dissociation is often linked to (severe or continued) trauma and other impactful, negative life events. Numerous studies focused on the negative consequences of dissociative responses during the trauma have found that peritraumatic dissociation was associated with an increased risk of developing PTSD. A review even indicated peritraumatic dissociation as one of the main risk factors for PTSD development (Ozer, Best, Lipsey, & Weiss, 2003). In this chapter, we address the link between dissociation and trauma. Overall, we stress that experiencing dissociation during stressful or life-threatening traumatic events is quite normal, and may even be functional. When the dissociative feelings endure after the event, however, they may interfere with the emotional processing of the trauma and thus hinder recovery. We discuss several forms of dissociation, describe the impact of dissociation on trauma recovery, and present several interventions for overcoming dissociation in the aftermath of a trauma.

WHAT IS DISSOCIATION?

Before discussing possible implications of dissociation, we need to clarify the concept. Unfortunately, well over a century after Pierre Janet introduced the term in the late 1900s, there is still no coherent conceptualization.

---

[1]This case represents a mixture of various clients whom we have seen in our clinical work who have experienced posttraumatic stress disorder and dissociation. Any resemblance to a specific individual is purely coincidental.

This lack of a uniformly accepted definition seriously hinders the systematic investigation of its impact. The fifth edition of the *Diagnostic and Statistical Manual of Mental Disorders* (DSM-5; American Psychiatric Association, 2013) describes dissociative disorders as characterized by a "disruption . . . in the normal integration of consciousness, memory, identity, emotion, perception, body representation, motor control, and behavior." Linda's consciousness was affected when she asked herself whether the abuse had really happened. In 1996, Nijenhuis, Spinhoven, Van Dyck, Van der Hart, and Vanderlinden introduced the term "somatoform dissociation" to describe dissociative symptoms that are manifested in somatic (bodily) rather than cognitive phenomena, thus delineating the disintegration of the somatoform components of experiences, as illustrated by Linda's perception problems, and her analgesia and tonic immobility during the sexual assaults. This broadening of the phenomena that can be interpreted as dissociation is also apparent in the *International Classification of Diseases* (World Health Organization, 1992), where conversion disorders—including the type with disintegrated motor functions—are categorized as dissociative disorders. Because both cognitive and motor dissociative symptoms have been found to be related to trauma, we will use this expanded definition of dissociation in this chapter.

Theoretical Models

In an attempt to clarify the construct, several authors have tried to categorize the different phenomena that are considered to be dissociative (Allen, 2001; Holmes et al., 2005; Kennedy et al., 2004; Nijenhuis, Spinhoven, Vanderlinden, van Dyck, & van der Hart, 1998), which has resulted in several distinct categorizations. It is beyond the scope of this chapter to discuss them all, which is why we will restrict ourselves to the dichotomous categorization that the majority of recent conceptualizations use, as it is not just descriptive but also based on distinct underlying mechanisms. The two types of dissociation in this dichotomy have been recognized by several authors (Allen, 2001; Brown, 2002; Cardeña, 1994; Holmes et al., 2005; Putnam, 1997) and are usually referred to as *detachment* and *compartmentalization*.

Detachment refers to experiences that concern an altered state of consciousness in which one feels detached from one's body, sense of self, or the world around one. Examples of detachment states are depersonalization, derealization, and emotional numbing. Linda felt emotionally numb during the assaults, and afterward in a dream-like state, not really living in this world, all indicative of derealization. Feeling "like a robot" showed that Linda also experienced depersonalization. The neurophysiological profile of detachment is assumed to be characterized by left prefrontal (top-down) inhibition of the amygdala, along with an activation of right prefrontal attentional systems, resulting in a lack of emotional coloring and increased alertness, respectively (Sierra & Berrios, 1998).

Compartmentalization refers to experiences involving "a deficit in the ability to deliberately control processes that would normally be amenable to such control" (Holmes et al., 2005, p. 7). The individual experiences an inability to bring normally accessible information into conscious awareness (like in dissociative amnesia), to deliberately move (like in conversion paralysis), or to stop movement (like in conversion seizures). Other examples of compartmentalization are sensory loss or pseudohallucinations and forms of somatoform dissociation. Because of its many distinct symptoms, it is unclear whether compartmentalization is characterized by one core neurophysiological profile. Studies on neural correlates of hypnotically induced compartmentalization symptoms (mainly analgesia and pain perception) suggest an interference with frontal integrative functions that involve the awareness of perceptual stimulation (Kallio, Revonsuo, Hamalainen, Markela, & Gruzelier, 2001). Moreover, there is some evidence that hypnotically induced catalepsy (i.e., compartmentalization) causes an alteration in mental motor representations (Roelofs, van Galen, Keijsers, & Hoogduin, 2002). Also, a positron emission tomography (PET) study showed a state of total body catalepsy to be related to a deactivation of primary visual and (less significantly) primary auditory areas, which may reflect a shift in selective attention away from external stimuli and toward internal sensations (Grond, Pawlik, Walter, Lesch, & Heiss, 1995).

Tonic Immobility

An example of compartmentalization that is highly relevant when it comes to trauma is tonic immobility. Widely studied in animals, tonic immobility is an involuntary defense response that is triggered in situations that involve intense fear and physical restraint, that is, when there is no (perceived) possibility of "flight or fight"(Gallup, 1977). It is characterized by profound motor inhibition (immobility), lack of vocalization, catalepsy or tremors, eye closure, and analgesia with evidence of a preserved awareness of the surroundings (Marks, 1987). The widely used phrases "scared stiff" or "frozen with fear" show that the experience of inhibition in response to highly frightening situations is seen in humans as well (Marx, Forsyth, Gallup, Fuse, & Lexington, 2008). Tonic immobility is commonly seen as a reaction to sexual assault and was first known as "rape-induced paralysis" (Burgess & Holmstrom, 1976). Prevalence rates of 37% during rape to 52.5% during childhood sexual abuse have been reported (Fuse, Forsyth, Marx, Gallup, & Weaver, 2007; Heidt, Marx, & Forsyth, 2005). Linda also showed tonic immobility during the sexual assaults: she felt as if she was frozen and could not move. In addition to sexual assault, other traumatic or highly threatening situations, such as armed robbery, can trigger tonic immobility as well, in both women and men (Abrams, Carleton, Taylor, & Asmundson, 2009; Fiszman et al., 2008; Galliano, Noble, Travis, & Puechl, 1993). Theoretical models have been suggested to explain tonic immobility reactions and understand it as a cascade of defense responses to fearful situations (e.g., Bracha, 2004; Schauer & Elbert, 2010) following thwarted fight-or-flight reactions.

Now that we have defined dissociation, in the next section, we try to answer the question whether dissociation is normal or an indication of psychopathology.

IS DISSOCIATION NORMAL OR PATHOLOGICAL?

Although Janet considered dissociation to be a discontinuous psychopathological phenomenon that is present in patients with psychiatric disorders and absent in healthy individuals (Putnam, 1989), dissociation is now widely agreed to be a continuous phenomenon, ranging from common, "harmless" dissociative symptoms to dissociative disorders (Ross, 1996).

Prevalence

Nonpathological dissociation is known to be quite common, having a lifetime prevalence of 26–74% in the general population (Hunter, Sierra, & David, 2004). With respect to detachment, nearly everyone has on occasion daydreamed, lost attention for external stimuli when reading an interesting book, or has experienced a déjà-vu. Benign forms of compartmentalization are quite common as well. For example, some people become mute in stressful situations, while others are unable to remember normally easily retrievable information (e.g., the name of their favorite writer) when under pressure. In a study on transient forms of compartmentalization in a nonclinical sample, we found that a substantial proportion of people (19.2%) reported tonic immobility (i.e., compartmentalization) in reaction to stressful or traumatic situations. Furthermore, almost one in three "experienced" tonic immobility during anxious dreams and nightmares (De Kleine & van Minnen, 2013). Experimental studies also found that even mild stressors induced tonic immobility in nonclinical populations (Schmidt, Richey, Zvolensky, & Maner, 2008).

However, although dissociative experiences are common to some extent and can be seen as normal, the other end of the continuum involves psychopathological dissociation, for example, in the form of dissociative disorders. Pathological dissociation can be assessed with the Dissociative Experiences Scale (DES; Carlson & Putnam, 1993). Pathological dissociation is common among psychiatric patients, with rates ranging between 5.4 and 12.7% in a randomly selected sample of psychiatric inpatients

(Modestin & Erni, 2004; Spitzer et al., 2006). In several specific diagnostic groups, such as in patients with eating disorders, PTSD, personality disorder, and schizophrenia, the prevalence tends to be higher, even as high as 48% (Spitzer et al., 2006; Waller, Ohanian, Meyer, Everill, & Rouse, 2001). Depersonalization is the most common dissociative symptom among psychiatric patients; 80% of inpatients reportedly suffer from it (Medford, Sierra, Baker, & David, 2005). Other dissociative disorders, like amnesia or dissociative identity disorder, are unknown or rare (below 10%; Ross, Duffy, & Ellason, 2002) and controversial. The main controversy involves the question of whether one can forget strong, emotionally traumatic events: some argue that one can, while others think it highly unlikely (for more information about the controversies about trauma and memory, see, among other authors Lilienfeld & Lynn, 2003; McNally, 2003).

Stress Dependence

Dissociation can thus refer to both a normal phenomenon and a psychopathological syndrome and it has been posited that it may be functional in certain situations, most specifically at the time of the stressful or traumatic event. Relevant to trauma, we know that dissociative symptoms are often triggered in highly emotional states. Indeed, in patients with dissociative disorders like depersonalization disorder (Simeon, Knutelska, Nelson, & Guralnik, 2003) or conversion disorder (Roelofs, Spinhoven, Sandijck, Moene, & Hoogduin, 2005), it was found that severe life stressors preceded the onset of symptoms, indicating that the dissociation was, at least partly, induced by stress and anxiety. Hunter, Phillips, Chalder, Sierra, and David (2003) furthermore state that there is compelling evidence that dissociation is closely linked to anxiety disorders, especially panic disorder, based on the similarity between depersonalization disorder and anxiety symptoms, the neurobiological similarities between the two disorders, and the high levels of mutual comorbidity. And, as stated earlier, also in healthy individuals even relatively mild anxiety-provoking stressors (e.g., increased CO_2 intake) can induce dissociative feelings (Schmidt et al., 2008). Taken together, dissociation is a reaction to or an epiphenomenon of a stressful emotional response. But why? What is its function?

Function

Detachment is thought to be part of a biological defense mechanism that minimizes anxiety during extreme threat. In that way, detachment serves as a protection device, regulating stress levels and thereby protecting the individual against an extreme emotional response. Another function of dissociation is that the sense of time is lost. For instance, dissociative window staring during prolonged travel can make the journey more endurable. Linda also lost track of time during the assaults, potentially to make them more bearable.

Tonic immobility may also function as a protective defense mechanism. In animals, tonic immobility responses are sometimes referred to as "playing dead," which behavior may serve to evade the attention of the predator. Similarly, sexual offenders may lose interest when their victims "play dead" in reaction to the sexual attack (Burgess & Holmstrom, 1976). Also, the autonomic physiological responses during tonic immobility, such as decreased blood pressure and heart rate, may prevent trauma victims from bleeding to death in case of severe injuries, emphasizing the survival function of dissociative reactions during trauma (Marx et al., 2008). Dissociation may also help alleviate or numb feelings of pain, for instance, during a visit to the dentist. Linda also reported that she felt no pain when her stepfather was penetrating her, which probably served to help her to endure the abuse.

In sum, it is good to keep in mind that although dissociation can take pathological forms and can be dysfunctional, dissociation is also a normal and functional reaction to stressful, highly emotional, or traumatic events. From an evolutionary perspective, dissociation during stress and trauma serves survival, underscoring its protective value. Despite that, it is often believed that people who show sustained dissociation during and after the trauma run a higher risk of developing psychopathology in the longer term, more specifically PTSD. In the next section, we look at the evidence for this assumption.

DISSOCIATION AND DEVELOPMENT OF PTSD

Peritraumatic Dissociation

Peritraumatic dissociation refers to dissociative symptoms that occur during or briefly after the traumatic event and is thought to negatively influence the process of overcoming the trauma. In this vein, several studies have linked peritraumatic dissociation to later PTSD development. Theoretically, dissociation is thought to affect the encoding and storage of trauma information during and after the trauma. More specifically, it is theorized that dissociation prevents information from being fully stored into autobiographical memory and instead results in vivid and sensory-rich memory fragments (Brewin & Saunders, 2001; van der Kolk & van der Hart, 1989).

Detachment

A meta-analysis (Ozer et al., 2003) indeed confirmed peritraumatic dissociation (defined as detachment) to be a strong predictor of PTSD. However, many of the studies included in these meta-analysis suffered from methodological shortcomings, for instance, by having retrospective designs and a lack of control for confounds. These aspects are particularly problematic in this context because recall of peritraumatic dissociation has been shown to be unstable over time and highly related with changes in PTSD symptoms (Marshall & Schell, 2002; Zoellner, Sacks, & Foa, 2001). Some studies failed to control for initial PTSD symptoms, making it unclear to what extent peritraumatic dissociation might act as an independent predictor of PTSD (Candel & Merckelbach, 2004). Also, most of the research on peritraumatic dissociation involved clinical field studies, and only very few studies used an experimental design to directly manipulate dissociation, hindering inferences about causality. In fact, in various studies, the effect of peritraumatic dissociation disappeared when confounding factors such as initial PTSD symptoms were controlled (e.g., Hagenaars, van Minnen, & Hoogduin, 2007). Moreover, a recent meta-analysis including prospective studies only (n = 17) demonstrated that in the majority of cases there was no or only weak predictive power for peritraumatic dissociation (van der Velden & Wittmann, 2008), with only half of the studies (n = 3) with positive results indicating that peritraumatic dissociation was an independent predictor of PTSD.

To gather more information about causality, a few experimental studies manipulated dissociation during analogue trauma and investigated the development of PTSD symptoms. The results are inconclusive. Manipulations of dissociation in terms of detachment did predict intrusion development in some studies (Holmes, Brewin, & Hennessy, 2004; Regambal & Alden, 2009), but not in others (Holmes & Steel, 2004).

Compartmentalization

As was the case with detachment, the predictive power of compartmentalization disappeared after controlling for initial PTSD symptoms (Hagenaars, van Minnen, & Hoogduin, 2007). In several studies tonic immobility reactions during trauma were found to be related to PTSD symptom development (Abrams et al., 2009; Bovin, Jager-Hyman, Gold, Marx, & Sloan, 2008; Heidt et al., 2005; Rizvi, Kaysen, Gutner, Griffin, & Resick, 2008; Rocha-Rego et al., 2009), but again, not all studies were well controlled, and the exact mechanism is unknown.

Interestingly, one study experimentally manipulated compartmentalization (dissociative tonic immobility) during a trauma film. It was found that dissociation led to increased intrusion levels relative to a free-to-move control condition. However, to separate movement from dissociation, an extra control condition was included in which participants were instructed to not move during the viewing, while no dissociation was induced. With this control, peritraumatic nonmovement, and not dissociation, was found to have increased the development of intrusions (Hagenaars, van Minnen, Holmes, Brewin, & Hoogduin, 2008).

In all, although a relationship with later PTSD development has been found several times, prospective and well-controlled studies failed to show high predictive power for peritraumatic dissociation. Possibly, previous findings were clouded by methodological issues such as retrospective designs and not controlling for confounding variables. What is more, in several studies, peritraumatic dissociation was found to be related to the severity of the experienced threat and subjective-rated fear levels. Together, these results suggest that, instead of being an independent predictor of PTSD, peritraumatic dissociation should be considered an epiphenomenon of peritraumatic distress (see also Fikretoglu et al., 2006) and thus occurring as a result of or in the context of severe threat and extreme emotions (Bernat, Ronfeldt, Calhoun, & Arias, 1998; Friedman, 2000). These findings are in line with the assumptions that dissociation is not a psychopathological, but rather a normal and functional reaction to increased stress. In Linda's case, it would hence seem opportune to educate her about her peritraumatic dissociative reactions by telling her they were normal and even functional in that they helped her survive the threatening events. Yet, although peritraumatic dissociation is normal, functional, and can even be life-saving, it may at some point become dysfunctional.

Sustained Dissociation

While some trauma survivors only experience dissociation during the event, others may continue to feel dissociative feelings well after the trauma. Such sustained dissociation can be dysfunctional as it does not allow adequate emotional processing of the event. For trauma processing to be successful, the feelings of dissociation should fade away within the first weeks after the trauma or at least have become intermittent with only occasional activation of trauma-related emotions. After the abuse had stopped, Linda continued feeling numb and remained unable to feel any negative or positive emotions. Both (sustained) detachment and compartmentalization have been associated with the development of PTSD (Briere, Scott, & Weathers, 2005; Hagenaars et al., 2007) and are also part of the diagnostic symptoms. As a PTSD criterion, amnesia can, for instance, be classified as compartmentalization, while PTSD-related numbing symptoms could be catalogued as detachment. Various studies moreover found that PTSD patients show elevated levels of sustained dissociation, especially after repeated and cumulative traumatization (Cloitre et al., 2009; Hagenaars, Fisch, & van Minnen, 2011).

Theoretically, sustained dissociation after a trauma affects PTSD development by hindering adequate processing of trauma information. For example, dissociation may inhibit adequate elaboration of the event and its sequelae over time, which, along with appraisals, is thought to be necessary for the trauma to be placed into context (Ehlers & Clark, 2000). Additionally, dissociation is related to avoidant coping styles, and avoidance is known to be related to both the development and the maintenance of PTSD (Ehlers & Clark, 2000; Foa & Kozak, 1986; van Minnen & Hagenaars, 2010). Dissociation has also been linked to various factors that contribute to the experience of stress and anxiety, such as neuroticism and frustration tolerance (Modestin, Lotscher, & Erni, 2002), factors that in turn have been found to predict PTSD (Ehlers & Clark, 2000; Ozer et al., 2003).

Empirically, few studies have tested the predictive power of sustained dissociation, but those that did found it to be stronger than peritraumatic dissociation (Briere et al., 2005). However, as no study controlled for the dissociation-related factors, it is not clear whether sustained dissociation is an independent predictor of PTSD or rather an expression of increased distress in those that were vulnerable to begin with (e.g., individuals scoring high on neuroticism). It could, accordingly, be explained to Linda that her dissociative responses at the time the sexual assaults took place were quite normal, but that her persistent dissociative tendencies in relation to these stressful childhood events are more pathological and that it is especially important to address these in therapy and to learn how to diminish or overcome them, given that sustained dissociation, as opposed to peritraumatic dissociation, can be influenced and changed. In the following section, we discuss several interventions aimed at preventing or reducing sustained dissociation.

INTERVENTIONS TO MANAGE SUSTAINED DISSOCIATION

There are several approaches to reducing the (sustained) occurrence of post-trauma dissociation and to promoting an adequate processing of the traumatic events. These include psychoeducation to help the trauma survivor to understand dissociation, preventing sustained dissociation by addressing the factors that induce dissociation, that is, reducing stress and substance abuse and improving sleep quality, as well as cognitive-behavioral interventions directly aimed at the dissociative symptoms, or at the psychopathology associated with the trauma or the dissociation, such as acute stress disorder or PTSD.

Understanding Dissociation: Psychoeducation

The occurrence of dissociative symptoms can be distressing by themselves. Peritraumatic tonic immobility can be particularly frightening and harmful given that it often engenders feelings of guilt and shame. Linda felt both guilty and ashamed because she had not actively resisted her stepfather during the sexual assaults. As a result, she perceived herself as a weak person and thought that it was her fault that the assaults happened. These appraisals can lead to distorted cognitions about one's self or the world (Ehlers & Clark, 2000), including self-blame. In their turn, guilt and self-blame have been related to less recovery from trauma (Frazier, 1990; Ullman, 1997). Psychoeducation with an emphasis on the involuntary nature of defense reactions and the survival function of dissociation may help trauma survivors to overcome these feelings. To stress their adaptive function, it is especially helpful to explain tonic immobility reactions to threat and how they serve survival purposes.

Psychoeducation may also be useful for the survivor's social network. In many cases, survivors will be asked questions like "Why didn't you run away?" or "Why didn't you scream for help?," or say "If it had been me, I would have hit him." Like survivors, the social support system is also unfamiliar with adaptive responses to severe threats. As a result of their questions and their implications that the victim did not act aptly during the trauma, the survivor's self-blame and guilt may be intensified, negatively affecting potentially beneficial social support. One study illustrates this well. McCaul, Veltum, Boyechko, and Crawford (1990) gave college students nine different rape scenarios, with the reports mainly differing in the way the victim had reacted to the assault. Notably, the less the victim had fought back or resisted in the scenario, the more the students blamed the victim. Because we know that social support, especially when it is trauma-related, is very important in preventing posttraumatic stress symptoms, it is crucial to also include the survivor's social network when explaining the adaptive functions of dissociation.

In addition to explaining peritraumatic dissociative reactions, trauma survivors need to be educated about "trauma replay"—that is, that they will probably show the same dissociative reactions when they are confronted with reminders of the trauma. Linda still showed symptoms of tonic immobility when she was reminded of her childhood experiences by watching television shows about sexual abuse. It is important for survivors to be prepared for this phenomenon, and to know that these are natural and normal reactions and no indication of "weakness" or "madness."

Preventing Dissociation: Promoting Stress Management, Improving Sleep Quality, and Reducing Substance Use

Some of the factors known to increase symptoms of dissociation are stress, poor sleep quality, and substance use (dependence or abuse). In trying to prevent or help survivors overcome feelings of dissociation in the aftermath of trauma, it is only logical to also address these factors. Next, we elaborate on these three factors and describe therapeutic techniques.

Promoting Stress Management

Because stress can increase symptoms of dissociation, it is advisable for trauma survivors to learn to reduce stress. However, because typical relaxation exercises require a focus on internal cues (e.g., breathing or flexing and relaxing muscles), it is likely that dissociative symptoms will increase rather than decrease (see also Hunter et al., 2003; Medford et al., 2005). To prevent this from happening, more active forms of relaxation, such as walking, making jigsaw puzzles, swimming, or reading are recommended, where the focus is more external. Looking at our clinical case, since Linda's dissociative problems were worst at night, she could be advised to go for a walk in the evenings. Exercise may have an extra beneficial effect, as there is some experimental evidence from an animal model of PTSD suggesting that physical exercise reduced tonic immobility during or after trauma (Hendriksen, Prins, Olivier, & Oosting, 2010). Since stress can provoke dissociative feelings and individuals with dissociative tendencies are likely to respond with dissociation to stress (Kihlstrom, 2005), it is essential for trauma survivors suffering from these debilitating symptoms to learn to manage stressful situations better. They should be advised to find out what causes them to feel stressed and search for ways to deal with the stress. Often, stress levels can be reduced by making changes in the living situation, relational status, work conditions, or social surroundings, for instance, by temporarily cutting working hours, avoiding stress-inducing parties, and accepting household help. It is important to bear in mind though that some survivors may avoid these situations out of fear or because they trigger traumatic memories: the avoidant behavior helps them maintain stress-related symptoms rather than reduce them. In Linda's case, skipping school activities seems inopportune; instead, her mother could be advised to be flexible to the school's demands on her during busy exam weeks so as not to add to her stress.

Improving Sleep Quality

We probably all know the sensation that, with a lack of sleep, the world seems distant and that if feels as if you are living in a haze. After a sleep deprivation of 36 hours, healthy undergraduates reported dissociative symptoms (Giesbrecht, Merckelbach, Burg, Cima, & Simeon, 2008), and several studies linked self-reported sleep anomalies to self-reported dissociation manifestations (Giesbrecht & Merckelbach, 2006; Watson, 2001). This relationship is also found in clinical populations. Patients with depersonalization disorder, for instance, experienced a worsening of symptoms when they felt tired (Hunter, Baker, Phillips, Sierra, & David, 2005). Sleep disruptions often occur after experiencing a traumatic event, with many victims reporting difficulty falling asleep or waking up. The occurrence of nightmares may also negatively affect sleep. Linda avoided going to sleep, and it is quite possible that her dissociative symptoms were, to a degree, maintained by the resultant lack of sleep, either directly, by causing dissociation, or indirectly, by lowering her stress threshold and diminishing her stress-coping abilities. Normally, sleep problems following a traumatic event are transient, but in some they persist. Persistent posttrauma sleep disturbances may be indicative of psychopathology. Koren, Arnon, Lavie, and Klein (2002) found that disturbed sleep occurring 1 month after trauma exposure was a significant predictor of PTSD diagnosis 12 months later.

In theory, trauma survivors suffering from persistent dissociative symptoms might then benefit from psychological interventions aimed at improving their quality of sleep. This was exactly what Krakow and colleagues (2002) put to the test. They offered 66 adults with PTSD a sleep-targeted therapy 10 months after the Cerro Grande Fire from which they were rescued. The intervention comprised sleep hygiene, that is, improving sleep habits (e.g., no alcohol before bedtime or daytime naps), stimulus control therapy (using the bed for sleeping only and not for watching TV or reading), sleep restriction (setting an allowable time in bed, based on the patient's average sleep time), and cognitive restructuring (see Espie, 2006, for an overview of cognitive-behavioral techniques in overcoming insomnia and sleep problems). The program improved both the sleep problems and PTSD symptoms, including the dissociative symptoms. Linda would then best be advised not to postpone going to bed, but instead to set fixed bedtimes. Linda deferred going to bed because it reminded her of the sexual abuse.

Reducing Substance Use

Associations between trauma exposure or PTSD and substance dependence and abuse have been consistently found in both community and clinical samples (Cougle, Bonn-Miller, Vujanovic, Zvolensky, & Hawkins, 2011; Kessler et al., 1997; Kilpatrick et al., 2000). Of those with lifetime PTSD, 32.7% report substance dependence or abuse (Sledjeski, Speisman, & Dierker, 2008). Vice versa, of those with lifetime alcohol dependence, twice as many people as in the normal population suffer from lifetime PTSD (Kessler et al., 1997). It is suggested that people use substances to help them cope with their trauma-related symptoms. Linda mentioned that she used alcohol to overcome her hypervigilance, resulting in more dissociative symptoms. Empirical studies about motivations for alcohol and drug use in PTSD patients supported this coping hypothesis (Dixon, Leen-Feldner, Ham, Feldner, & Lewis, 2009; Jacobsen, Southwick, & Kosten, 2001; Potter, Vujanovic, Marshall-Berenz, Bernstein, & Bonn-Miller, 2011; Ullman, Filipas, Townsend, & Starzynski, 2006).

Thus, trauma-exposed individuals are at higher risk of substance misuse, with both alcohol and street drugs (e.g., cannabis, ecstasy, LSD) known to have dissociative properties. In healthy individuals, feelings of depersonalization or derealization following intoxication with alcohol and or drugs are common, while for a substantial proportion of patients diagnosed with depersonalization disorder, the onset of their symptoms falls within a short period of illicit drug use (Medford et al., 2003). Besides triggering them, substances tend to also exacerbate dissociative feelings. In depersonalization disorder patients, both alcohol and drugs have been found to do so (Simeon et al., 2003). Linda's sense of numbness was also raised when she had taken too much alcohol. What is more, research has shown that trauma survivors have a heightened risk of a subsequent trauma, often referred to as "revictimization" (Messman-Moore & Long, 2003). This relationship is found to be partially mediated by risk-taking inclinations, such as alcohol-related and sexual risk behaviors (Testa, Hoffman, & Livingston, 2010), which stresses the importance of limiting alcohol and drug use in the aftermath of a trauma.

Besides alcohol and recreational drugs, a large proportion of trauma survivors use benzodiazepines to manage their trauma-associated symptoms (van Minnen, Arntz, & Keijsers, 2002). However, the use of benzodiazepine also has various downsides. First, benzodiazepine use was linked to poorer processing of the traumatic event (van Minnen et al., 2002), thereby maintaining PTSD symptoms. Second, the effects of benzodiazepines resemble those of dissociative symptoms, especially in terms of their numbing effects. In conclusion, because of their sedating effects and the overlap with dissociation symptoms, the use of benzodiazepines and all other sedating substances should be advised against, in particular in trauma survivors with dissociative tendencies.

Reducing Sustained Dissociation: Cognitive-Behavioral Interventions

Little is known about the psychological treatment of dissociative symptoms or disorders, and randomized controlled trials are scarce in this field. However, available treatment programs may help us to develop strategies promoting recovery from sustained, trauma-related dissociative symptoms or enhancement of coping skills. Recently, several cognitive-behavioral therapy (CBT) programs for detachment symptoms have been developed. In an open study Hunter and colleagues (2003) reported the results of CBT in 21 patients with depersonalization disorder. Their manualized program shows great resemblance to existing treatment protocols for panic disorder and included reinterpreting dissociative symptoms in a nonthreatening way, limiting avoidance and safety behavior, and reducing symptom monitoring. This approach led to significant improvement of both dissociative symptoms and related psychopathology. In their model, the authors assume that patients falsely interpret their dissociative symptoms as a harmful rather than as a normal reaction to stress, emotions, and/or lack of sleep. As a result, initial stress and anxiety levels will increase even more, as will the dissociative tendencies. In the same line of reasoning, Goldstein and colleagues (2010) conducted a randomized controlled pilot trial on the effects of CBT for dissociative seizures (a subtype of conversion disorder and a manifestation of compartmentalization). Their 12-session program comprised psychoeducation, attention refocusing, exposure *in vivo* assignments, and cognitive restructuring (Goldstein, Deale, Mitchell-O'Malley, Toone, & Mellers, 2004). The authors reported a significantly higher symptom reduction compared to the reduction obtained with standard medical care (Goldstein et al., 2010).

Derived from these treatment programs, in the aftermath of trauma, survivors can best be advised to not avoid situations or interoceptive (bodily) cues that might evoke dissociative symptoms, but instead approach the challenges. It can be explained to them that in most cases dissociation is connected with stress levels and that dissociative sensations can fluctuate along with the changes in perceived stress. To illustrate that dissociative symptoms can come and go, and that they can be actively induced, one could invite them to do interoceptive exposure exercises, such as staring at a wall, looking in a mirror, or breathing fast and superficially, all activities that are known to increase stress and dissociative phenomena (see also Craske & Barlow, 2008). The exercises may help them gain some sense of control and a better understanding of where these feelings come from. Also, *in vivo* exposure may be recommended in terms of exercises by which they expose themselves to situations they normally avoid out of fear of inducing dissociative manifestations. Finally, they may be persuaded to engage in "behavioral experiments" in which they are encouraged to challenge their (dysfunctional) beliefs about dissociation.

With interoceptive exposure the individual's attention is explicitly drawn to the dissociative manifestations with the goal to first intensify them and thereby educate the patient about the harmlessness of those feelings, to eventually achieve stress reduction. However, when the immediate goal is to reduce dissociation, the best option would be to help the patient focus his or her attention toward external stimuli and thus away from the dissociative symptoms. Task focusing, customarily part of CBT programs for social phobia (Bögels, Mulkens, & De Jong, 1997), may also be considered, given that patients with depersonalization disorder reported the technique had reduced their dissociative symptoms, while self- or symptom focusing had exacerbated them (Simeon et al., 2003). Typically, patients are first instructed to focus on themselves, after which they are invited to direct their attention to a cognitively demanding task, for instance, ordering number cards. As a rule, they will experience the difference in that the self-focus task will increase and the card-ordering task will decrease their symptoms. Since Linda suffered from depersonalization episodes during her schooldays, she may be encouraged to try to focus on her schoolwork rather than on her bodily sensations.

Another approach that promotes a shift from internal to external cues and that is based on the exploitation of the five senses is called "grounding." Grounding techniques are commonly used in clinical CBT care to train coping skills for dissociative symptoms (Linehan, 1993). Basically, the method aims to help the individual to "connect with the present" and focus on the here-and-now, as opposed to feeling numb and detached from the self and the world. There are several grounding techniques, but most utilize the senses. One may, for example, ask the patient to pick out and name three different things he or she sees in the room, to next name three different things he or she physically feels (e.g., the texture of the chair), and to lastly describe three different things he or she hears. This technique helped Linda fall asleep. Instead of focusing on her symptoms and fears, she learned to focus on neutral, external cues. Alternatively, one can use objects with distinct tactile properties (e.g., a rock or stress ball). Patients can be asked to hold an object in their hands and focus on its properties. They can then be instructed to find an object that they can carry with them (e.g., in a pocket). Although obviously deliberate self-harm is not an adequate means to learn to deal with dissociation, more benign forms of self-inflicted bodily sensations can effectively diminish dissociative feelings. One may have the patient hold an ice cube in his or her hand, or have him or her put a hand in icy water, for instance. Another option is to ask the patient to wear an elastic band around the wrist; pulling the band will give a sharp pang of pain that may help him or her to stay focused on the present.

There are some indications that mindfulness-based approaches combining task-focusing elements and grounding techniques focusing on the senses could also be helpful in overcoming dissociation, especially emotional numbing (Follette, Palm, & Pearson, 2006; Kimbrough, Magyari, Langenberg, Chesney, & Berman, 2010; Thompson & Waltz, 2010). Examples of mindfulness exercises are attentional breathing, easy yoga exercises, the "body scan," mindful tooth brushing or mindful walking (for more information, see Orsillo & Roemer, 2011).

Treating Trauma-Related Psychopathology

Although some manifestations of trauma-related symptoms, such as reexperiencing, avoidance, and increased arousal are quite normal in the direct aftermath of a trauma, sustained and severe dissociation might be an indication of dissociation- or trauma-related psychopathology. For both acute stress disorder (ASD) and PTSD trauma-focused cognitive-behavioral treatments and exposure-based programs in particular are found to be effective in reducing all PTSD-associated symptoms, including numbing and dissociation (Bryant, Friedman, Spiegel, Ursano, & Strain, 2010; Powers, Halpern, Ferenschak, Gillihan, & Foa, 2010). Unfortunately, in clinical decision making, ASD and PTSD patients who suffer from (severe) dissociative symptoms are less likely to be referred for trauma-focused treatment, the reason being that effective treatment is thought to be complicated or hindered by the dissociative symptoms, even though there is little empirical evidence to support this belief. Hagenaars and colleagues (2010) examined the effects of dissociation (detachment) on treatment outcome of exposure therapy for PTSD. Pretreatment dissociative symptoms (trait dissociation, depersonalization, and emotional numbing) were found *not to predict* treatment outcome. As opposed to the widely held clinical view that dissociation is a contraindication, this study revealed that even patients suffering from severe dissociation benefited from exposure treatment. What is more, although the standard exposure treatment was offered, without any modifications for dissociative symptoms, dissociative symptoms also decreased significantly during treatment. Linda received 12 sessions of prolonged exposure (a variant of trauma-focused exposure therapy) for her PTSD, and as a result not only her PTSD symptoms, among which were nightmares and hyperarousal, had declined significantly, but so had her feelings of detachment, depersonalization, and derealization.

As for compartmentalization, there is some indication that tonic immobility negatively affects treatment outcome (Fiszman et al., 2008; Lanius et al., 2010; Lima et al., 2010). Yet, as with detachment symptoms, when baseline PTSD symptoms are controlled for, the predictive value of tonic immobility seems to disappear (van Minnen, Hagenaars, & De Kleine, 2010), making it more likely that, rather than being an independent predictor of treatment outcome, tonic immobility is related to PTSD symptom severity. Several clinical cases have even shown that it is possible to treat PTSD patients successfully when they also suffer from severe compartmentalization symptoms such as conversion mutism (Rothbaum & Foa, 1991) or conversion paralysis (Hendriks, de Kleine, van Rees, Bult, & van Minnen, 2010).

The above-mentioned PTSD studies all used standardized CBT programs that were not adapted to patients scoring high on dissociation measures. All trauma-focused treatments include confrontation with the traumatic memory and are thereby stress-inducing by nature. As mentioned earlier, people with dissociative tendencies are likely to respond to stress with dissociation (Kihlstrom, 2005), and they are hence likely to also do so during the exposure. But how do you cope with dissociation during the exposure sessions? Emotional processing theory (Foa & Kozak, 1986) posits that fear activation is necessary to effectively treat anxiety disorders. Factors that impede fear activation would, logically, have a negative impact on treatment outcome. Dissociative symptoms, such as numbing, can interfere with fear activation. Some studies showed that, when dissociation occurs, patients are likely to respond with high subjective fear levels (Griffin, Resick, & Mechanic, 1997; Hagenaars et al., 2010), but with low physiological stress (Griffin et al., 1997), which may indicate that the complete fear structure is not activated, potentially negatively affecting the treatment results. Still, in the Hagenaars and colleagues (2010) study where no explicit techniques were employed to reduce dissociation, dissociative patients who responded with high subjective levels of fear did improve to the same degree as those without dissociation reporting lower fear levels. Nevertheless, the manual for prolonged exposure (Foa, Hembree, & Rothbaum, 2007) prescribes several techniques to regulate anxiety levels, although these are not unique for dissociative patients but general, standard procedures to help the patient adequately process the traumatic memory. These techniques are described below.

As previously stated, dissociative symptoms are most likely to occur when anxiety levels are high. In most cases, patients are fully capable of noticing the onset of dissociation and indicate this to the therapist, for example, by raising a finger. When conducting imaginal exposure, the first step for the therapist would then be to reduce the anxiety by reducing the vividness of the traumatic memory, hence lowering the emotional response. Here it may be beneficial to instruct the patient to use the past tense and third-person singular (as opposed to the present tense and first person) during the narrations, or to project the sequence of events on a wall "as if you are watching a movie," and to keep the eyes open. For most patients, these techniques suffice, but when they do not, the therapist could incorporate grounding exercises. Again, after the patient has signaled that he or she is starting to feel dissociated, the therapist can pause the exposure exercise and start a grounding exercise. It is recommended to have an indexing method at hand to quantify the severity of the dissociative symptoms, for example, by having the patient rate current manifestations on a scale from 0 to 10. If the dissociative sensations have diminished after the grounding exercise, exposure can be resumed. There is no hard-and-fast rule as to what constitutes an acceptable level of dissociation for exposure to be continued. In general, it is advisable to explain the rationale of exposure to the patient prior to the exposure, stressing that to some extent he or she can dissociate during the exposure, but that it is important that he or she remain able to learn things from it. The patient can then be asked before the start of a session to indicate the level of dissociation (0–10) he or she thinks he or she can handle and at which point learning is likely to be impeded.

In conclusion, in addition to or instead of cognitive-behavioral interventions directly addressing dissociative symptoms, CBT programs aimed at reducing dissociation- or trauma-related psychopathology, such as ASD and PTSD, are similarly appropriate for reducing dissociative tendencies. In case dissociation prevents the patient from experiencing the fear levels deemed appropriate for adequate trauma processing, simple dissociation-reducing strategies to modify anxiety levels or "grounding" exercises can be applied.

SUMMARY AND CLINICAL RECOMMENDATIONS

Taking all things together, the information described in this chapter showed that dissociation and trauma are closely linked and that dissociation may take various forms. Several key points have been raised:

1. *Dissociation is a common and normal experience in the immediate aftermath of trauma.* Symptoms of dissociation can manifest themselves at a *cognitive* level and also on a more *somatic* level, but typically occur in combination. Generally, two types of dissociation are distinguished: *detachment* and *compartmentalization*, and both can occur during and after a traumatic event. Although the two phenomena are quite common and considered typical and even functional responses to severe threat and stress, not many people are familiar with the symptoms, which is why it is highly relevant to *educate* survivors about dissociation in the aftermath of a trauma. Because dissociation during or some time after the trauma is normal and not indicative of psychopathology, no specific interventions are needed at that stage.

2. *Persistent dissociation may impair recovery and initial intervention should focus on factors that may mitigate dissociation.* However, when a trauma survivor continues feeling dissociated regularly, this may hinder him or her to emotionally process the trauma, which does warrant attention. The first line of intervention, then, is to prevent symptoms from being sustained any further by influencing the factors that are known to be connected with dissociative tendencies. Trauma survivors should be advised to learn to manage or lower *stress* levels, to make sure they *sleep* well, and to refrain from using any sedating *substances*.

3. *Continued persistent dissociation may be responsive to reducing avoidance of, and instead approaching, situations and cues that initiate dissociation and shifting focus to external cues.* If they continue to feel dissociated, *cognitive-behavioral interventions* that specifically aim to reduce dissociation may be called for. During therapy, survivors should be advised *to not avoid* situations or interoceptive cues that tend to initiate dissociative feelings but instead approach them. Facing these triggers will help them to understand how dissociation works, thereby giving them more control over their responses: the dissociation and avoidance behavior will not be

maintained, decreasing the risk of sustained symptoms leading to psycho-pathology. Learning to cope with dissociation also requires a greater *focus on external cues*. This may be achieved by simple *task-focusing* exercises and exercises exploiting *the senses*, which may help trauma survivors over-come situations in which they tend to become overwhelmed, prompting dissociative responses.

4. *Treatment for trauma-related psychopathology, particularly cogni-tive-behavioral interventions, reduce dissociation*. Finally, if despite these interventions dissociation persists or other symptoms become apparent, screening for *trauma-related psychopathology*, for instance, acute stress disorder and posttraumatic stress disorder, is recommended. There are highly effective *cognitive-behavioral treatments* available for both condi-tions that have been shown to also significantly reduce symptoms of dis-sociation.

REFERENCES

Abrams, M. P., Carleton, R. N., Taylor, S., & Asmundson, G. J. (2009). Human tonic immobility: Measurement and correlates. *Depression and Anxiety, 26*(6), 550–556.

Allen, J. G. (2001). *Traumatic relationships and serious mental disorders*. New York: Wiley.

American Psychiatric Association. (2013). *Diagnostic and statistical manual of mental disorders* (5th ed.). Arlington, VA: Author.

Bernat, J. A., Ronfeldt, H. M., Calhoun, K. S., & Arias, I. (1998). Prevalence of traumatic events and peritraumatic predictors of posttraumatic stress symp-toms in a nonclinical sample of college students. *Journal of Traumatic Stress, 11*(4), 645–664.

Bögels, S. M., Mulkens, S., & De Jong, P. J. (1997). Task concentration training and fear of blushing. *Clinical Psychology and Psychotherapy, 4*(4), 251–258.

Bovin, M. J., Jager-Hyman, S., Gold, S. D., Marx, B. P., & Sloan, D. M. (2008). Tonic immobility mediates the influence of peritraumatic fear and perceived inescapability on posttraumatic stress symptom severity among sexual assault survivors. *Journal of Traumatic Stress, 21*(4), 402–409.

Bracha, H. (2004). Freeze, flight, fight, fright, faint: Adaptationist perspectives on the acute stress response spectrum. *CNS Spectrums, 9*(9), 679–685.

Brewin, C. R., & Saunders, J. (2001). The effect of dissociation at encoding on intrusive memories for a stressful film. *British Journal of Medical Psychology, 74*(4), 467–472.

Briere, J., Scott, C., & Weathers, F. (2005). Peritraumatic and persistent disso-ciation in the presumed etiology of PTSD. *American Journal of Psychiatry, 162*(12), 2295–2301.

Brown, R. J. (2002). The cognitive psychology of dissociative states. *Cognitive Neuropsychiatry, 7*(3), 221–235.

Bryant, R. A., Friedman, M. J., Spiegel, D., Ursano, R., & Strain, J. (2010). A review of acute stress disorder in DSM-5. *Depression and Anxiety, 28*(9), 802–817.

Burgess, A. W., & Holmstrom, L. L. (1976). Coping behavior of the rape victim. *American Journal of Psychiatry, 133*(4), 413–418.

Candel, I., & Merckelbach, H. (2004). Peritraumatic dissociation as a predictor of posttraumatic stress disorder: A critical review. *Comprehensive Psychiatry, 45*(1), 44–50.

Cardeña, E. (1994). The domain of dissociation. In S. J. Lynn & J. W. Rhue (Eds.), *Dissociation: Clinical and theoretical perspectives* (pp. 15–31). New York: Guilford Press.

Carlson, E. B., & Putnam, F. W. (1993). An update on the Dissociative Experiences Scale. *Dissociation, 6*, 16–27.

Cloitre, M., Stolbach, B. C., Herman, J. L., van der Kolk, B., Pynoos, R., Wang, J., et al. (2009). A developmental approach to complex PTSD: Childhood and adult cumulative trauma as predictors of symptom complexity. *Journal of Traumatic Stress, 22*(5), 399–408.

Cougle, J. R., Bonn-Miller, M. O., Vujanovic, A. A., Zvolensky, M. J., & Hawkins, K. A. (2011). Posttraumatic stress disorder and cannabis use in a nationally representative sample. *Psychology of Addictive Behaviors, 25*(3), 554–558.

Craske, M. G., & Barlow, D. H. (2008). Panic disorder and agoraphobia. In D. H. Barlow (Ed.), *Clinical handbook of psychological disorders: A step-by-step treatment manual* (4th ed., pp. 1–64). New York: Guilford Press.

De Kleine, R. A., & van Minnen, A. (2013). *Susceptibility to tonic immobility: Fright in stressful situations and anxious dreams.* Manuscript in preparation.

Dixon, L. J., Leen-Feldner, E. W., Ham, L. S., Feldner, M. T., & Lewis, S. F. (2009). Alcohol use motives among traumatic event-exposed, treatment-seeking adolescents: Associations with posttraumatic stress. *Addictive Behaviors, 34*(12), 1065–1068.

Ehlers, A., & Clark, D. M. (2000). A cognitive model of posttraumatic stress disorder. *Behaviour Research and Therapy, 38*(4), 319–345.

Espie, C. A. (2006). *Overcoming insomnia and sleep problems: A self-help guide using cognitive behavioral techniques.* London: Robinson.

Fikretoglu, D., Brunet, A., Best, S., Metzler, T., Delucchi, K., Weiss, D. S., et al. (2006). The relationship between peritraumatic distress and peritraumatic dissociation: an examination of two competing models. *Journal of Nervous and Mental Disease, 194*(11), 853–858.

Fiszman, A., Mendlowicz, M. V., Marques-Portella, C., Volchan, E., Coutinho, E. S., Souza, W. F., et al. (2008). Peritraumatic tonic immobility predicts a poor response to pharmacological treatment in victims of urban violence with PTSD. *Journal of Affective Disorders, 107*(1–3), 193–197.

Foa, E. B., Hembree, E. A., & Rothbaum, B. O. (2007). *Prolonged exposure therapy for PTSD: Emotional processing of traumatic experiences: Therapist guide.* New York: Oxford University Press.

Foa, E. B., & Kozak, M. J. (1986). Emotional processing of fear: Exposure to corrective information. *Psychological Bulletin, 99*(1), 20–35.

Follette, V., Palm, K. M., & Pearson, A. N. (2006). Mindfulness and trauma: Implications for treatment. *Journal of Rational-Emotive and Cognitive Behavior Therapy, 24*(1), 45–61.

Frazier, P. A. (1990). Victim attributions and post-rape trauma. *Journal of Personality and Social Psychology, 59*(2), 298–304.

Friedman, M. J. (2000). What might the psychobiology of posttraumatic stress disorder teach us about future approaches to pharmacotherapy? *Journal of Clinical Psychiatry, 61*(Suppl. 7), 44–51.

Fuse, T., Forsyth, J., Marx, B., Gallup, G., & Weaver, S. (2007). Factor structure of the Tonic Immobility Scale in female sexual assault survivors: An exploratory and confirmatory factor analysis. *Journal of Anxiety Disorders, 21*(3), 265–283.

Galliano, G., Noble, L. M., Travis, L. A., & Puechl, C. (1993). Victim reactions during rape/sexual assault: A preliminary study of the immobility response and its correlates. *Journal of Interpersonal Violence, 8*(1), 109–114.

Gallup, G. G. (1977). Tonic immobility: The role of fear and predation [Special issue]. *Psychological Record, 27*, 41–61.

Giesbrecht, T., & Merckelbach, H. (2006). Dreaming to reduce fantasy?: Fantasy proneness, dissociation, and subjective sleep experiences. *Personality and Individual Differences, 41*(4), 697–706.

Giesbrecht, T., Merckelbach, H., Burg, L. T., Cima, M., & Simeon, D. (2008). Acute dissociation predicts rapid habituation of skin conductance responses to aversive auditory probes. *Journal of Traumatic Stress, 21*(2), 247–250.

Goldstein, L. H., Chalder, T., Chigwedere, C., Khondoker, M. R., Moriarty, J., Toone, B. K., et al. (2010). Cognitive-behavioral therapy for psychogenic non-epileptic seizures: A pilot RCT. *Neurology, 74*(24), 1986–1994.

Goldstein, L. H., Deale, A. C., Mitchell-O'Malley, S. J., Toone, B. K., & Mellers, J. D. (2004). An evaluation of cognitive behavioral therapy as a treatment for dissociative seizures: A pilot study. *Cognitive and Behavioral Neurology, 17*(1), 41–49.

Griffin, M. G., Resick, P. A., & Mechanic, M. B. (1997). Objective assessment of peritraumatic dissociation: Psychophysiological indicators. *American Journal of Psychiatry, 154*(8), 1081–1088.

Grond, M., Pawlik, G., Walter, H., Lesch, O. M., & Heiss, W. D. (1995). Hypnotic catalepsy-induced changes of regional cerebral glucose metabolism. *Psychiatry Research: Neuroimaging, 61*(3), 173–179.

Hagenaars, M. A., Fisch, I., & van Minnen, A. (2011). The effect of trauma onset and frequency on PTSD-associated symptoms. *Journal of Affective Disorders, 132*, 192–199.

Hagenaars, M. A., van Minnen, A., Holmes, E., Brewin, C. R., & Hoogduin, K. A. (2008). The effect of hypnotically induced somatoform dissociation on the development of intrusions after an aversive film. *Cognition and Emotion, 22*(5), 944–963.

Hagenaars, M. A., van Minnen, A., & Hoogduin, K. A. (2007). Peritraumatic psychological and somatoform dissociation in predicting PTSD symptoms: A prospective study. *Journal of Nervous and Mental Disease, 195*(11), 952–954.

Hagenaars, M. A., van Minnen, A., & Hoogduin, K. A. L. (2010). The impact of dissociation and depression on the efficacy of prolonged exposure treatment for PTSD. *Behaviour Research and Therapy, 48*(1), 19–27.

Heidt, J., Marx, B., & Forsyth, J. (2005). Tonic immobility and childhood sexual abuse: A preliminary report evaluating the sequela of rape-induced paralysis. *Behaviour Research and Therapy, 43*(9), 1157–1171.

Hendriks, L., de Kleine, R., van Rees, M., Bult, C., & van Minnen, A. (2010). Feasibility of brief intensive exposure therapy for PTSD patients with childhood sexual abuse: A brief clinical report. *European Journal of Psychotraumatology, 1,* 5626.

Hendriksen, H., Prins, J., Olivier, B., & Oosting, R. S. (2010). Environmental enrichment induces behavioral recovery and enhanced hippocampal cell proliferation in an antidepressant-resistant animal model for PTSD. *PLoS ONE, 5*(8), e11943.

Holmes, E., Brewin, C. R., & Hennessy, R. G. (2004). Trauma films, information processing, and intrusive memory development. *Journal of Experimental Psychology: General, 133*(1), 3–22.

Holmes, E., Brown, R., Mansell, W., Fearon, R., Hunter, E. C. M., Frasquilho, F., et al. (2005). Are there two qualitatively distinct forms of dissociation?: A review and some clinical implications. *Clinical Psychology Review, 25*(1), 1–23.

Holmes, E., & Steel, C. (2004). Schizotypy: A vulnerability factor for traumatic intrusions. *Journal of Nervous and Mental Disease, 192*(1), 28–34.

Hunter, E. C. M., Baker, D., Phillips, M., Sierra, M., & David, A. (2005). Cognitive-behaviour therapy for depersonalisation disorder: An open study. *Behaviour Research and Therapy, 43*(9), 1121–1130.

Hunter, E. C. M., Phillips, M. L., Chalder, T., Sierra, M., & David, A. S. (2003). Depersonalisation disorder: A cognitive-behavioural conceptualisation. *Behaviour Research and Therapy, 41*(12), 1451–1467.

Hunter, E. C. M., Sierra, M., & David, A. S. (2004). The epidemiology of depersonalisation and derealisation. *Social Psychiatry and Psychiatric Epidemiology, 39*(1), 9–18.

Jacobsen, L. K., Southwick, S. M., & Kosten, T. R. (2001). Substance use disorders in patients with posttraumatic stress disorder: A review of the literature. *American Journal of Psychiatry, 158*(8), 1184–1190.

Kallio, S., Revonsuo, A., Hamalainen, H., Markela, J., & Gruzelier, J. (2001). Anterior brain functions and hypnosis: A test of the frontal hypothesis. *International Journal of Clinical and Experimental Hypnosis, 49*(2), 95–108.

Kennedy, F., Clarke, S., Stopa, L., Bell, L., Rouse, H., Ainsworth, C., et al. (2004). Towards a cognitive model and measure of dissociation. *Journal of Behavior Therapy and Experimental Psychiatry, 35*(1), 25–48.

Kessler, R. C., Crum, R. M., Warner, L. A., Nelson, C. B., Schulenberg, J., & Anthony, J. C. (1997). Lifetime co-occurrence of DSM-III-R alcohol abuse and dependence with other psychiatric disorders in the National Comorbidity Survey. *Archives of General Psychiatry, 54*(4), 313–321.

Kihlstrom, J. F. (2005). Dissociative disorders. *Annual Review of Clinical Psychology, 1*(1), 227–253.

Kilpatrick, D. G., Acierno, R., Saunders, B., Resnick, H. S., Best, C. L., & Schnurr, P. P. (2000). Risk factors for adolescent substance abuse and dependence: Data from a national sample. *Journal of Consulting and Clinical Psychology, 68*(1), 19–30.

Kimbrough, E., Magyari, T., Langenberg, P., Chesney, M., & Berman, B. (2010).

Mindfulness intervention for child abuse survivors. *Journal of Clinical Psychology, 66*(1), 17–33.

Koren, D., Arnon, I., Lavie, P., & Klein, E. (2002). Sleep complaints as early predictors of posttraumatic stress disorder: A 1-year prospective study of injured survivors of motor vehicle accidents. *American Journal of Psychiatry, 159*(5), 855–857.

Krakow, B. J., Melendrez, D. C., Johnston, L. G., Clark, J. O., Santana, E. M., Warner, T. D., et al. (2002). Sleep dynamic therapy for Cerro Grande Fire evacuees with posttraumatic stress symptoms: A preliminary report. *Journal of Clinical Psychiatry, 63*(8), 673–684.

Lanius, R. A., Vermetten, E., Loewenstein, R. J., Brand, B., Schmahl, C., Bremner, J., et al. (2010). Emotion modulation in PTSD: Clinical and neurobiological evidence for a dissociative subtype. *American Journal of Psychiatry, 167*(6), 640–647.

Lilienfeld, S. O., & Lynn, S. J. (2003). Dissociative identity disorder: Multiple personalities, multiple controversies. In S. O. Lilienfeld, S. J. Lynn, & J. M. Lohr (Eds.), *Science and pseudoscience in clinical psychology* (pp. 109–142). New York: Guilford Press.

Lima, A. A., Fiszman, A., Marques-Portella, C., Mendlowicz, M. V., Coutinho, E. S., Maia, D. C., et al. (2010). The impact of tonic immobility reaction on the prognosis of posttraumatic stress disorder. *Journal of Psychiatric Research, 44*(4), 224–228.

Linehan, M. M. (1993). *Skills training manual for treating borderline personality disorder.* New York: Guilford Press.

Marks, I. M. (1987). *Fears, phobias, and rituals: Panic, anxiety, and their disorders.* New York: Oxford University Press.

Marshall, G. N., & Schell, T. L. (2002). Reappraising the link between peritraumatic dissociation and PTSD symptom severity: Evidence from a longitudinal study of community violence survivors. *Journal of Abnormal Psychology, 111*(4), 626–636.

Marx, B. P., Forsyth, J. P., Gallup, G. G., Fuse, T., & Lexington, J. M. (2008). Tonic immobility as an evolved predator defense: Implications for sexual assault survivors. *Clinical Psychology: Science and Practice, 15*(1), 74–90.

McCaul, K. D., Veltum, L. G., Boyechko, V., & Crawford, J. J. (1990). Understanding attributions of victim blame for rape: Sex, violence, and foreseeability. *Journal of Applied Social Psychology, 20*(1), 1–26.

McNally, R. J. (2003). *Remembering trauma.* Cambridge, MA: Harvard University Press.

Medford, N., Baker, D., Hunter, E., Sierra, M., Lawrence, E., Phillips, M. L., et al. (2003). Chronic depersonalization following illicit drug use: A controlled analysis of 40 cases. *Addiction, 98*(12), 1731–1736.

Medford, N., Sierra, M., Baker, D., & David, A. S. (2005). Understanding and treating depersonalisation disorder. *Advances in Psychiatric Treatment, 11*(2), 92–100.

Messman-Moore, T. L., & Long, P. J. (2003). The role of childhood sexual abuse sequelae in the sexual revictimization of women: An empirical review and theoretical reformulation. *Clinical Psychology Review, 23*(4), 537–571.

Modestin, J., & Erni, T. (2004). Testing the dissociative taxon. *Psychiatry Research, 126*(1), 77–82.

Modestin, J., Lotscher, K., & Erni, T. (2002). Dissociative experiences and their correlates in young non-patients. *Psychology and Psychotherapy: Theory, Research and Practice, 75*(1), 53–64.

Nijenhuis, E. R., Spinhoven, P., Vanderlinden, J., van Dyck, R., & van der Hart, O. (1998). Somatoform dissociative symptoms as related to animal defensive reactions to predatory imminence and injury. *Journal of Abnormal Psychology, 107*(1), 63–73.

Nijenhuis, E. R., Spinhoven, P., Van Dyck, R., Van Der Hart, O., & Vanderlinden, J. (1996). The development and psychometric characteristics of the Somatoform Dissociation Questionnaire (SDQ-20). *Journal of Nervous and Mental Disease, 184*(11), 688–694.

Orsillo, S. M., & Roemer, L. (2011). *The mindful way through anxiety: Break free from chronic worry and reclaim your life.* New York: Guilford Press.

Ozer, E. J., Best, S. R., Lipsey, T. L., & Weiss, D. S. (2003). Predictors of posttraumatic stress disorder and symptoms in adults: A meta-analysis. *Psychological Bulletin, 129*(1), 52–73.

Potter, C. M., Vujanovic, A. A., Marshall-Berenz, E. C., Bernstein, A., & Bonn-Miller, M. O. (2011). Posttraumatic stress and marijuana use coping motives: The mediating role of distress tolerance. *Journal of Anxiety Disorders, 25*(3), 437–443.

Powers, M. B., Halpern, J. M., Ferenschak, M. P., Gillihan, S. J., & Foa, E. B. (2010). A meta-analytic review of prolonged exposure for posttraumatic stress disorder. *Clinical Psychology Review, 30*(6), 635–641.

Putnam, F. W. (1989). Pierre Janet and modern views of dissociation. *Journal of Traumatic Stress, 2*(4), 413–429.

Putnam, F. W. (1997). *Dissociation in children and adolescents: A developmental perspective.* New York: Guilford Press.

Regambal, M. J., & Alden, L. E. (2009). Pathways to intrusive memories in a trauma analogue paradigm: A structural equation model. *Depression and Anxiety, 26*(2), 155–166.

Rizvi, S. L., Kaysen, D., Gutner, C. A., Griffin, M. G., & Resick, P. A. (2008). Beyond fear: The role of peritraumatic responses in posttraumatic stress and depressive symptoms among female crime victims. *Journal of Interpersonal Violence, 23*(6), 853–868.

Rocha-Rego, V., Fiszman, A., Portugal, L. C., Garcia Pereira, M., de Oliveira, L., Mendlowicz, M. V., et al. (2009). Is tonic immobility the core sign among conventional peritraumatic signs and symptoms listed for PTSD? *Journal of Affective Disorders, 115*(1–2), 269–273.

Roelofs, K., Spinhoven, P., Sandijck, P., Moene, F. C., & Hoogduin, K. A. L. (2005). The impact of early trauma and recent life-events on symptom severity in patients with conversion disorder. *Journal of Nervous and Mental Disease, 193*(8), 508–514.

Roelofs, K., van Galen, G. P., Keijsers, G. P., & Hoogduin, C. A. (2002). Motor initiation and execution in patients with conversion paralysis. *Acta Psychologica, 110*(1), 21–34.

Ross, C. A. (1996). Epidemiology of dissociation in children and adolescents: Extrapolations and speculations. *Child and Adolescent Psychiatric Clinics of North America, 5*(2), 273–284.

Ross, C. A., Duffy, C. M., & Ellason, J. W. (2002). Prevalence, reliability and validity of dissociative disorders in an inpatient setting. *Journal of Trauma and Dissociation, 3*(1), 7–17.

Rothbaum, B. O., & Foa, E. B. (1991). Exposure treatment of PTSD concomitant with conversion mutism: A case study. *Behavior Therapy, 22*(3), 449–456.

Schauer, M., & Elbert, T. (2010). Dissociation following traumatic stress. *Zeitschrift für Psychologie/Journal of Psychology, 218*(2), 109–127.

Schmidt, N., Richey, J., Zvolensky, M., & Maner, J. (2008). Exploring human freeze responses to a threat stressor. *Journal of Behavior Therapy and Experimental Psychiatry, 39*(3), 292–304.

Sierra, M., & Berrios, G. E. (1998). Depersonalization: Neurobiological perspectives. *Biological Psychiatry, 44*(9), 898–908.

Simeon, D., Knutelska, M., Nelson, D., & Guralnik, O. (2003). Feeling unreal: A depersonalization disorder update of 117 cases. *Journal of Clinical Psychiatry, 64*, 990–997.

Sledjeski, E., Speisman, B., & Dierker, L. (2008). Does number of lifetime traumas explain the relationship between PTSD and chronic medical conditions?: Answers from the National Comorbidity Survey—Replication (NCS-R). *Journal of Behavioral Medicine, 31*(4), 341–349.

Spitzer, C., Barnow, S., Grabe, H. J., Klauer, T., Stieglitz, R.-D., Schneider, W., et al. (2006). Frequency, clinical and demographic correlates of pathological dissociation in Europe. *Journal of Trauma and Dissociation, 7*(1), 51–62.

Testa, M., Hoffman, J. H., & Livingston, J. A. (2010). Alcohol and sexual risk behaviors as mediators of the sexual victimization–revictimization relationship. *Journal of Consulting and Clinical Psychology, 78*(2), 249–259.

Thompson, B. L., & Waltz, J. (2010). Mindfulness and experiential avoidance as predictors of posttraumatic stress disorder avoidance symptom severity. *Journal of Anxiety Disorders, 24*(4), 409–415.

Ullman, S. E. (1997). Attributions, world assumptions, and recovery from sexual assault. *Journal of Child Sexual Abuse: Research, Treatment, and Program Innovations for Victims, Survivors, and Offenders, 6*(1), 1–19.

Ullman, S. E., Filipas, H. H., Townsend, S. M., & Starzynski, L. L. (2006). Correlates of comorbid PTSD and drinking problems among sexual assault survivors. *Addictive Behaviors, 31*(1), 128–132.

van der Kolk, B. A., & van der Hart, O. (1989). Pierre Janet and the breakdown of adaptation in psychological trauma. *American Journal of Psychiatry, 146*(12), 1530–1540.

van der Velden, P. G., & Wittmann, L. (2008). The independent predictive value of peritraumatic dissociation for PTSD symptomatology after type I trauma: A systematic review of prospective studies. *Clinical Psychology Review, 28*(6), 1009–1020.

van Minnen, A., Arntz, A., & Keijsers, G. P. J. (2002). Prolonged exposure in patients with chronic PTSD: Predictors of treatment outcome and dropout. *Behaviour Research and Therapy, 40*(4), 439–457.

van Minnen, A., & Hagenaars, M. A. (2010). Avoidance behaviour of patients with posttraumatic stress disorder: Initial development of a questionnaire, psychometric properties and treatment sensitivity. *Journal of Behavior Therapy and Experimental Psychiatry, 41*(3), 191–198.

van Minnen, A., Hagenaars, M. A., & De Kleine, R. A. (2010, November). *Prolonged exposure therapy for PTSD in patients with dissociative and/or conversion symptoms.* Paper presented at the annual conference of the Association for Behavioral and Cognitive Therapies, San Francisco.

Waller, G., Ohanian, V., Meyer, C., Everill, J., & Rouse, H. (2001). The utility of dimensional and categorical approaches to understanding dissociation in the eating disorders. *British Journal of Clinical Psychology, 40*(4), 387–397.

Watson, D. (2001). Dissociations of the night: Individual differences in sleep-related experiences and their relation to dissociation and schizotypy. *Journal of Abnormal Psychology, 110*(4), 526–535.

World Health Organization. (1992). Chapter 5: Mental and behavioral disorders, diagnostic criteria and diagnostic guidelines. *International classification of disorders: Clinical descriptions and diagnostic guidelines (ICD-10).* Geneva: World Health Organization, Divison of Mental Health.

Zoellner, L. A., Sacks, M. B., & Foa, E. B. (2001). Stability of emotions for traumatic memories in acute and chronic PTSD. *Behaviour Research and Therapy, 39*(6), 697–711.

Chapter 11

Avoidance

Lori A. Zoellner, Elizabeth H. Marks,
Janie J. Jun, *and* Hillary L. Smith

Ande, a 36-year-old African American woman, was brutally raped in her home. In the middle of the night, a perpetrator, a tall Hispanic male, broke a bathroom window and crawled into her house. She awoke with the masked perpetrator standing next to her bed holding a knife. He told her that if she made a noise, he would kill her and her kids sleeping in the room next door. He then gagged her and repeatedly raped her. He left her tied up in the bed, but left the kids unharmed. After Ande reported the rape to the police, she was taken to the local emergency room, and a victim's assistance officer suggested that she contact our center. She then had a friend go to her house, board up the window, and get clothes for her and the kids. Ande moved into her mother's house because she couldn't bear to go back to "that place." In the days following the event, no matter what she did she couldn't get the image of the masked man out of her mind. Even things in her mother's home that were similar to her own furnishings (e.g., similar photographs to those in her home) reminded her of the incident and made her paralyzed by fear. Every time she saw the perpetrator's masked face in her mind, she was overwhelmed with intense fear and disgust. She tried to keep busy by going back to work, cleaning her mother's house, and focusing on her kids. However, the more she tried not to think about the rape, the more the memories seemed to haunt her. She also couldn't bring herself to go back to the house but also worried that she couldn't sell it and move to another place. The police caught the perpetrator when he was attempting to break into another house. Nevertheless, she was still afraid. After talking with her mom, they devised a plan where they would go back to the home together at different times during the day, working to improve the home's security and fixing the window. They started going back to the home at night and eventually spent the night together there. Ande decided to buy a new bed and moved her bedroom into another room in the house. They also completely changed the color and furnishings in the old bedroom, turning it into a family game room. After a while, she moved back into the house with her family. Although it was initially hard, when she was barraged by thoughts or images of that night, she allowed herself to experience them and tried not to block whatever emotions came along with the thoughts. She also reached out to her mom when these things happened and honestly shared what she was thinking and feeling. Three months after the rape, she was doing well and didn't need treatment for posttraumatic stress disorder (PTSD).[1]

Ande is a clear example of how recovery, even after a horrific event, can occur without professional intervention. Despite her fear, Ande was able to take the steps she needed to take to help her recover, eventually resuming her preassault roles and activities. Yet, we see in this example the profound tendency to avoid activities, situations, and places that remind the survivor of the trauma. Avoidance not only minimizes encounters with reminders of the trauma, but also potentially minimizes the likelihood of the trauma reoccurring. The avoidance patterns that develop after trauma exposure are highly related to the characteristics of the event itself and, even within a specific type of event, may be highly idiosyncratic. Thus, events that share common features often have similar patterns of avoidance, though variations exist based on a trauma survivor's own experiences. For example, individuals who have been in a motor vehicle accident may tend to avoid driving or riding in a car, specific types of roads such as highways, or specific driving conditions such as driving in the dark or in the rain. There also may be avoidance that is very specific to an individual's accident, such as avoiding having a passenger in the car, listening to the radio, or letting someone talk to the driver. Regardless of the type of traumatic event, both common and idiographic patterns of avoidance often emerge very soon after trauma exposure.

Avoidance soon after the trauma helps decrease fear and panic but also has profound consequences for the trauma survivor. Although Ande's

---

[1]This case represents a mixture from several clients whom we have seen in our clinical work. Case details have been altered to conceal client identities and any resemblance to a specific individual is purely coincidental.

avoidance was localized to specific trauma-related stimuli, it is easy to imagine how her avoidance could generalize to other stimuli such as being afraid to leave the house alone, keeping her kids close to her at all times, and being afraid of men. The long-term consequences of avoidance can be highly detrimental, restricting a trauma survivor's ability to function in the world, limiting his or her activities and interests, and leading to further depression. Many trauma survivors resonate with the analogy that trauma-related fear and avoidance feels like "living in a cave." This analogy is à propos in that a cave provides safety from danger and shelter from storms but at the same time is a dark, cold, and generally lifeless place.

It is no surprise that avoidance is a symptom of PTSD. When Ande approached rather than avoided feared but generally safe situations, she started feeling better and her initial posttrauma reactions never developed into chronic PTSD. In this chapter, we first broadly define trauma-related avoidance and discuss the theoretical underpinnings of avoidance in the animal and human fear literatures. Next, we examine forms of avoidance focusing on cognitive avoidance, experiential avoidance, and behavioral avoidance. Finally, we discuss implications for enhancing natural recovery, prevention, and clinical treatment.

THEORETICAL UNDERPINNINGS OF AVOIDANCE

Probably the most straightforward model for understanding persistent emotional reactions to a traumatic event is one that focuses on classical, or Pavlovian, conditioning. In classical conditioning, real danger leads to the development of learned danger signals. This model of fear conditioning is incredibly well studied in both the animal and human literatures. The typical paradigm used to study classical conditioning in animals uses a brief foot shock as an unconditioned stimulus (US) to elicit an unconditioned response of fear (UCR). The foot shock is then paired with a neutral stimulus such as a tone, called the conditioned stimulus (CS). The animal eventually responds to this neutral stimulus in the same way it did to the original unconditioned stimulus, which becomes a conditioned response (CR) of fear (CS → CR). This same pairing of previously neutral stimuli with an aversive event also occurs during trauma exposure. Previously neutral situations, places, or things (e.g., sights, sounds, people) develop the ability to elicit reexperiencing of the trauma memory and acute physiological reactivity. Most likely, the stimuli that are avoided are CSs; they have the ability to elicit a fear reaction. In our example, anything Ande associated with her home (CS), such as her furnishings and the bed, brought back memories of the night she was raped and how afraid for her life she was (CR).

"Two-factor" theory explicitly brings in the role of avoidance, incorporating both classical and operant conditioning principles in the learning and maintenance of fear. This model was originally formulated by Mowrer (1939, 1947) and extended to PTSD by Keane, Fairbank, Caddell, and Zimering (1989). Specifically, after classical conditioning occurs, there is a motivation to escape the CS. This escape reduces the CR (i.e., fear), which in turn reinforces the escape response. Thus, fears acquired through classical conditioning are thought to be maintained by the fear-reducing properties of avoidance behavior. In extending this model to fear responding after trauma exposure, Keane and colleagues argued that serial presentation of different CSs prior to the US, higher-order conditioning processes (i.e., conditioned fear response evoked by a previously neutral stimulus after this neutral stimulus is paired with a stimulus that has been previously conditioned), and stimulus generalization (i.e., the transfer of a learned response from one stimulus to another) result in the pervasive patterns of avoidance seen in chronic PTSD. In other words, there are many CSs associated with the traumatic event itself and other neutral stimuli that were not present during the trauma that can easily develop the ability to elicit fear responses, leading to avoidance to reduce the fear responding. Taken together, these additions to the two-factor model are thought to better capture the stable avoidance and widespread fear responding to trauma-related cues seen in PTSD.

This conceptualization is intuitively appealing, as it is clear in our example that Ande avoided her own home. Similar furnishings in her mother's home had the ability to reactivate her fear, and while she avoided these things, her reactions persisted. When she returned to her home and approached other trauma reminders (i.e., mitigating avoidance), her trauma-related reactions began to abate. However, the critical role of avoidance in maintaining fear responding has been called into question. The specific emphasis on avoidance reinforcement by means of fear reduction was questioned when it was discovered that feedback from escaping a warning signal (i.e., a CS) is not important when it would already be avoided by innate escape behaviors that serve to protect the organism (Bolles, 1969, 1972). In other words, avoidance is acquired easily and rapidly if the required response resembles an innate, natural defensive behavior. If the response is not an innate defensive behavior, avoidance is then dependent on feedback from warning signals and is much more difficult to learn (Bolles, 1972). Bolles (1970, 1972) termed these innate defensive behaviors "species-specific defense reactions" (SSDRs), arguing that all species have built-in behaviors that serve to protect them from danger in the world. Avoidance is a readily learned SSDR because it is an innate and highly effective flight response, removing the organism from a dangerous situation. Another example of a SSDR is freezing, where there is literally an absence of all movement except for vital functions such as respiration. In humans, freezing, termed "tonic immobility," can occur before, during, or immediately after trauma exposure (see Marx, Forsyth, Gallup, Fusé, & Lexington,

2008; Zoellner, 2008). Notably, and crucial to the clinical understanding of avoidance, natural SSDRs are guided by classical conditioning learning about environmental cues rather than operant learning reinforced by their consequences (Bouton, 2007).

In summary, avoidance does not necessarily maintain fear by reinforcing principles. Avoidance patterns naturally and rapidly develop because avoidance is an innate response (i.e., an SSDR) to danger in humans. The clinical application of this is fairly straightforward. Trauma survivors can easily grasp these concepts and often find them refreshing, namely the idea that avoidance is something that is an in-built, natural desire and can easily be developed after trauma exposure. Similarly, clinicians need to understand how powerful this avoidance tendency is and how quickly and easily such patterns develop. This leads to a very straightforward application to facilitate natural recovery in the immediate aftermath of trauma exposure. If realistically safe situations, activities, and places can be approached rather than avoided, long-term patterns of avoidance will not develop.

EXTINCTION LEARNING

We now move to discuss the role of approaching avoided situations, activities, and places. Given that classical conditioning processes govern avoidant behavior, it is critical to understand the parameters of fear conditioning and its extinction. Older conceptualizations of fear reduction suggested that repeated exposure to the CS without the US erased the memory for the original pairing. For some trauma survivors, this erasure of the original conditioned learning is especially appealing because it suggests that it might be possible to return to a pretrauma state or that a "cure" for PTSD is plausible. In contrast, Bouton (1988, 1991, 2004; Bouton & Bolles, 1985) suggested that this fear reduction process, termed extinction, does not in fact erase original learning but rather creates new learning.

Extinction, sometimes referred to in the clinical literature as "habituation," refers to the process of repeated presentation of the CS without the US. This isolated CS presentation results in a reduction of the ability of the CS to elicit the CR. Bouton (1988, 1991, 2004; Bouton & Bolles, 1985) argued that extinction results in the acquisition of an inhibitory association that suppresses activation of the CR. Thus, instead of erasing the excitatory CS → CR association, during extinction, a new inhibitory association between the CS and the CR develops. Considerable research examining the return of fear (i.e., renewal, reinstatement, and spontaneous recovery) shows the persistence of this CS → CR association. Furthermore, Bouton argues that this new inhibitory association acquired during extinction is highly dependent on context (i.e., the environment in which the learning takes place) in a way that initial fear conditioning is not. Specifically, conditioning to a CS in one context will easily transfer to other contexts. By contrast, a shift from the context in which extinction occurred will often lead to a "renewal" of conditioned responding. Such findings indicate that both memories of conditioning and extinction are maintained after extinction and are available for retrieval if prompted by the appropriate retrieval cues. Accordingly, memory for extinction is viewed both as new and as fragile inhibitory learning, directly competing against a strong, excitatory memory for conditioning. This has implications for understanding trauma reactions: learning to be afraid is easy but learning to not be afraid after learning to be afraid is hard. Furthermore, if erasure of the original conditioning is not possible, the old fear learning persists even after fear reduction has occurred through natural recovery or successful treatment and can be relatively easily reactivated by previous trauma reminders or retraumatization. In this view, an ultimate "cure" is not possible; trauma survivors will periodically have trauma-related reactions, even after acute fear and anxiety decrease over time, naturally or therapeutically. Linking this to our example of Ande, she will always have the memories of what happened and related associations that can provoke anxiety or fear as part of her long-term memory. These long-term memories will be more or less available for retrieval depending on the various contexts (e.g., what she does, what she thinks about).

The Role of Higher Cortical Processes in Extinction

At a systems level, it is now well accepted that the underlying circuitry in extinction learning includes the amygdala, prefrontal cortex, and hippocampus (Anderson & Insel, 2006), with studies highlighting the role of the ventromedial prefrontal cortex (vmPFC) in recall of fear extinction and the hippocampus in contextual modulation (Milad, Rauch, Pitman, & Quirk, 2006; Rauch, Shin, & Phelps, 2006; Sotres-Bayon, Cain, & LeDoux, 2006). The amygdala is responsible for the processing of emotional reactions such as fear, the prefrontal cortex is associated with executive functioning and higher cortical processing, and the hippocampus functions to help consolidate information from short-term to long-term memory. One of the well-replicated findings in the PTSD literature is that individuals with PTSD have decreased vmPFC activation and increased amygdala activation compared to those without PTSD (e.g., Francati, Vermetten, & Bremner, 2007).

As discussed above, extinction is thought to result in the acquisition of an inhibitory association that suppresses activation of the CR. From years of animal research, it is commonly accepted that this inhibitory extinction learning directly involves the prefrontal cortex, with extinction learning involving the medial prefrontal cortex and extinction recall being mediated by the infralimbic cortex (see Quirk & Beer, 2006, for a review). Furthermore, failure to activate the vmPFC, specifically the infralimbic region, may underlie extinction deficits (Kim, Jo, Kim, Kim, & Choi, 2010). There is emerging information in humans showing converging evidence. Using a conditioning and extinction paradigm, Phelps and colleagues (Phelps, Delgado, Nearing, & LeDoux, 2004) reported that activation of the subgenual anterior cingulate in the vmPFC predicted successful extinction recall and was also associated with amygdala activation. Similarly, at a morphological level, greater thickness of the vmPFC, specifically the medial orbitofrontal cortex, has been strongly associated with better extinction retention (Milad et al., 2005; Milad, Orr, Pitman, & Rauch, 2005). Extending this further to examine activation of the vmPFC, Milad and colleagues (2006) reported that higher activation in both the vmPFC and the hippocampus were strongly associated with the strength of the extinction recall. Taken together, the growing animal and human literature implicate higher cortical processes in extinction learning. Furthermore, consistent with this finding, individuals with PTSD show functional and morphological abnormalities in the perigenual prefrontal cortex (Bremner, 2002; Rauch et al., 2003; Shin et al., 2004), arguing that extinction circuits may be compromised in PTSD (Mahan & Ressler, 2012). Taken together, learning not to be afraid is dependent on the prefrontal cortex, which is associated with executive functioning and inhibition.

Accordingly, because extinction learning is inhibitory in nature and context-dependent, many researchers are specifically examining ways to promote inhibitory, prefrontal cortex functioning in trauma-exposed individuals with PTSD, particularly during the fear reduction process. These strategies employ targeted drugs including methylene blue, D-cycloserine, glucocorticoids, and yohimbine paired with exposure therapy (e.g., Hofmann, 2007), brain stimulation of the dorsolateral prefrontal cortex (e.g., Boggio et al., 2010), and other strategies to enhance vmPFC functioning such as cognitive training in attentional bias modification (e.g., Browning, Holmes, Murphy, Goodwin, & Harmer, 2010). At the present time, no large clinical trials applying these strategies to PTSD have been conducted, so the clinical application of these approaches is still unknown. Existing empirically supported interventions should accordingly take precedence over these novel approaches, particularly given that many trauma survivors have not received these first-line treatments or have not tried them at an adequate dosage. Nevertheless, the specific targeting of enhancing inhibitory prefrontal cortex functioning, particularly during systematic and repeated approaching of trauma reminders as done in exposure therapy, may be an exciting next step in facilitating natural recovery, preventing PTSD development, and treating chronic PTSD.

Relevant Extinction Parameters

Typically, avoidance is addressed through either *in vivo* (i.e., in life) exposure to trauma reminders or imaginal exposure to the trauma memory, using repeated and prolonged exposure to the feared stimuli. Usually easier exposures are addressed first (e.g., memory of traumatic event, with little focus on specific content; wearing a skirt) while more difficult exposures (e.g., scariest or most difficult parts of the trauma memory; talking to a stranger at a bar) are approached after successful, repeated practice of the easier ones. As discussed above, the goal is to develop a new, inhibitory CS → CR association, through repeated presentation of the CS in the absence of the US. Thus, a successful exposure provides information that is incompatible with the original CS → US and the learned CS → CR associations. This learning of new associations is also apparent in cognitive therapy approaches, where expectancies for aversive events are altered through discussion and logical empiricism rather than necessarily through direct experience, though cognitive experiments routinely utilize direct exposure.

Fear Activation and Fear Reduction

Years of research in both animals and humans have helped to identify common principles yielding better extinction. Emotional processing theory (Foa & Kozak, 1986) highlighted the role of fear activation (i.e., the experience of anxiety at the onset of the exposure), in-session habituation (i.e., fear reduction within an exposure session), and between-session habituation (i.e., fear reduction between exposure sessions) as components of successful emotional processing during exposure therapy. Consistent with this theory, both fear activation (e.g., Foa, Riggs, Massie, & Yarczower, 1995; Jaycox, Foa, & Moral, 1998; Pitman, Orr, Altman, & Longpre, 1996) and between-session habituation (e.g., Jaycox et al., 1998; Rauch, Foa, Furr, & Filip, 2004; van Minnen & Hagenaars, 2010) have been associated with better PTSD treatment outcome. Thus, a good exposure should elicit anxiety, but over repeated sessions of exposure this anxiety should decrease.

However, in other anxiety disorders, a growing body of research shows successful exposure treatment despite the lack of between-session habituation (see Craske et al., 2008). Instead of experiencing anxiety reduction during repeated exposures, the individual's anxiety does not abate but his or her symptoms eventually decrease. This has been termed "distress tolerance." Based on the inhibitory model discussed above, it may be that, although the anxiety is not abating, the person is still learning the new inhibitory association. Specifically, he or she learns to tolerate the presence of the CS and that the US will not occur in the presence of the CS. This is encouraging for both individuals who are approaching trauma-related fears and therapists who are helping them. Even if anxiety reduction is not occurring during or between sessions, critical information is still being learned (i.e., the feared consequence is not occurring) that should facilitate recovery.

Manipulation of Context and CSs

Although less well-studied than the parameters of fear activation and fear reduction, new learning during exposure to avoided situations, activities, and memories may be enhanced by manipulating the presentation of various CSs and contexts. If extinction learning is dependent on contextual cues from the environment, then one obvious clinical implication is to conduct exposure in a variety of contexts, particularly those a person is likely to experience in his or her daily life. Time, specifically spacing between exposures, may also act as a temporal form of context that can be varied. Thus, for Ande, it would be critical to ascertain the variety of contexts (e.g., nighttime, being alone) that activate the CS → CR association and make sure that exposure to the CSs (e.g., her house, tall men) occurs in these salient contexts. Ande, like many trauma survivors, did this on her own without any formal therapeutic intervention encouraging this behavior.

Similarly, identification of and exposure to a variety of CSs should facilitate the development of inhibitory learning. Variability of CSs may provide more robust extinction learning (e.g., Rowe & Craske, 1998). For example, if a trauma survivor has problems talking with men, talking to a variety of different men as opposed to practicing with the same man will yield much better inhibitory learning. This idea has been further expanded in the examination of multiple conditioned excitors, where individual CSs are extinguished separately and then combined together for additional extinction trials (Rescorla, 2006). This form of compound extinction could potentially yield stronger, longer lasting inhibitory learning. Clinically, a variant of this form of compound exposure is often used in both cognitive and virtual reality exposure therapy. During behavioral experiments, related CSs (e.g., salient sounds, images, or smells) are incorporated into *in vivo* or imaginal exposures (e.g., Ehlers et al., 2003; Rothbaum, Hodges, Ready, Graap, & Alarcon, 2001). The enhanced efficacy of compound stimulus presentations has not been evaluated with trauma survivors. It may be that the advantage of this form of compound presentation is not necessarily in enhancing short-term symptom reduction but in preventing the return of fear months or years later.

Safety Signals

In contrast, conditioned inhibitors (i.e., conditioned stimuli that signal the absence of the US) have the potential to impair new inhibitory learning (e.g., McConnell & Miller, 2010). Notably, individuals with PTSD show impairments in the ability to learn new conditioned inhibitors, having difficulty using cues in the environment to inhibit anxiety reactions (e.g., Jovanovic, Kazama, Bachevalier, & Davis, 2012). More colloquially, these conditioned inhibitors are typically called "safety signals," which help to assure the trauma survivor that the feared consequence will not occur again. Safety signals can be things such as having another person present, carrying a cell phone, or carrying a weapon. For example, for a woman who was raped after a drug was placed in her alcoholic drink, never letting a drink leave her hand may be a safety signal that allows her to drink, whereas avoiding drinking altogether may be an avoidance behavior. The line between safety signals and avoidance behaviors is not always entirely clear. Regardless, it usually is not necessary to determine which is which but rather to recognize that neither conditioned inhibitors nor avoidance behaviors are helpful because they prevent an opportunity to learn the new inhibitory association. Although safety signals may initially be used to help a trauma survivor engage in various activities, to enhance extinction learning, the use of these safety signals should eventually decrease over repeated exposures.

Alternatively, some safety signals may be appropriate and adaptive (e.g., for a motor vehicle accident survivor, carrying a cell phone while driving alone), and for this reason, not directly targeted. However, if the person can never drive alone without a charged cell phone in normal, safe circumstances, then this behavior would be a target for change. Some have even extended this argument for the adaptive nature of safety signals further, suggesting the use of multiple conditioned inhibitors during exposure (Massad & Hulsey, 2006). The idea here is that using cues for inhibition of fear during exposure will facilitate approach to avoided situations, provide more cues for the new extinction learning, and potentially make it less likely for later return of fear. In this way, safety signals could serve as retrieval cues for the new learning, potentially attenuating the effects of shifting contexts (e.g., Brooks & Bouton, 1993). This may be exactly what Ande was doing when she made changes to her home by increasing its security, repainting it, and changing her bedroom into a game room. Using these safety signals may have helped Ande to move back and resume her life in her house.

Given these very discrepant recommendations, it is not surprising that the animal and human literatures on conditioned inhibitors at present are not conclusive as to whether conditioned inhibitors consistently enhance or impair new inhibitory learning and return of fear (e.g., Lovibond, Davis, & O'Flaherty, 2000; Lovibond & Shanks, 2002). It may be that conditioned inhibitors associated with the initial fear learning are detrimental to later extinction, whereas new conditioned inhibitors, though more difficult to learn, may be helpful in providing retrieval cues to facilitate extinction and prevent later return of fear. This is an important area for future study that has clear clinical implications for the recovery of trauma survivors.

SUMMARY

Systematic and repeated approaching of avoided, but safe, situations, as Ande did by returning to her house, is one of the best ways to address avoidance. Notably, learning to not be afraid is more difficult than learning to be afraid. A variety of strategies such as enhancing prefrontal cortex functioning, repeated approaching of feared activities (with or without fear reduction), varying the cues and context during exposure, and paying attention to safety signals may help facilitate development of new inhibitory learning to not be afraid and help mitigate later return of fear.

FORMS OF AVOIDANCE:
COGNITIVE, EXPERIENTIAL, AND BEHAVIORAL

Up to this point, we have focused on avoidance as largely a unitary construct, assuming that avoidance of activities and things are similar to avoidance of emotions and cognitions. The symptoms of PTSD (American Psychiatric Association, 2013) explicitly include efforts to avoid thoughts, feelings, or conversations associated with the trauma and efforts to avoid activities, places, or people that arouse recollections of the trauma. Notably, these avoidance symptoms of PTSD, in factor-analytic studies, typically emerge as a single avoidance factor (e.g., Yufik & Simms, 2010), arguing for their similarity rather than their differences. In this next section, we focus on the empirical literature examining three forms of avoidance, namely cognitive, experiential, and behavioral avoidance, and specific clinical implications for each type of avoidance.

Cognitive Avoidance

Cognitive avoidance includes a variety of strategies such as thought suppression (i.e., trying hard to push thoughts out of the mind) or distraction (i.e., actively trying not to think thoughts by keeping the mind constantly occupied with other things) in order to avoid negative, intrusive thoughts or recollections about a traumatic event (e.g., Ehlers & Clark, 2000). This form of avoidance includes both avoidance of images and thoughts. In our example with Ande, she experienced persistent intrusive images and thoughts of the perpetrator that evoked intense fear and disgust. The more she tried to avoid these images and thoughts, the more they seemed to emerge and haunt her.

Information-processing theories (e.g., Foa, Huppert, & Cahill, 2006; Horowitz, 1997) suggest that intrusive thoughts and reexperiencing of the event occur as a by-product of the trauma survivor trying to incorporate his or her traumatic experiences into his or her preexisting cognitive networks. Accordingly, intrusions are thought to be part of the natural recovery process and ought to decline as the survivor integrates the experience into his or her life. However, individuals with PTSD may negatively appraise these intrusive symptoms as signs of losing control or going crazy, motivating them to engage in cognitive avoidance. This in turn is thought to prevent the elaboration and reappraisal of the trauma memory, further maintaining the symptoms (Ehlers & Clark, 2000). In fact, in several prospective studies, greater initial cognitive avoidance was one of the best predictors of higher future PTSD symptom severity (e.g., Aaron, Zaglul, & Emery, 1999; Ehlers, Mayou, & Bryant, 1998; Tiet et al., 2006; Trickey, Siddaway, Meiser-Stedman, Serpell, & Field, 2012).

One strategy that trauma survivors may use to avoid trauma-related thoughts and images is thought suppression. Thought suppression is thought to lead to a paradoxical increase in intrusion frequency (Wegner, Schneider, Carter, & White, 1987). Wegner and colleagues (Wegner, 1994; Wegner & Erber, 1992) proposed a two-part mechanism of thought suppression. In his model, there is first a conscious search for a distractor to replace the thought or image to be suppressed. At the same time, an "automatic" scan of consciousness for traces of the to-be-suppressed target occurs to see whether efforts of suppression have failed or not. This process inadvertently leads the distractor to be associated with the to-be-suppressed thought. Thus, once suppression efforts cease, a "rebound effect" occurs due to the greater number of stimuli cuing the target. Though this effect is generally well established (e.g., Abramowitz, Tolin, & Street, 2001; Wenzlaff & Wegner, 2000), it is not clear that individuals with PTSD have more problems associated with thought suppression than those without PTSD; some experimental studies have shown increased paradoxical effects in individuals with PTSD for suppression of trauma-related thoughts while others have not (e.g., Aikins et al., 2009; Amstadter & Vernon, 2006; Beck, Gudmundsdottir, Palyo, Miller, & Grant, 2006; Shipherd & Beck, 2005). The varied findings may be due to methodological differences, such as discrepancies in thought control and suppression instructions, timing of assessments, and the nature of the target thoughts.

Another common cognitive avoidance strategy is distraction. Several cross-sectional studies have shown an association between greater distraction efforts and higher PTSD symptomatology (e.g., Pietrzak, Harpaz-Rotem, & Southwick, 2011; Scarpa, Wilson, Wells, Patriquin, & Tanaka, 2009; Steil & Ehlers, 2000). However, other studies have found that increased levels of distraction are not always associated with greater PTSD severity (e.g., Bennett, Beck, & Clapp, 2009; Reynolds & Wells, 1999), suggesting that distraction may at times serve as an adaptive coping strategy. It has been suggested that using positive images, thoughts, or activities as distractors may actually aid in reducing PTSD symptoms (Bennett et al., 2009), though it is unclear if this is a helpful long-term strategy. Better experimental and prospective research is needed to investigate when distraction is adaptive and when it is not (see Rodriguez & Craske, 1993).

Several studies have sought to directly manipulate factors related to cognitive avoidance and examined their impact on intrusions. Using a distress-film paradigm in psychologically healthy individuals, visuospatial distraction tasks (i.e., complex spatial key tapping, clay modeling, and playing a video game) either during the film or immediately after reduce the frequency of later intrusions (e.g., Bourne, Frasquilho, Roth, & Holmes, 2010; Brewin & Saunders, 2001; Holmes, Brewin, & Hennessy, 2004; Holmes, James, Coode-Bate, & Deeprose, 2009; Stuart, Holmes, & Brewin, 2006). However, there are mixed findings as to whether verbal-interference distraction tasks, such as counting out-loud backward by threes or reading irrelevant materials, decrease or increase later intrusions (e.g., Bourne et al., 2010; Ehring, Fuchs, & Kläsener, 2009; Ehring, Szeimies, & Schaffrick, 2009; Holmes et al., 2004; Krans, Näring, Becker, & Holmes, 2009), suggesting that the modality of the distraction task may be important. A distraction task that utilizes central executive functioning that is presented during or soon after trauma exposure may interfere with encoding of the trauma memory in an adaptive manner, reducing subsequent intrusions (Holmes et al., 2009). Thus, cognitive avoidance during or soon after trauma exposure may act as a preventive measure shifting how the traumatic memory is encoded. However, when individuals engage in cognitive avoidance later on, it may become costly and ineffective in reducing intrusions and PTSD symptoms. No studies of visuospatial distraction in the prevention of PTSD immediately after trauma exposure have been conducted to date.

In summary, cognitive avoidance in the short term, as seen in thought suppression, may either increase the frequency of intrusions or, as seen in distraction, may minimize distress from intrusions or even decrease their frequency. The implication for PTSD prevention, whether to encourage or discourage the use of distraction strategies immediately after trauma exposure, is simply not known. On the other hand, in the long term, cognitive avoidance may contribute to the maintenance of the fear and PTSD symptoms. Interventions typically directly target cognitive avoidance by encouraging patients to identify and confront the triggers and intrusive thoughts in order to reappraise them and reduce the sense of current threat. The challenge for clinicians may be in identifying the ways the patient is avoiding cognitions and evaluating whether it is effective or maladaptive. Some methods will be overt (e.g., not willing to speak of thoughts and feelings, keeping busy, constantly listening to music or TV, drinking), while other methods are covert and subtle (e.g., changing the topic of conversation, ruminating on a particular thought, using sarcasm or humor). Thus, the clinician should aim to change negative appraisals of intrusions and target specific cognitive avoidance strategies (Steil & Ehlers, 2000).

Experiential Avoidance

Experiential avoidance is a psychological process in which one attempts to modify both the form and frequency of unpleasant internal experiences (Hayes, Wilson, Gifford, Follette, & Strosahl, 1996). The process arises from an unwillingness to endure negative emotions (e.g., guilt, sadness) or bodily states (e.g., nausea, hot flashes). In order to avoid such experiences, individuals use a variety of strategies like substance abuse, distraction, or self-injury to escape unwanted feelings. In order to decrease the frequency of negative internal experiences, individuals engage in both automatic avoidance strategies, like emotional numbing, as well as more deliberate strategies, like situational avoidance (Foa et al., 1995). Experiential avoidance is usually defined very similarly to emotional avoidance and is often used interchangeably (e.g., Feldner, Zvolensky, Eifert, & Spira, 2003; Karekla, Forsyth, & Kelly, 2004). In our example, Ande initially engaged in experiential avoidance by trying to block her feelings through a variety of strategies including distraction and overt situational avoidance.

Experiential avoidance is thought to function paradoxically; avoidance of distressing internal states fails to reduce distress and instead leads to higher levels of subjective distress and emotional reactivity (e.g., Campbell-Sills, Barlow, Brown, & Hofmann, 2006; Karekla et al., 2004). In PTSD, individuals who avoid negative emotions posttrauma report higher levels of psychological distress, more PTSD symptoms, and lower life satisfaction compared to less experientially avoidant individuals (e.g., Kashdan & Kane, 2011; Kumpula, Orcutt, Bardeen, & Varkovitzky, 2011; Plumb, Orsillo, & Luterek, 2004). More specifically, higher levels of experiential avoidance have been found to predict greater symptom severity above and beyond other constructs like peritraumatic dissociation (Marx & Sloan, 2005). In cross-sectional studies, increased experiential avoidance reduced the observed relationship between trauma exposure and more frequent PTSD symptoms (Shenk, Putnam, & Noll, 2012) and between anxiety sensitivity and more frequent PTSD symptoms (Pickett, Bardeen, & Orcutt, 2011). In sum, experiential avoidance appears to play an important role in PTSD, which is not surprising given its strong correlation with both general psychological distress and anxiety-related symptomatology (Kashdan, Barrios, Forsyth, & Steger, 2006).

Very few studies have systematically examined the direct targeting of experiential avoidance in the prevention and treatment of PTSD. As discussed earlier, distress tolerance, the ability to be persistent in an activity despite distress, is something that is often developed over the course of repeatedly approaching trauma-related reminders. Indeed, it has been argued that distress tolerance is part of the inhibitory learning that occurs during exposure (Craske et al., 2008). Some have sought to directly target experiential avoidance through specific interventions employing mindfulness and acceptance strategies. Acceptance and commitment therapy (ACT) is a behavioral therapy based in acceptance and mindfulness principles, with the overarching therapeutic goals being decreased experiential avoidance and increased quality of life (Hayes, Strosahl, & Wilson, 1999). Mindfulness promotes awareness of feelings and perhaps, more importantly, teaches individuals to refrain from judging or changing their feelings (Kabat-Zinn, 1990). A review of treatment studies for anxiety and depression suggests the efficacy of mindfulness-based interventions (Hofmann, Sawyer, Witt, & Oh, 2010). In a noncontrolled, small sample study of war veterans seeking treatment for PTSD and depression, mindfulness-based stress reduction was shown to reduce PTSD symptom severity (Kearney, McDermott, Malte, Martinez, & Simpson, 2012). Similarly, using ACT, two case studies showed improvement in PTSD symptoms (Batten & Hayes, 2005; Twohig, 2009). Although encouraging, to date, no large-scale, randomized control trials of mindfulness-based interventions for PTSD exist, either comparing to wait list or, more importantly, comparing to existing PTSD interventions. Although most all empirically supported treatments for PTSD target experiential avoidance to some degree, incorporating mindfulness techniques is one possible augmentation strategy to directly target experiential avoidance (e.g., Becker & Zayfert, 2001; Thompson & Waltz, 2010).

An important limitation of studying experiential avoidance is how we measure the construct itself. Because emotions are private internal experiences, our measurements of emotional engagement are largely subjective and largely rely on retrospective report. Individuals who are experientially avoidant likely have more difficulty expressing feelings related to the trauma (e.g., Tull & Roemer, 2003), which makes assessing experiential avoidance challenging.

A variety of retrospective reporting measures exist to assess experiential avoidance, including measures of acceptance (e.g., Hayes, 2000), mindfulness (e.g., Lau et al., 2006), distress tolerance (e.g., Simons & Gaher, 2005), and emotion regulation (e.g., Gratz & Roemer, 2004). Unfortunately, retrospective self-reports say very little about an individual's ability to actually successfully experience emotion, as it is biased by current mood and memory effects. Convergent validity of these measures with more objective, observable measures of in-the-moment experiences of emotion or avoidance such as physiological activation, brain wave patterns seen through electroencephalogram readings, or brain region activation seen through functional magnetic resonance imaging are typically lacking and are needed. Another issue with self-report measures is that they are often highly face-valid. Although this is a strength in terms of content validity, it is also a weakness when trying to compare the effectiveness of interventions that directly and indirectly target experiential avoidance. For example, the statement "I was more concerned with being open to my experiences than controlling or changing them" may simply assess buy-in or adherence to the tested interventions rather than actual change in experiential avoidance.

At the present time, it is unknown if experiential avoidance needs to be directly targeted or if there is an additive benefit of targeted interventions such as ACT or other mindfulness-based interventions directly aimed at reducing experiential avoidance above existing intervention approaches. This is all the more critical because existing interventions may also directly or indirectly target experiential avoidance, though existing self-report measures of experiential avoidance may not help in addressing differential intervention effects. An additional clinical implication that has not been discussed up to now is the role of actively seeking out positive emotional experiences following trauma exposure. Indeed, individuals with PTSD notably have deficits experiencing positive emotions (e.g., Litz, Orsillo, Kaloupek, & Weathers, 2000). These deficits, coupled with the frequent onset of depression after trauma, suggest that an intentional "seeking out" of positive experiences to increase emotional flexibility could prove to be beneficial in preventing symptom development or in treating these symptoms once they emerge. Indeed, there is preliminary evidence for the utility of behavioral activation strategies, which target increasing activities that cultivate a sense of accomplishment and those associated with pleasure in the treatment of PTSD and depression (e.g., Nixon & Nearmy, 2011; Strachan, Gros, Ruggiero, LeJuez, & Acierno, 2012). This work builds on the idea that individuals with PTSD must repeatedly seek out positive experiences in order to gradually expand their emotional range to include more positive, desirable emotions. This might include encouraging a trauma survivor to pursue new and previously enjoyed hobbies.

Behavioral Avoidance

Behavioral avoidance is the deliberate effort to avoid trauma-related activities, situations, things, or people to escape triggers that arouse distressing and unwanted recollections of a traumatic event or to prevent the traumatic event from reoccurring. Avoidant coping is a related construct characterized by behaviors that orient away from a stressor or one's reaction to it. This construct, coming more directly from the stress and coping literature, is part of an approach–avoidance dimension of handling stress (see Roth & Cohen, 1986). In contrast with avoidant coping style, an approach coping style is characterized by an orientation toward the stressor. This dimension of approach and avoidant coping is reminiscent of Horowitz's (1976) trauma stress–response model of intrusion and denial, where the trauma survivor is motivated to protect the ego from the power of the traumatic stressor through strategies like emotional numbing, not thinking about the event, and avoiding reminders of the trauma. Notably, in this framework and within Roth and Cohen's (1986) framework, approach and avoidance are not considered mutually exclusive and an individual can rapidly shift between styles. In our example, Ande responded to the trauma by immediately avoiding her home; she sent her friend to the house to board up the broken window and moved in with her mother, all the while steering clear of the home she once treasured. Yet, later on, her response to the trauma is characterized by approach, where Ande made efforts to slowly and systematically confront her fear by visiting the house with her mother and improving home security.

The literature presents a wealth of evidence linking behavioral avoidance or avoidant coping to the development and severity of PTSD symptomology (e.g., Ehlers et al., 1998; Harvey & Bryant, 1998; Lawrence, Fauerbach, & Munster, 1996; Schuettler & Boals, 2011; Schuster, Park, & Frisman, 2011; Valentiner, Foa, Riggs, & Gershuny, 1996). Indeed, there are a number of prospective studies (ranging from 4 months to 2 years postbaseline assessment) demonstrating that initial behavioral avoidance is predictive of future PTSD symptom severity, even after controlling for trauma and immediate posttrauma reactions (e.g., Benotsch et al., 2000), type of trauma (e.g., Valentiner et al., 1996), intrusive thoughts (e.g., Ehlers et al., 1998), and initial PTSD severity (e.g., Benotsch et al., 2000; Dunmore, Clark, & Ehlers, 2000; Solomon, Mikulincer, & Avitzur, 1988; Valentiner et al., 1996). Notably, there is some evidence that avoidant coping actually mediates the relationship between previous trauma exposure and subsequent psychological symptom severity (e.g., Schuster et al., 2011), and initial PTSD symptom severity is associated with future behavioral avoidance (Tiet et al., 2006).

The strong predictive value of behavioral avoidance argues that targeting such avoidance is important in preventing the development of PTSD. Behavioral avoidance and avoidant coping is most directly targeted through *in vivo* exposure. That said, as seen with our example of Ande, it is not clear that a direct therapeutic intervention is always needed to address trauma-related avoidance, and it may be that simple encouragement or psychoeducation to approach rather than avoid reminders and feared, but safe, situations may facilitate natural recovery on its own. This echoes the common advice to figuratively get back on the proverbial horse and return to normalcy as much as possible following trauma exposure. *In vivo* exposure is one of the components in empirically supported interventions used for the prevention of chronic PTSD (e.g., Bryant, Harvey, Dang, Sackville, & Basten, 1998) and the treatment of chronic PTSD (e.g.,

Brom, Kleber, & Defares,1989; Foa et al., 2005; Paunovic & Öst, 2001). Notably, one-session interventions focusing on reducing behavioral avoidance have been remarkably effective in treating PTSD in earthquake survivors (e.g., Başoğlu, M., Şalcioğlu, Livanou, Kalender, & Acar, 2005). Further examination of the data in this study (Başoğlu, Şalcioğlu, & Livanou, 2007) highlighted the role of an increased sense of control associated with reduction in avoidance, which suggests that live exposure to fear cues designed to enhance sense of control might be sufficient for recovery from PTSD.

In contrast, in a dismantling study, successful treatment for chronic PTSD does not need to directly target behavioral avoidance via *in vivo* exposure (e.g., Bryant et al., 2008). Other empirically supported interventions for chronic PTSD do not directly target behavioral avoidance and similarly show lasting benefits for trauma survivors (e.g., Ironson, Freund, Strauss, & Williams, 2002; Marks, Lovell, Noshirvani, Livanou, & Thrasher, 1998; Resick, Nishith, Weaver, Astin, & Feuer, 2002). That said, across most intervention trials, change in behavioral avoidance is often poorly assessed, usually relying solely on two interview or self-report questions from the DSM-IV (American Psychiatric Association, 2000) or DSM-5 (American Psychiatric Association, 2013) (C1 and C2) symptoms of PTSD. In other anxiety disorders, behavioral avoidance is often directly measured through behavioral approach tasks (i.e., having the person attempt the feared task and measuring behavioral, subjective, and physiological outcomes) or through the use of much more detailed avoidance self-report measures. This form of detailed and systematic assessment of avoidance behaviors is now becoming more common in the PTSD field (e.g., van Minnen & Hagenaars, 2010). Better assessment of behavioral avoidance will help determine whether various interventions similarly impact behavioral avoidance or not and whether shifts in avoidance mediate change in these therapies.

Despite the fact that behavioral avoidance is so readily referred to and accepted as a clear construct in the literature, the research lacks a satisfying distinction between effortful and habitual behavioral avoidance. Although effortful avoidance implies that the trauma survivor is cognizant of his or her behavior, habitual avoidance becomes engrained in routine over years and is more difficult to identify and address. This form of avoidance becomes habit over time, and its link to the trauma often becomes obscure to the trauma survivor (e.g., in survivors of child abuse, never talking about their childhood). Clinically, for patients where there has been considerable time between trauma exposure and PTSD treatment, habitual avoidance may impede the construction of a list of avoided situations, making the clinician think the avoidance is less severe than it actually is. Furthermore, once identified, approaching these habitually avoided situations may be more difficult than anticipated for the trauma survivor.

SUMMARY AND CLINICAL RECOMMENDATIONS

Avoidance is common following trauma exposure. As seen in our example, Ande's avoidance took several forms: clear behavioral avoidance of the home where the assault occurred; cognitive avoidance of images and thoughts of the trauma including attempts at suppressing the thoughts and distracting herself through focusing on her kids and housework; and experiential avoidance of the fear and disgust she felt during and after the rape. Over time, Ande chose to gradually approach the things she was afraid of, going back to her home, making changes to the security and appearance of the home, and allowing herself to share her thoughts and feelings with her mother. Although this process was difficult, the mere shift in perspective and action facilitated her recovery without formal therapeutic intervention. Undoubtedly, targeting avoidance in the immediate aftermath of trauma exposure and in those with chronic PTSD facilitates recovery. To summarize key points:

1. Avoidance develops easily and rapidly after trauma exposure because it is an innate behavior designed to protect us as humans from future danger (i.e., a species-specific defense reaction).

2. Avoidance persists, largely not due to its ability to reduce anxiety, but because it is an innate defense strategy. This strategy operates more on classical conditioning principles than on principles of reinforcement.

3. Understanding principles of learning to inhibit fear through extinction is particularly relevant in addressing trauma-related avoidance. Although fear is easy to learn and persists over time, learning not to be afraid is a form of inhibitory learning that is dependent on environmental cues and relatively difficult to retrieve. Accordingly, some return of fear even after successful recovery is likely to occur for many trauma survivors, though not necessarily a reemergence of the PTSD per se.

4. Principles that facilitate extinction of fear are relevant in addressing trauma-related avoidance. Increasing inhibitory prefrontal cortex functioning, activating anxiety during exposure, promoting anxiety reduction or distress tolerance, varying triggers and environmental contexts, and manipulating safety signals are all potential strategies to enhance inhibitory learning and prevent return of fear.

5. Careful assessment of avoidance needs to examine and address cognitive, experiential, and behavioral forms of avoidance. Each of these forms of avoidance may interfere with long-term recovery posttrauma, though they may be adaptive in the short term.

6. Addressing avoidance through approaching feared but safe activities, situations, and places has the potential to be an effective

intervention in and of itself to reduce the likelihood of developing PTSD after trauma exposure and successfully treat chronic PTSD.

Of all of the principles that facilitate recovery, targeting avoidance and facilitating approach to realistically safe but feared thoughts, feelings, conversations, activities, places, and people has some of the most potential for helping the trauma survivor make the necessary adjustments to life after trauma exposure and build the life he or she desires to live. Undoubtedly, for the trauma survivor, approaching rather than avoiding is distressing, and learning not to be afraid does not occur easily. It takes a strong commitment on the part of the trauma survivor and the therapist who works with him or her. It also takes repetition, even in the face of apparent setbacks. As said at the beginning of this chapter, avoidance is like living in a cave. Though safe and sheltered, helping the trauma survivor to come out of this cave is crucial to create or rebuild a life worth living.

ACKNOWLEDGMENTS

Preparation of this chapter was supported in part by a grant to Lori A. Zoellner (No. R01MH66347, Principal Investigator).

REFERENCES

Aaron, J., Zaglul, H., & Emery, R. E. (1999). Posttraumatic stress in children following acute physical injury. *Journal of Pediatric Psychology, 24,* 335–343.

Abramowitz, J. S., Tolin, D. F., & Street, G. P. (2001). Paradoxical effects of thought suppression: A meta-analysis of controlled studies. *Clinical Psychology Review, 21,* 683–703.

Aikins, D. E., Johnson, D. C., Borelli, J. L., Klemanski, D. H., Morrissey, P. M., Benham, T. L., et al. (2009). Thought suppression failures in combat PTSD: A cognitive load hypothesis. *Behaviour Research and Therapy, 47,* 744–751.

American Psychiatric Association. (2000). *Diagnostic and statistical manual of mental disorders* (DSM-IV-TR). Washington DC: Author.

American Psychiatric Association. (2013). *Diagnostic and statistical manual of mental disorders* (DSM-5). Arlington, VA: Author.

Amstadter, A. B., & Vernon, L. L. (2006). Suppression of neutral and trauma targets: Implications for posttraumatic stress disorder. *Journal of Traumatic Stress, 19,* 517–526.

Anderson, K. C., & Insel, T. R. (2006). The promise of extinction research for the prevention and treatment of anxiety disorders. *Biological Psychiatry, 60,* 319–321.

Başoğlu, M., Şalcioğlu, E., Livanou, M., Kalender, D., & Acar, G. (2005). Single-session behavioral treatment of earthquake-related posttraumatic stress disorder: A randomized waiting list controlled trial. *Journal of Traumatic Stress, 18*, 1–11.

Batten, S. V., & Hayes, S. C. (2005). Acceptance and commitment therapy in the treatment of comorbid substance abuse and posttraumatic stress disorder. *Clinical Case Studies, 4*, 246–262.

Beck, J. G., Gudmundsdottir, B., Palyo, S. A., Miller, L. M., & Grant, D. M. (2006). Rebound effects following deliberate thought suppression: Does PTSD make a difference? *Behavior Therapy, 37*, 170–180.

Becker, C. B., & Zayfert, C. (2001). Integrating DBT-based techniques and concepts to facilitate exposure treatment for PTSD. *Cognitive and Behavioral Practice, 8*, 107–122.

Bennett, S. A., Beck, J. G., & Clapp, J. D. (2009). Understanding the relationship between posttraumatic stress disorder and trauma cognitions: The impact of thought control strategies. *Behaviour Research and Therapy, 47*, 1018–1023.

Benotsch, E. G., Brailey, K., Vasterling, J. J., Udo, M., Constans, J. I., & Stuker, P. B. (2000). War zone stress, personal and environmental resources, and PTSD symptoms in Gulf War veterans: A longitudinal perspective. *Journal of Abnormal Psychology, 109*, 205–213.

Boggio, P. S., Rocha, M., Oliveira, M. O., Fecteau, S., Cohen, R. B., Campanhã, C., et al. (2010). Noninvasive brain stimulation with high-frequency and low-intensity repetitive transcranial magnetic stimulation treatment for posttraumatic stress disorder. *Journal of Clinical Psychiatry, 71*, 992–999.

Bolles, R. C. (1969). Avoidance and escape learning: Simultaneous acquisition of different responses. *Journal of Comparative and Physiological Psychology, 68*, 90–99.

Bolles, R. C. (1970). Species specific defense reactions and avoidance learning. *Psychological Review, 7*, 32–48.

Bolles, R. C. (1972). *Psychology of learning and motivation* (Vol. 6). New York: Academic Press.

Bourne, C., Frasquilho, F., Roth, A. D., & Holmes, E. A. (2010). Is it mere distraction?: Peritraumatic verbal tasks can increase analogue flashbacks but reduce voluntary memory performance. *Journal of Behavior Therapy and Experimental Psychiatry, 41*, 316–324.

Bouton, M. E. (1988). Context and ambiguity in the extinction of emotional learning: Implications for exposure therapy. *Behaviour Research and Therapy, 26*, 137–149 .

Bouton, M. E. (1991). Context and retrieval in extinction and in other examples of interference in simple associative learning. In L. Dachowski & C. F. Flaherty (Eds.), *Current topics in animal learning: Brain, emotion, and cognition* (pp. 25–53). Hillsdale, NJ: Erlbaum.

Bouton, M. E. (2004). Context and behavioral processes in extinction. *Learning and Memory, 11*, 485–494.

Bouton, M. E. (2007). *Learning and behavior: A contemporary synthesis.* Sunderland, MA: Sinauer Associates.

Bouton, M. E., & Bolles, R. C. (1985). Contexts, event-memories, and extinction. In P. D. Balsam & A. Tomie (Eds.), *Context and learning* (pp. 133–166). Hillsdale, NJ: Erlbaum.

Bremner, J. D. (2002). *Does stress damage the brain?: Understanding trauma-related disorders from a neurological perspective.* New York: Norton.

Brewin, C., & Saunders, J. (2001). The effect of dissociation at encoding on intrusive memories for a stressful film. *British Journal of Medical Psychology, 74,* 467–472.

Brom, D., Kleber, R., & Defares, P. (1989). Brief psychotherapy for posttraumatic stress disorders. *Journal of Consulting and Clinical Psychology, 57,* 607–612.

Brooks, D. C., & Bouton, M. E. (1993). Time and context effects on performance in a Pavlovian discrimination reversal. *Journal of Experimental Psychology: Animal Behavior Processes, 19,* 165–179.

Browning, M., Holmes, E. A., Murphy, S. E., Goodwin, G. M., & Harmer, C. J. (2010). Lateral prefrontal cortex mediates the cognitive modification of attention bias. *Biological Psychiatry, 67,* 919–925.

Bryant, R., Harvey, A., Dang, S., Sackville, T., & Basten, C. (1998). Treatment of acute stress disorder: A comparison of cognitive behavioral therapy and supportive counseling. *Journal of Consulting and Clinical Psychology, 66,* 862–866.

Bryant, R. A., Moulds, M. L., Guthrie, R. M., Dang, S. T., Mastrodomenico, J., Nixon, R. D. V., et al. (2008). A randomized controlled trial of exposure therapy and cognitive restructuring for posttraumatic stress disorder. *Journal of Consulting and Clinical Psychology, 76,* 695–703.

Campbell-Sills, L., Barlow, D. H., Brown, T. A., & Hofmann, S. G. (2006). Effects of suppression and acceptance on emotional responses of individuals with anxiety and mood disorders. *Behaviour Research and Therapy, 44,* 1251–1263.

Craske, M., Kircanski, K., Zelikowsky, M., Mystkowski, J., Chowdhury, N., & Baker, A. (2008). Optimizing inhibitory learning during exposure therapy. *Behavior Research and Therapy, 46,* 5–27.

Dunmore, E., Clark, D., & Ehlers, A. (2000). A prospective investigation of the role of cognitive factors in persistent posttraumatic stress disorder (PTSD) after physical or sexual assault. *Behavior Research and Therapy, 39,* 1063–1084.

Ehlers, A., & Clark, D. M. (2000). A cognitive model of posttraumatic stress disorder. *Behaviour Research and Therapy, 38,* 319–345.

Ehlers, A., Clark, D. M., Hackmann, A., McManus, F., & Fennell, M. (2005). Cognitive therapy for post-traumatic stress disorder: Development and evaluation. *Behaviour Research and Therapy, 43,* 413–431.

Ehlers, A., Clark, D. M., Hackmann, A., McManus, F., Fennell, M., Herbert, C., et al. (2003). A randomized controlled trial of cognitive therapy, a self-help booklet, and repeated assessments as early interventions for posttraumatic stress disorder. *Archives of General Psychiatry, 60,* 1024–1032.

Ehlers, A., Mayou, R. A., & Bryant, B. (1998). Psychological predictors of chronic posttraumatic stress disorder after motor vehicle accidents. *Journal of Abnormal Psychology, 107,* 508–519.

Ehlers, A., & Steil, R. (1995). Maintenance of intrusive memories in posttraumatic stress disorder: A cognitive approach. *Behavioural and Cognitive Psychotherapy, 23,* 217–249.

Ehring, T., Fuchs, N., & Kläsener, I. (2009). The effects of experimentally induced rumiation versus distraction on analogue posttraumatic stress symptoms. *Behavior Therapy, 40,* 403–413.

Ehring, T., Szeimies, A., & Schaffrick, C. (2009). An experimental analogue study into the role of abstract thinking in trauma-related rumination. *Behaviour Research and Therapy, 47,* 285–293.

Feldner, M. T., Zvolensky, M. J., Eifert, G. H., & Spira, A. P. (2003). Emotional avoidance: An experimental test of individual differences and response suppression using biological challenge. *Behaviour Research and Therapy, 41,* 403–411.

Foa, E. B., Hembree, E. A., Cahill, S. P., Rauch, S. A. M., Riggs, D. S., Feeny, N. C., et al. (2005). Randomized trial of prolonged exposure for posttraumatic stress disorder with and without cognitive restructuring: Outcome at academic and community clinics. *Journal of Consulting and Clinical Psychology, 73,* 953–964.

Foa, E. B., Huppert, J. D., & Cahill, S. P. (2006). Emotional processing theory: An update. In B. O. Rothbaum (Ed.), *Pathological anxiety: Emotional processing in etiology and treatment* (pp. 3–24). New York: Guilford Press.

Foa, E. B., & Kozak, M. J. (1986). Emotional processing of fear: Exposure to corrective information. *Psychological Bulletin, 99,* 20–35.

Foa, E. B., Riggs, D. S., Massie, E. D., & Yarczower, M. (1995). The impact of fear activation and anger on the efficacy of exposure treatment for posttraumatic stress disorder. *Behavior Therapy, 26,* 487–499.

Francati, V., Vermetten, E., & Bremner, J. D. (2007). Functional neuroimaging studies in posttraumatic stress disorder: Review of current methods and findings. *Depression and Anxiety, 24,* 202–218.

Gratz, K. L., & Roemer, L. (2004). Multidimensional assessment of emotion regulation and dysregulation: Development, factor structure, and initial validation of the difficulties in emotion regulation scale. *Journal of Psychopathology and Behavioral Assessment, 26,* 41–54.

Harvey, A., & Bryant, R. (1998). The relationship between acute stress disorder and posttraumatic stress disorder: A prospective evaluation of motor vehicle accident survivors. *Journal of Consulting and Clinical Psychology, 66,* 507–512.

Hayes, S. C. (2000). *The Acceptance and Action Questionnaire.* Reno, NV: Author.

Hayes, S. C., Strosahl, K. D., & Wilson, K. G. (1999). *Acceptance and commitment therapy: An experiential approach to behavior change.* New York: Guilford Press.

Hayes, S. C., Wilson, K. G., Gifford, E. V., Follette, V. M., & Strosahl, K. (1996). Experiential avoidance and behavioral disorders: A functional dimensional approach to diagnosis and treatment. *Journal of Consulting and Clinical Psychology, 64,* 1152–1168.

Hofmann, S. G. (2007). Enhancing exposure-based therapy from a translational research perspective. *Behaviour Research and Therapy, 45,* 1987–2001.

Hofmann, S. G., Sawyer, A. T., Witt, A. A., & Oh, D. (2010). The effect of mindfulness-based therapy on anxiety and depression: A meta-analytic review. *Journal of Consulting and Clinical Psychology, 78,* 169–183.

Holmes, E. A., Brewin, C. R., & Hennessy, R. G. (2004). Trauma films, information processing, and intrusive memory development. *Journal of Experimental Psychology: General, 133,* 3–22.

Holmes, E. A., James, E. L., Coode-Bate, T., & Deeprose, C. (2009). Can playing the computer game "Tetris" reduce the build-up of flashbacks for trauma?: A proposal from cognitive science. *PLoS One, 4,* e4153.

Horowitz, M. J. (1976). *Stress response syndromes.* Oxford, UK: Jason Aronson.

Horowitz, M. J. (1997). *Stress response syndromes: PTSD, grief, and adjustment disorders* (3rd ed.). Lanham, MD: Jason Aronson.

Ironson, G., Freund, B., Strauss, J. L., & Williams, J. (2002). Comparison of two treatments for traumatic stress: A community-based study of EMDR and prolonged exposure. *Journal of Clinical Psychology, 58,* 113–128.

Jaycox, L. H., Foa, E. B., & Moral, A. R. (1998). Influence of emotional engagement and habituation on exposure therapy for PTSD. *Journal of Consulting and Clinical Psychology, 66,* 185–192.

Jovanovic, T., Kazama, A., Bachevalier, J., & Davis, M. (2012). Impaired safety signal learning may be a biomarker of PTSD. *Neuropharmacology, 62,* 695–704.

Kabat-Zinn, J. (1990). *Full catastrophe living: Using the wisdom of your body and mind to face stress, pain, and illness.* New York: Guilford Press.

Karekla, M., Forsyth, J. P., & Kelly, M. M. (2004). Emotional avoidance and panicogenic responding to a biological challenge procedure. *Behavior Therapy, 35,* 725–746.

Kashdan, T. B., Barrios, V., Forsyth, J. P., & Steger, M. F. (2006). Experiential avoidance as a generalized psychological vulnerability: Comparisons with coping and emotion regulation strategies. *Behaviour Research and Therapy, 44,* 1301–1320.

Kashdan, T. B., & Kane, J. Q. (2011). Post-traumatic distress and the presence of post-traumatic growth and meaning in life: Experiential avoidance as a moderator. *Personality and Individual Differences, 50,* 84–89.

Keane, T. M., Fairbank, J. A., Cadell, J. M., & Zimering, R. T. (1989). Implosive (flooding) therapy reduces symptoms of PTSD in Vietnam combat veterans. *Behavior Therapy, 20,* 245–260.

Kearney, D. J., McDermott, K., Malte, C., Martinez, M., & Simpson, T. L. (2012). Association of participation in a mindfulness program with measures of PTSD, depression and quality of life in a veteran sample. *Journal of Clinical Psychology, 68,* 101–116.

Kim, S. C., Jo, Y. S., Kim, I. H., Kim, H., & Choi, J. S. (2010). Lack of medial prefrontal cortex activation underlies the immediate extinction deficit. *Journal of Neuroscience, 30,* 832–837.

Krans, J., Näring, G., Becker, E. S., & Holmes, E. A. (2009). Intrusive trauma memory: A review and functional analysis. *Applied Cognitive Psychology, 23,* 1076–1088.

Kumpula, M. J., Orcutt, H. K., Bardeen, J. R., & Varkovitzky, R. L. (2011). Peritraumatic dissociation and experiential avoidance as prospective predictors of posttraumatic stress symptoms. *Journal of Abnormal Psychology, 120,* 617–627.

Lau, M. A., Bishop, S. R., Segal, Z. V., Buis, T., Anderson, N. D., Carlson, L., et al. (2006). The Toronto Mindfulness Scale: Development and validation. *Journal of Clinical Psychology, 62,* 1445–1146.

Lawrence, J., Fauerbach, J., & Munster, A. (1996). Early avoidance of traumatic stimuli predicts chronicity of intrusive thoughts following brain injury. *Behavior Research and Therapy, 34,* 643–646.

Litz, B. T., Orsillo, S. M., Kaloupek, D., & Weathers, F. (2000). Emotional processing in posttraumatic stress disorder. *Journal of Abnormal Psychology, 109,* 26–39.

Lovibond, P. F., Davis, N. R., & O'Flaherty, A. S. (2000). Protection from extinction in human fear conditioning. *Behaviour Research and Therapy, 38,* 967–983.

Lovibond, P. F., & Shanks, D. R. (2002). The role of awareness in Pavlovian conditioning: Empirical evidence and theoretical implications. *Journal of Experimental Psychology: Animal Behavior Processes, 28,* 3–26.

Mahan, A. L., & Ressler, K. J. (2012). Fear conditioning, synaptic plasticity and the amygdala: Implications for posttraumatic stress disorder. *Trends in Neuroscience, 35,* 24–35.

Marks, I. M., Lovell, K., Noshirvani, H., Livanou, M., & Thrasher, S. (1998). Treatment of posttraumatic stress disorder by exposure and/or cognitive restructuring: A controlled study. *Archives of General Psychiatry, 55,* 317–325.

Marx, B. P., Forsyth, J. P., Gallup, G. G., Fusé, T., & Lexington, J. M. (2008). Tonic immobility as an evolved predator defense: Implications for sexual assault survivors. *Clinical Psychology: Science and Practice, 15,* 74–90.

Marx, B. P., & Sloan, D. M. (2005). Peritraumatic dissociation and experiential avoidance as predictors of posttraumatic stress symptomatology. *Behaviour Research and Therapy, 43,* 569–583.

Massad, P. M., & Hulsey, T. L. (2006). Exposure therapy renewed. *Journal of Psychotherapy Integration, 16,* 417–428.

McConnell, B. L., & Miller, R. R. (2010). Protection from extinction provided by a conditioned inhibitor. *Learning and Behavior, 38,* 68–79.

Milad, M. R., Orr, S. P., Pitman, R. K., & Rauch, S. L. (2005). Context modulation of memory for fear extinction in humans. *Psychophysiology, 42,* 456–464.

Milad, M. R., Quinn, B. T., Pitman, R. K., Orr, S. P., Fischi, B., & Rauch, S. L. (2005). Thickness of ventromedial prefrontal cortex in humans is correlated with extinction memory. *Proceedings of the National Academy of Sciences of the United States of America, 102,* 10706–10711.

Milad, M. R., Rauch, S. L., Pitman, R. K., & Quirk, G. J. (2006). Fear extinction in rats: Implications for human brain imaging and anxiety disorders. *Biological Psychiatry, 73,* 61–71.

Mowrer, O. H. (1939). A stimulus–response analysis of anxiety and its role as a reinforcing agent. *Psychological Review, 46,* 553–565.

Mowrer, O. H. (1947). On the dual nature of learning: A re-interpretation of "conditioning" and "problem-solving." *Harvard Educational Review, 17,* 102–148.

Nixon, R. D. V., & Nearmy, D. M. (2011). Treatment of comorbid posttraumatic stress disorder and major depressive disorder: A pilot study. *Journal of Traumatic Stress, 24,* 451–455.

Paunovic, N., & Öst, L. G. (2001). Cognitive-behavior therapy vs. exposure therapy in the treatment of PTSD in refugees. *Behaviour Research and Therapy,*
39, 1183–1197.

Phelps, E. A., Delgado, M. R., Nearing, K., & LeDoux, J. E. (2004). Extinction
learning in humans: Role of the amygdala and vmPFC. *Neuron, 43,* 897–905.

Pickett, S. M., Bardeen, J. R., & Orcutt, H. K. (2011). Experiential avoidance as a
moderator of the relationship between behavioral inhibition system sensitivity and posttraumatic stress symptoms. *Journal of Anxiety Disorders, 25,*
1038–1045.

Pietrzak, R. H., Harpaz-Rotem, I., & Southwick, S. M. (2011). Cognitive-behavioral coping strategies associated with combat-related PTSD in treatment-
seeking OEF–OIF veterans. *Psychiatry Research, 189*(2), 251–258.

Pitman, R. K., Orr, S. P., Altman, B., & Longpre, R. E. (1996). Emotional processing
and outcome of imaginal flooding therapy in Vietnam veterans with chronic
posttraumatic stress disorder. *Comprehensive Psychiatry, 37,* 409–418.

Plumb, J. C., Orsillo, S. M., & Luterek, J. A. (2004). A preliminary test of the
role of experiential avoidance in post-event functioning. *Journal of Behavior*
Therapy and Experimental Psychiatry, 35, 245–257.

Quirk, G. J., & Beer, J. S. (2006). Prefrontal involvement in the regulation of emotion: Convergence of rat and human studies. *Current Opinion in Neurobiol-*
ogy, 16, 723–727.

Rauch, S. A., Foa, E. B., Furr, J. M., & Filip, J. C. (2004). Imagery vividness and
perceived anxious arousal in prolonged exposure treatment for PTSD. *Journal*
of Traumatic Stress, 17, 461–465.

Rauch, S. L., Shin, L. M., & Phelps, E. A. (2006). Neurocircuitry models of posttraumatic stress disorder and extinction : Human neuroimaging research—
Past, present, and future. *Biological Psychiatry, 60,* 376–382.

Rauch, S. L., Shin, L. M., Segal, E., Pitman, R. K., Carson, M. A., McMullin, K.,
et al. (2003) Selectively reduced regional cortical volumes in posttraumatic
stress disorder. *NeuroReport, 14,* 913–916.

Rescorla, R. A. (2006). Deepened extinction from compound stimulus presentation. *Journal of Experimental Psychology: Animal Behavior Processes, 32,*
135–144.

Resick, P. A., Nishith, P., Weaver, T. L., Astin, M. C., & Feuer, C. A. (2002). A
comparison of cognitive-processing therapy with prolonged exposure and a
waiting condition for the treatment of chronic posttraumatic stress disorder
in female rape victims. *Journal of Consulting and Clinical Psychology, 70,*
867–879.

Reynolds, M., & Wells, A. (1999). The Thought Control Questionnaire—Psychometric properties in a clinical sample, and relationships with PTSD and
depression. *Psychological Medicine, 29,* 1089–1099.

Rodriguez, B. I., & Craske, M. G. (1993). The effects of distraction during exposure to phobic stimuli. *Behaviour Research and Therapy, 31,* 549–558.

Roth, S., & Cohen, L. J. (1986). Approach, avoidance, and coping with stress.
American Psychologist, 41, 813–819.

Rothbaum, B. O., Hodges, L. F., Ready, D., Graap, K., & Alarcon, R. D. (2001).
Virtual reality exposure therapy for Vietnam veterans with posttraumatic
stress disorder. *Journal of Clinical Psychiatry, 62,* 617–622.

Rowe, M. K., & Craske, M. G. (1998). Effects of varied-stimulus exposure training on fear reduction and return of fear. *Behaviour Research and Therapy, 36,* 719–734.

Şalcioğlu, M., Başoğlu, E., & Livanou, M. (2007). Effects of live exposure on symptoms of posttraumatic stress disorder: The role of reduced behavioral avoidance in improvement. *Behaviour Research and Therapy, 45,* 2268–2279.

Scarpa, A., Wilson, L. C., Wells, A. O., Patriquin, M. A., & Tanaka, A. (2009). Thought control strategies as mediators of trauma symptoms in young women with histories of child sexual abuse. *Behaviour Research and Therapy, 47,* 809–813.

Schuettler, D., & Boals, A. (2011). The path to posttraumatic growth versus posttraumatic stress disorder: Contributions of event centrality and coping. *Journal of Loss and Trauma, 16,* 180–194.

Schuster, J., Park, C. L., & Frisman, L. K. (2011). Trauma exposure and PTSD symptoms among homeless mothers: Predicting coping and mental health outcomes. *Journal of Social and Clinical Psychology, 30,* 887–904.

Shenk, C. E., Putnam, F. W., & Noll, J. G. (2012). Experiential avoidance and the relationship between child maltreatment and PTSD symptoms: Preliminary evidence. *Child Abuse and Neglect, 36,* 118–126.

Shin, L. M., Orr, S. P., Carson, M. A., Rauch, S. L., Macklin, M. L., Lasko, N. B., et al. (2004). Regional cerebral blood flow in the amygdala and medial prefrontal cortex during traumatic imagery in male and female vietnam veterans with PTSD. *Archives of General Psychiatry, 61,* 168–176.

Shipherd, J. C., & Beck, J. G. (2005). The role of thought suppression in posttraumatic stress disorder. *Behavior Therapy, 36,* 277–287.

Simons, J. S., & Gaher, R. M. (2005). The Distress Tolerance Scale: Development and validation of a self-report measure. *Motivation and Emotion, 9,* 83–102.

Solomon, Z., Mikulincer, M., & Avitzur, E. (1988). Coping, locus of control, social support, and combat-related posttraumatic stress disorder: A prospective study. *Journal of Personality and Social Psychology, 55,* 279–285.

Sotres-Bayon, F., Cain, C. K., & LeDoux, J. E. (2006). Brain mechanisms of fear extinction: Historical perspectives on the contribution of prefrontal cortex. *Biological Psychiatry, 60,* 329–336.

Steil, R., & Ehlers, A. (2000). Dysfunctional meaning of posttraumatic intrusions in chronic PTSD. *Behaviour Research and Therapy, 38,* 537–558.

Strachan, M., Gros, D. F., Ruggiero, K. J., Lejuez, C. W., & Acierno, R. (2012). An integrated approach to delivering exposure-based treatment for symptoms of PTSD and depression in OIF/OEF veterans: Preliminary findings. *Behavior Therapy, 43,* 560–569.

Stuart, A. D. P., Holmes, E. A., & Brewin, C. R. (2006). The influence of a visuospatial grounding task on intrusive images of a traumatic film. *Behaviour Research and Therapy, 44,* 611–619.

Thompson, B. L., & Waltz, J. (2010). Mindfulness and experiential avoidance as predictors of posttraumatic stress disorder avoidance and symptom severity. *Journal of Anxiety Disorders, 24,* 409–415.

Tiet, Q. Q., Rosen, C., Cavella, S., Moos, R. H., Finney, J. W., & Yesavage, J. (2006). Coping, symptoms, and functioning outcomes of patients with posttraumatic stress disorder. *Journal of Traumatic Stress, 19,* 799–811.

Trickey, D., Siddaway, A. P., Meiser-Stedman, R., Serpell, L., & Field, A. P. (2012). A meta-analysis of risk factors for post-traumatic stress disorder in children and adolescents. *Clinical Psychology Review, 32,* 122–138.

Tull, M. T., & Roemer, L. (2003). Alternative explanations of emotional numbing of posttraumatic stress disorder: An examination of hyperarousal and experiential avoidance. *Journal of Psychopathology and Behavioral Assessment, 25,* 147–154.

Twohig, M. P. (2009). Acceptance and commitment therapy for treatment-resistant posttraumatic stress disorder: A case study. *Cognitive and Behavioral Practice, 16,* 243–252.

Valentiner, D. P., Foa, E. B., Riggs, D. S., & Gershuny, B. S. (1996). Coping strategies and posttraumatic stress disorder in female victims of sexual and nonsexual assault. *Journal of Abnormal Psychology, 105,* 455–458.

van Minnen, A., & Hagenaars, M. A. (2010). Avoidance behaviour of patients with posttraumatic stress disorder: Initial development of a questionnaire, psychometric properties and treatment sensitivity. *Journal of Behavior Therapy and Experimental Psychiatry, 41,* 191–198.

Wegner, D. M. (1994). Ironic processes of mental control. *Psychological Review, 101,* 34–52.

Wegner, D. M., & Erber, R. (1992). The hyperaccessibility of suppressed thoughts. *Journal of Personality and Social Psychology, 63,* 903–912.

Wegner, D. M., Schneider, D. J., Carter, S. R., & White, T. L. (1987). Paradoxical effects of thought suppression. *Journal of Personality and Social Psychology, 53,* 5–13.

Wenzlaff, R. M., & Wegner, D. M. (2000). Thought suppression. *Annual Review of Psychology, 51,* 59–91.

Yufik, T., & Simms, L. J. (2010). A meta-analytic investigation of the structure of posttraumatic stress disorder symptoms. *Journal of Abnormal Psychology, 119,* 764–776.

Zoellner, L. A. (2008). Translational challenges with tonic immobility. *Clinical Psychology: Science and Practice, 15,* 98–101.

Chapter 12

Chronic Pain and Posttraumatic Stress Disorder

Gordon J. G. Asmundson, Lydia Gómez-Pérez,
and Mathew G. Fetzner

During a security patrol in Afghanistan, a light armored vehicle was hit with an improvised explosive device (IED) blast, killing its occupants. Jamie, a 26-year-old corporal on gunner duty, was standing in the turret of the light armored vehicle behind the one that was hit directly. Although sustaining significant wounds to both legs, Jamie was able to apply first aid to others in his group, after which all were medivaced to Kandahar Air Field for further medical attention and stabilization. Jamie was then sent for surgery in Germany and thereafter returned home and immediately entered and completed a physical rehabilitation program before resuming regular duties. Pain resulting from the injury persisted after completion of the physical rehabilitation program. Prior to deployment, his peers had known Jamie as an outgoing yet somewhat anxious person who was always conscientious about his health habits; but, since returning home, colleagues and family began commenting that he was even more anxious and health-focused than usual. When asked about this, Jamie stated that he was worried about his persistent pain, the potential of reinjury of his legs, and whether he would ever "get back to normal." He also stated that he was constantly "revved up" inside and worried that this might be related to some unknown disease process. He began to avoid most physical activity, especially physical training with members of his unit and leisure activities with his wife. He also reported sleep difficulties, poor concentration, disturbing recollections of the IED blast and its aftermath, jumpiness, feelings of frustration, and relationship difficulties with his partner. Even though he wanted his pain to stop, he reported that a part of him felt as if he deserved "to feel the hurt" because his actions, before and after the blast, contributed to the death of his friends.[1]

Posttraumatic stress disorder (PTSD) and clinically significant pain experiences, both acute and chronic, commonly co-occur in civilian and military populations (Asmundson, Coons, Taylor, & Katz, 2002; Beck & Clapp, 2011; Otis, Keane, & Kerns, 2003; Sharp & Harvey, 2001). The co-occurrence of PTSD and clinically significant pain is associated with a poorer prognosis, increased work and social impairment (Beckham et al., 1997), decreased potential for successful intervention (Wald, Taylor, & Fedoroff, 2004), and has a considerable negative financial impact to society in terms of work absenteeism as well as health care and insurance expenditures. Jamie's experience, derived from a composite of cases that we have seen subsequent to events that are potentially traumatic and painful, is illustrative of these empirical findings and underscores the multitude of considerations in understanding and treating co-occurring PTSD and clinically significant pain. The purposes of the present chapter are several fold. First, we review explanatory models concerning the co-occurrence of PTSD and clinically significant pain experiences. Since the focus of the explanatory models as well as the majority of empirical work has focused on chronic pain (i.e., pain persisting for a duration of greater than 3 months), the primary focus of this chapter is on the co-occurrence of PTSD and chronic pain. Second, we briefly review the current state of the art regarding the models, with a particular focus on several potentially modifiable maintenance and shared vulnerability factors for which there is accumulating evidence. Finally, we provide concrete and actionable clinical recommendations for treating individuals who present for treatment of both PTSD and chronic pain. Possible directions for future research are outlined throughout.

BASICS OF PTSD AND CHRONIC PAIN

PTSD is described in detail elsewhere in this volume. Here we highlight several features that are relevant to the co-occurrence of PTSD and chronic

---

[1]This case represents a mixture of details from several clients whom we have seen in our clinical work. Case details have been altered to conceal client identities and any resemblance to a specific individual is purely coincidental.

pain. Recent data indicate that approximately 10% of the general population will experience PTSD at some point during their lifetime (Seedat
& Stein, 2001); however, lifetime prevalence rates of PTSD exceed 50%
in certain "at-risk" groups (e.g., deployed military, police, emergency
responders, inner-city dwellers; American Psychiatric Association, 2013).
PTSD often follows a chronic course. The frequency and severity of
symptoms typically fluctuate over time, depending on a range of factors,
including the person's degree of exposure to subsequent stressors, which
can amplify or exacerbate symptoms (Taylor, 2006). PTSD-exacerbating
events may include everyday stressors, as well as stressors that are linked to
the person's trauma. The disorder is associated with a heightened risk for
developing other psychiatric disorders (e.g., anxiety disorders, mood disorders, substance use disorders; American Psychiatric Association, 2013) as
well as diminished physical health (Asmundson et al., 2002) and a variety
of general medical conditions (Sareen, Cox, Clara, & Asmundson, 2005),
including acute and chronic pain.

Acute pain (i.e., pain with a sudden onset, often stemming from tis-
sue damage) is adaptive in that it signals the potential of actual damage
and motivates action to limit damage and, in some cases, promote recovery (Wall, 1978). Acute pain experiences subside with physical recovery;
but, for some, acute pain transitions through a complex interaction of
biological, psychological, and social processes to become chronic (Katz,
McCartney, & Rashiq, 2008). Chronic pain is typically defined as pain
persisting longer than 3 months (International Association for the Study
of Pain, 1986). Available data indicate that approximately 20% of the
population living in Westernized countries experience current chronic
pain (e.g., Breivik, Collett, Ventafridda, Cohen, & Gallacher, 2006), making it one of the most common chronic health conditions. Unlike acute
pain, chronic pain is not adaptive (Turk & Rudy, 1988); indeed, for most
who experience it, chronic pain is associated with considerable emotional
distress, increased risk of developing psychiatric disorders (Asmundson
& Katz, 2009), impaired social and occupational function, as well as
increased medical service utilization (Gureje, Von Korff, Simon, & Gater,
1998).

It is now well established that PTSD and chronic pain are prevalent
conditions that are associated with significant personal and societal costs;
as such, each has been deemed a public health concern. The staggeringly
common co-occurrence of these conditions—and the impact this has on
individual suffering, treatment outcomes, and societal costs—has made
this an increasingly relevant area of mental health research. What seems
clear at this point is that the co-occurrence of PTSD and chronic pain is not
coincidental; that is, these conditions are related in some way that increases
the odds that they will co-occur.

MODELS

Over the past decade several explanatory models have been offered as heuristics to guide research and clinical practice. These include the mutual maintenance model (Sharp & Harvey, 2001), the shared vulnerability model (Asmundson et al., 2002), the triple vulnerability model (Otis et al., 2003), and the mutual perpetuating model (Liedl & Knaevelsrud, 2008). Each model differs with respect to degree of focus on risk (i.e., vulnerability) versus maintaining factors as well as specific paths of association; notwithstanding, all draw on tenets of empirically supported cognitive-behavioral models of PTSD (e.g., Ehlers & Clark, 2000; Foa, Steketee, & Rothbaum, 1989) and chronic pain (e.g., Asmundson, Norton, & Norton, 1999; Vlaeyen & Linton, 2000).

Maintenance Models

Sharp and Harvey (2001) proposed the mutual maintenance model to account for the co-occurrence of PTSD and chronic pain. Their model holds that various aspects of PTSD maintain symptoms of pain and, likewise, aspects of the chronic pain experience maintain symptoms of PTSD. Seven specific mechanisms of mutual maintenance—attentional and reasoning biases, anxiety sensitivity, reminders of trauma, avoidance, depression, perception of anxiety and pain, and limited adaptive coping strategies—are suggested as having potential impact along bidirectional pathways with distress, pain, PTSD, and disability. To illustrate, the model predicts that Jamie's leg pain serves as a persistent and anxiety-provoking reminder of the IED blast in which he was injured. The anxiety and other negative emotions he experiences in response to recalling details of the IED blast contribute, in turn, to his avoidance of physical and other activities. The longer Jamie remains inactive, the more likely he is to become physically deconditioned and, as a consequence, the more likely he is to experience additional pain. The model suggests that Jamie has, in essence, become trapped in a vicious cycle whereby his symptoms of PTSD and chronic pain interact to produce self-perpetuating distress and functional disability.

Liedl and Knaevelsrud (2008) have recently proposed the perpetual avoidance model, a variant of the mutual maintenance model that incorporates postulates of the cognitive model of PTSD (Ehlers & Clark, 2000) and the fear-avoidance model of musculoskeletal pain (Vlaeyen & Linton, 2000) to account for responsible mechanisms of association. The essence of these models is that if a traumatic or painful experience is appraised as threatening (e.g., as a situation that may never resolve), it may be dealt with in a maladadptive manner that perpetuates a vicious fear-avoidance cycle that, in turn, promotes continued emotional distress and functional disability. While the perpetual avoidance model differs from the mutual maintenance model in terms of specifics regarding proposed mechanisms, the basic premise that PSTD and pain symptoms are maintained through self-perpetuating vicious cycles is the same.

Shared Vulnerability Models

Several theorists (Asmundson et al., 2002; Asmundson & Taylor, 2006; Otis et al., 2003; Turk, 2002) extended the postulates of the Sharp and Harvey (2001) mutual maintenance model by positing that some of the proposed maintenance mechanisms may be more accurately conceptualized as shared vulnerability, or risk, factors for the development of co-occurring PTSD and chronic pain. As with the mutual maintenance and perpetual avoidance models, the shared vulnerability models differ in subtle ways; yet, the basic premise of each is similar. To illustrate, our shared vulnerability model (Asmundson et al., 2002; Asmundson & Katz, 2009; Asmundson & Taylor, 2006) posits that individual difference factors predispose people to develop PTSD and chronic pain when exposed to certain environmental conditions; more specifically, the model suggests that the interaction of a genetically based psychological vulnerability to respond to stimuli with fear (e.g., high anxiety sensitivity, selective attention for threat), a lowered physiological threshold for alarm reactions to stressors (i.e., activation of physiological processes that prepare one to fight, flee, or freeze), and instigating stressful events (e.g., traumatic incident, injury) all influence negative emotional responses, their consequences (e.g., increased arousal, avoidance, increase in frequency of intrusive thoughts), and explain the development of PTSD and chronic pain. The triple vulnerabilities posited by Otis and colleagues (2003)—generalized biological vulnerability, a sense of uncontrollability over events and personal response to them, and a specific psychological vulnerability to focus on anxiety—map closely onto our shared vulnerability model.

The shared vulnerability models further posit that co-occurring PTSD and chronic pain are most likely to develop in cases where vulnerable people are exposed to an event that is both traumatic and painful, since such experiences are likely to facilitate associations between the traumatic event and pain and increase the probability that each will serve as a persistent reminder of the other. This postulate is consistent with the mutual maintenance and perpetual avoidance models and further illustrates how vulnerability factors can also contribute to maintenance of these conditions.

Jamie was described as a somewhat anxious and health-conscientious individual prior to his involvement in the IED blast in which he was injured. Not only did the IED blast result in injury to Jamie's legs, it put him in a horrific situation where he witnessed the death of coworkers and had to administer first aid to minimize harm or save the lives of other coworkers while exposed and under possible threat of enemy fire. It is possible that his pre- and postinjury tendencies toward anxiety and attentional focus on health (or potential threats to health) reflect elevated levels of concern regarding the meaning of anxious arousal (i.e., anxiety sensitivity) and concerns about physical well-being (i.e., fear of pain or reinjury, health anxiety), both of which may denote vulnerability for developing various anxiety disorders and chronic health conditions subsequent to experiences like the IED blast and its immediate aftermath.

Heuristic Value of Models and Empirical Support

The maintenance and shared vulnerability models suggest that PTSD and chronic pain are most likely to develop subsequent to an event that is both traumatic and painful in a person who (1) is predisposed (or vulnerable) to respond to such an event with fear, (2) feels that the event and response to it is beyond his or her control, and (3) focuses on his or her arousal and responds to it as an indication of pending catastrophe. The models further suggest that reminders of the event (e.g., intrusive thoughts, thematically related events) and pain sensations can trigger additional anxiety and pain and, as such, serve to maintain symptoms and associated functional limitations. This basic understanding of the co-occurrence of PTSD and chronic pain has stimulated a growing area of empirical inquiry, including research that has informed our understanding of maintenance and vulnerability factors and associated clinical implications. Moreover, these models and mounting empirical evidence provide a foundation from which to develop early intervention strategies for people experiencing an event that is potentially traumatic and painful and treatment strategies for people presenting with both PTSD and chronic pain.

STATE OF THE ART ON MAINTENANCE
AND SHARED VULNERABILITY FACTORS

Recent comprehensive reviews of empirical findings related to postulates of the maintenance and shared vulnerability models are available elsewhere (e.g., Asmundson & Katz, 2009; Beck & Clapp, 2011; Liedl & Knaevelsrud, 2008). All models assume or explicitly identify an event that is potentially traumatic and painful. There is evidence to suggest that prior trauma history increases the risk of developing PTSD (Zatzick et al., 2002) as well as postinjury progression from acute to chronic pain (Young Casey, Greenberg, Nacassio, Harpin, & Hubbard, 2008). Characteristics of the precipitating event have also been shown to influence both PTSD and chronic pain; specifically, regardless of objective indices of severity, subjective appraisals of the event and associated injuries and pain predict PTSD symptom severity (Gabert-Quillen, Fallon, & Delahanty, 2011) and pain chronicity (Holmes et al., 2010). While more research is needed to understand the impact of former and reference events in the context of co-occurring PTSD and chronic pain, it is a focus on the proposed maintenance and shared vulnerability factors that may be fundamental to improving our understanding of co-occurrence.

As detailed by Beck and Clapp (2011), there are several proposed maintenance mechanisms that have yet to be systematically explored, including reminders of trauma, avoidance behavior, and increased demand on cognitive resources. This is also true of trait vulnerabilities beyond anxiety sensitivity (e.g., fear of pain, illness/injury sensitivity) and autonomic nervous system dysregulation. Rather than consider these understudied factors further, we instead highlight the maintenance and shared vulnerability factors for which there is mounting empirical evidence and actionable clinical recommendations—anxiety sensitivity, depressed mood and activity reduction, and attentional biases.

Anxiety Sensitivity

Anxiety sensitivity (i.e., fear of arousal-related sensations based on the belief that they may have harmful cognitive, physiological, or social consequences), a potentially heritable trait, has been associated with an increased sense of danger and fearful responding in potentially threatening situations. As noted above, it is possible that high levels of anxiety sensitivity are driving Jamie's pre- and postinjury tendencies toward anxiety and worries that his arousal (and, perhaps, pain) is indicative of disease. Anxiety sensitivity is elevated in patients with PTSD (Taylor, Koch, & McNally, 1992) and in some patients with chronic pain (Asmundson, Wright, & Hadjistavropoulos, 2000). It has also been shown to correlate positively with the PTSD symptoms (Federoff, Taylor, Asmundson, & Koch, 2000) and pain severity (Lang, Sorrell, Rodgers, & Lebeck, 2006), and to increase the risk of pain-related avoidance and disability following physical injury (Martin, McGrath, Brown, & Katz, 2007). Recent findings from a longitudinal study of postinjury anxiety sensitivity and PTSD symptoms indicate that immediate postinjury levels of anxiety sensitivity are predictive of subsequent PTSD symptom severity and that PTSD symptom severity predicts later levels of anxiety sensitivity (Marshall, Miles, & Stewart, 2010). This suggests that anxiety sensitivity may be both a shared vulnerability and a maintenance mechanism (also see Jakupcak et al., 2006) for PTSD. It has yet to be established whether elevated anxiety sensitivity precedes the development of chronic pain, becomes elevated as a consequence of chronic pain, or, as in the case of its associations with PTSD, both. Notwithstanding, the current state of the art suggests interventions designed to reduce anxiety sensitivity may be effective in the treatment of co-occurring PTSD and chronic pain.

Depressed Mood and Activity Reduction

Depression frequently co-occurs with PTSD (Beck, DeMond, Clapp, & Paylo, 2009) and chronic pain (Farmer Teh, Zaslavsky, Reynolds, & Cleary, 2010) and is identified as a potential maintenance factor in contemporary models of each of these conditions. Several recent studies have assessed depression in people with co-occurring PTSD and chronic pain (Jakupcak et al., 2006; Poundja, Fikretoglu, & Brunet, 2006), finding that depression plays a significant role in observed associations between PTSD and chronic pain (or general somatic complaints) in veteran military personnel. Structural equation modeling of data collected from consecutive referrals for treatment of chronic pain stemming from injury suggests unique pathways of influence, with PTSD directly influencing depression and depression directly and, through pain-related disability, indirectly influencing pain severity (Roth, Geisser, & Bates, 2008). The specific mechanism through which PTSD influences depression in people with chronic pain remains to be determined.

It seems plausible that PTSD symptoms influence mood such that a person is more likely to become mired in a self-perpetuating cycle where catastrophic thinking and fear promote inactivity and physical deconditioning and, as a consequence, further pain. Jamie was worried about a number of things, including the physical consequences of his arousal and pain, and was avoiding most physical activity. It is possible that his avoidance behavior effectively reduced the concerning arousal and pain sensations in the short term; however, if persistent, avoidance of physical activity has potential for leading to diminished physical conditioning, increased arousal and pain during necessary activity, and, in turn, further avoidance behavior. This is consistent with the model proposed by Liedl and Knaevelsrud (2008), and stems directly from the fear-avoidance model of chronic pain (Asmundson et al., 1999; Vlaeyen & Linton, 2000). Interventions designed to reduce pain-related catastrophizing and fearful responding and increase activity may prove effective in treating co-occurring PTSD and chronic pain.

Attentional Biases

It is well established that people with various forms of anxiety-related psychopathology selectively attend to threat-related stimuli that represent their primary concern (Bar-Haim, Lamy, Pergamin, Bakerman-Kranenburg, &

van IJzendoorn, 2007); for example, people with social anxiety disorder direct attention to social threat stimuli rather than other threat or neutral stimuli. It has been suggested that such attentional biases act as both vulnerability and maintenance mechanisms for various psychopathologies (Mathews & MacLeod, 2002; Williams, Mathews, & MacLeod, 1996), probably as a function of decision-making and resource allocation processes (Mogg & Bradley, 1998). Whereas there is a generally consistent body of evidence indicative of attentional biases for trauma-related stimuli in people with PTSD, findings remain equivocal for chronic pain; in short, there is conflicting evidence about whether people with chronic pain selectively attend to pain-related threat stimuli (Asmundson & Katz, 2009). There has been only one published investigation of the nature of attentional biases in people who, like Jamie, have co-occurring PTSD and pain. Beck, Freeman, Shipherd, Hamblen, and Lackner (2001) used the emotional Stroop task, finding that people with co-occurring PTSD and pain had attentional biases for both pain- and accident-related stimuli, whereas those with pain and no PTSD showed bias only toward pain-related stimuli. These findings, despite being reported over a decade ago, await replication. Notwithstanding, the findings suggest that emerging strategies designed to modify selective attentional biases for threat stimuli and thereby reduce symptom severity may be effective in the treatment of co-occurring PTSD and chronic pain.

CLINICAL STRATEGIES AND RECOMMENDATIONS

Without careful assessment and case conceptualization, it is often the case that only one of PTSD or chronic pain is the focus of treatment. Co-occurrence is often overlooked because those working in mental health settings with people presenting with anxiety disorders do not routinely screen for chronic pain, and those working in pain clinics do not routinely screen for PTSD. As a consequence, the focus of treatment is typically either PTSD or pain, not both. Comprehensive assessment and case conceptualization facilitate effective intervention. It is beyond the scope of this chapter to provide a detailed synopsis of assessment strategies and tools for PTSD, chronic pain, and their co-occurrence. Assessment of PTSD is described elsewhere in this volume. Likewise, numerous authors (e.g., Dworkin et al., 2005; Thorn, 2004) have described pain assessment. We (Asmundson, McMillan, & Carleton, 2011) have recently provided guidelines to facilitate time-efficient yet reasonably comprehensive pain assessment in people presenting to anxiety disorder clinics. This, in essence, involves reviewing available medical records, conducting a brief clinical interview, and collecting supplemental information from prospective monitoring and select self-report measures (see Asmundson et al.,

2011) to glean information regarding pain severity and stability, location of pain, attitudes and beliefs about pain, pain-specific emotional distress (i.e., fear, anxiety, mood changes), pain-related coping styles, and pain-related functional capacity. The latter is particularly important given that some people with chronic pain function well despite their pain, whereas others do not.

There have been a limited number of studies on the impact of treatment strategies targeting PTSD in people with co-occurring PTSD and chronic pain. Some findings suggest that pain symptoms can interfere with PTSD treatment by negatively impacting a person's ability to fully engage in important aspects of treatment (e.g., muscle spasms and associated pain may interfere with concentration or discourage continuing participation; Koch & Taylor, 1995; Taylor et al., 2001; Wald et al., 2004). Findings from other studies indicate that PTSD treatment can be effective in reducing PTSD symptom severity despite presence of pain; however, it remains inconclusive whether such treatment has a positive impact on pain severity (Beck, Coffey, Foy, Keane, & Blanchard, 2009; Shiperd et al., 2007) or not (Shiperd, Beck, Hamblen, Lackner, & Freeman, 2003). It also remains to be determined whether treating PTSD has a positive influence on pain-related functional limitations (Shiperd et al., 2003) or not (Muse, 1986). Our clinical experience has also been mixed, with pain severity intermittently impeding progress with PTSD treatment in some cases, or diminishing coincidental with reduction of PTSD symptoms and overall gains in functional ability in others. To the best of our knowledge, there is a dearth of published studies on the positive or negative effects of evidence-based pain management strategies—such as pharmacotherapy (Kroenke, Krebs, & Bair, 2009), cognitive-behavioral therapy (CBT; Morley, Williams, & Hussain, 2008), and multidisciplinary rehabilitation (Guzman et al., 2001)—on PTSD; although, several investigators have noted that CBT-based pain management has minimal impact on symptoms of PTSD (Muller et al., 2009; Muse, 1986). In short, the available literature suggests that it may be insufficient to treat only one of either PTSD or pain in people who experience these conditions together.

Aside from a treatment-as-usual approach for one of either PTSD (for those referred to mental health settings) or chronic pain (for those referred to pain clinics) in a person presenting with both, there are several clinical strategies that stem from general postulates of the maintenance and shared vulnerability models as well as from the state of the art regarding anxiety sensitivity, depression and activity limitations, and attentional biases. These strategies can be classified as falling roughly into categories of early intervention, integrated treatment, and treatment specific to maintenance and shared vulnerability mechanisms. Despite holding promise, all of the following strategies require further empirical evaluation.

Early Intervention

No early therapeutic interventions have been specifically designed to prevent the development of co-occurring PTSD and chronic pain. The results of the studies examining the usefulness of existing early intervention for the independent occurrence of these conditions are mixed. Application of psychological debriefing, such as critical incident stress debriefing, to prevent PTSD development after a potentially traumatic event has been criticized (Litz, Gray, Bryant, & Adler, 2002) for failure to demonstrate therapeutic benefit or for resulting in worse mental health outcomes than no intervention (Deahl et al., 2000; Mayou, Ehlers, & Hobbs, 2000; Rose, Brewin, Andrews, & Kirk, 1999). A more promising strategy is to screen people for vulnerability for posttrauma psychopathology, symptoms of PTSD (or acute stress disorder), and impaired functioning and, for those screening positive, implement brief CBT (O'Donnell, Bryant, Creamer, & Carty, 2008). Early intervention methods for chronic pain, on the other hand, have been largely supported in contemporary literature (Rosenfeld, Gunnarsson, & Borenstein, 2000); for example, individuals participating in programs designed to restore preinjury functioning through graded physical activity soon after injury have been found to improve indices of health care utilization, medication use, and self-reported pain variables when compared to individuals left untreated (Gatchel et al., 2003). It seems reasonable to speculate that, in cases similar to those of Jamie, an early intervention strategy incorporating both graded physical activity and therapy for significant posttrauma psychological symptoms would circumvent the development and maintenance of co-occurring PTSD and chronic pain. Such an approach, however, remains to be empirically evaluated.

There may also be some potentially beneficial pharmacologically based early interventions for co-occurring PTSD and chronic pain. Indeed, as a means of blunting acute pain experiences and possibly interrupting memory consolidation and associated fear conditioning (Morgan, Krystal, & Southwest, 2003), opioid analgesics (e.g., morphine) might be applied in the immediate aftermath of an event that is both painful and traumatic. Preliminary research has shown that, despite side effects that can mimic trauma-related anxiety (e.g., derealization, depersonalization, irritability, concentration difficulties), such an approach is effective in reducing PTSD symptom severity (Bryant, Creamer, O'Donnell, Silove, & McFarlane, 2009) and reduces risk of developing PTSD (Holbrook, Galarneau, Dye, Quinn, & Dougherty, 2010). Whether these observed effects are a function of interrupted memory consolidation and diminished fear conditioning, reduction of pain severity interrupting activation of shared vulnerability mechanisms and associated reduction of risk for

PTSD, or some combination thereof, remains to be determined; but, as an early intervention for presentations similar to that of Jamie, the effects appear promising.

Although preliminary, the above-mentioned finding suggest that early interventions (i.e., as soon after a traumatic and painful event as feasible) that aggressively target both emotional and behavioral reactions to both trauma and pain may effectively prevent development of one or both of PTSD and chronic pain; that is, these early interventions may prevent acute stress reactions and acute pain from progressing to a point where they become maladaptive. By encouraging confrontation of potentially threatening situations and adaptive coping, such interventions should, in theory, prevent a person from becoming mired in the vicious self-perpetuating cycles that characterize PTSD, chronic pain, and their co-occurrence. Longitudinal studies are needed to determine whether this speculation will be empirically supported.

Integrated Treatment

Given the multitude of issues faced by individuals affected by co-occurring PTSD and chronic pain, contemporary thought consistently advocates for multidisciplinary and integrated treatment options (Clark, Bair, Buckenmaier, Girinda, & Walker, 2007; McGreary, Moore, Vriend, Peterson, & Gatchel, 2011; Wald et al., 2004). While the focus of various proposed integrated programs differ to some degree, they share in common a focus on integrating components of evidence-based treatments for PTSD (e.g., Resick, Monson, & Rizvi, 2008; van Etten & Taylor, 1998) and for chronic pain (e.g., Morley et al., 2008) into an approach that seamlessly attempts to improve psychological well-being and reduce pain-related functional limitations. There are several published descriptions of these integrated approaches. For example, Otis, Kean, Kerns, Monson, and Scioli (2009) have developed a program comprising 12 sessions targeting psychoeducation, cognitive restructuring, emotion regulation strategies (e.g., progressive muscle relaxation), exposure, activity planning, and other issues pertinent to both PTSD and chronic pain. Similarly, McGeary and colleagues (2011) describe a program, based on that of Otis and colleagues (2009), that appears to more strongly emphasize provision of abbreviated prolonged exposure for traumatic stress within the context of an interdisciplinary pain management program. Only preliminary data are available regarding the effectiveness of these and similar integrated programs. These preliminary findings are encouraging, indicating improvements in pain severity, perceived disability, and emotional distress (Otis et al., 2009; Smeeding, Bradshaw, Kumpfer, Trevithick, & Stoddard, 2011).

RECOMMENDATIONS TARGETING MAINTENANCE
AND SHARED VULNERABILITY MECHANISMS

The models proposed to explain the co-occurrence of PTSD and chronic pain posit a variety of mechanisms of mutual maintenance and shared vulnerability, several of which represents possible targets for intervention. Below we highlight three treatment strategies that appear to have promise in addressing mutual maintenance and shared vulnerability factors. These include interoceptive exposure, activity management, and attention modification. Each of these treatment strategies stems from systematic evidence supporting effectiveness in reducing either PTSD symptoms or aspects of chronic pain and, in some instances, observed effectiveness in clinical cases such as that of Jamie. Systematic evaluation in the early stages following a potentially traumatic and painful event (i.e., as a means of early intervention) and in people who have PTSD and chronic pain remains unexplored; as such, these are important avenues of future investigation.

Interoceptive Exposure

Exposure therapy (e.g., prolonged exposure, graded *in vivo* exposure) produces therapeutic effects relative to comparison strategies for PTSD symptoms (e.g., Rothbaum, Hodges, Ready, Graap, & Alacron, 2001; Rothbaum & Schwartz, 2002) and pain and associated functional limitations (Bailey, Carleton, Vlaeyen, & Asmundson, 2010). Indeed, there is mounting evidence that exposure therapy alone may be as effective or more effective than exposure therapy with a cognitive restructuring element because similar cognitive changes are mediated by exposure alone (Hofmann, 2008). There are, however, cases in which these treatment strategies are either not well tolerated or not effective. Consequently, investigators have sought innovative applications of CBT that might prove to be effective alternatives in these cases. Treatment strategies based on the principle of interoceptive exposure (IE)—exposure to feared bodily sensations associated with arousal—appear to hold considerable promise. IE also works on the premise that one must face the things one fears in order to overcome fear; specifically, IE reduces fear of arousal-related sensations, or anxiety sensitivity, by helping people discover that these sensations may be discomforting but that they do not have harmful consequences.

As applied to PTSD, IE protocols typically comprise exercises proven effective for inducing arousal in the context of panic disorder or elevated health anxiety (e.g., hyperventilation to induce breathless and racing heart, shaking head side to side to induce dizziness and depersonalization, stationary running to induce racing heart and chest tightness; Taylor, 2006). IE typically begins with screening for medical conditions that may contraindicate certain IE exercises, identification of a few (i.e., two to four) specific exercises that provoke arousal in the person, performing these exercises repeatedly with the therapist present, and then again repeatedly as homework. IE exercises are brief, requiring only a few minutes each; consequently, five trials of each of several exercises can be performed in a treatment session and as daily homework. Progress can be monitored by having the person rate and graph maximum distress during each trial of each selected exercise. Recent findings suggest that IE may derive its effectiveness in reducing PTSD symptoms not only by exposing patients to discomforting arousal-related sensations (Wald & Taylor, 2005, 2007), but also via triggering of trauma-related memories and images (Wald & Taylor, 2008); that is, IE may be effective in treating PTSD through reduction of anxiety sensitivity and as an unconventional form of trauma-related imaginal exposure.

There is also preliminary evidence that IE, performed in standard fashion as described above, may be effective in the management of pain. For example, to test the hypothesis that IE would be effective in reducing fear of pain, Watt, Stewart, Lefaivre, and Uman (2006) randomly assigned women with either high or low levels of anxiety sensitivity to receive a nonspecific treatment or three 1-hour sessions of CBT, the final session comprising IE using running as the exposure exercise. Findings indicated, as predicted, that the single session of IE led to significant reductions in fear of pain from pre- to posttreatment in women with high pretreatment anxiety sensitivity. Pain severity was not assessed. More recently, Flink, Nicholas, Boersma, and Linton (2009) compared the effectiveness of IE to relaxation/distraction (each practiced a minimum of 15 minutes twice daily for 3 weeks) in reducing pain severity and pain-related distress in six people with chronic pain using a multiple baseline cross-over design. Pain severity remained unchanged, or increased, in all but one person from pre- to posttreatment; however, improvements in pain acceptance and reductions in pain-related functional limitations and pain catastrophizing were observed from pre- to posttreatment and generally maintained at follow-up. Contrary to expectations, neither treatment had a distinct advantage over the other. Although Flink and colleagues described this study as an evaluation of IE, it might be more accurately conceptualized as a comparison of acceptance of pain versus relaxation/distraction; specifically, by only instructing participants to "calmly focus their attention on their pain sensations" (p. 724), their IE protocol is not consistent with standard IE protocols (i.e., those designed to specifically elicit feared sensations). Effectiveness of standard IE protocols remains to be determined in people with chronic pain.

We have previously suggested that IE may be effective in treating people with co-occurring PTSD and chronic pain (Asmundson & Katz, 2009; Asmundson & Taylor, 2006). As described in more detail below, we used IE in Jamie's treatment plan. This approach is predicated on the assumption that targeting the shared vulnerability—anxiety sensitivity in this case—will reduce severity of symptoms of both PTSD and chronic pain. Wald and colleagues (Wald, Taylor, Chiri, & Sica, 2010) recently evaluated this idea in a case series of four people with PTSD and chronic pain following involvement in motor vehicle accidents. Treatment comprised four sessions of standard IE and eight sessions of trauma-related exposure. The results suggest that, despite having some residual PTSD and return of pain symptoms at 3-month follow-up, this treatment approach was generally effective. IE reduced PTSD symptom severity; however, it was most effective in reducing anxiety sensitivity as well as pain severity and related functional limitations. Trauma-related exposure was more effective than IE in reducing PTSD symptom severity (especially avoidance); however, it was associated with increases in pain severity and related functional limitations. The reductions in anxiety sensitivity as a result of IE are consistent with the hypothesis that the treatment targets fear of arousal sensations. Wald and colleagues (2010) speculate that this reduction in fear of arousal may contribute to reductions in physiological arousal, including muscle tension, and thereby reduce pain severity and associated functional limitations. Another possibility is that IE reduces anxiety sensitivity, which promotes corresponding reductions in fear of pain, which, in turn, reduces catastrophic interpretations of pain sensations and associated functional limitations. While the specific mechanism of action remains to be determined, and fine-tuning is needed to maximize effectiveness, these preliminary findings indicate IE as a promising intervention for people presenting with co-occurring PTSD and chronic pain.

Activity Management

Physical activity has been shown to reduce depressive symptoms among those with major depressive disorder (Goodwin, 2003) and anxiety sensitivity among both depressed and anxious individuals (Smits et al., 2008). In short, the available evidence suggests that physical activity has a beneficial impact on mental health. Physical activity may initiate neurochemical changes similar to that of selective serotonin reuptake inhibitor (SSRI) medication (Chaouloff, 1997), reduce worry and anxiety (Bahrke & Morgan, 1978), interrupt social withdrawal (Hopko, Lejuez, Ruggiero, & Eifert, 2003), aid in development of a sense of mastery (Craft, 2005), and improve physical fitness (Stathopoulou, Powers, Berry, Smits, & Otto, 2006). Increased physical activity can be defined in many different ways; however, in this context this typically requires at least six exercise sessions for 20 minutes at 70% maximum heart rate over a 2-week period (Brouman-Fulks, Berman, Rabian, & Webster, 2004; Smits et al., 2008). Beyond a few small-scale preliminary investigations in adults (Manger & Motta, 2005) and children (Newman & Motta, 2007), both of which indicate promise, the impact of increased physical activity on PTSD remains relatively unexplored. In people with chronic pain, on the other hand, increased physical activity through exercise (Wright & Sluka, 2001) as well as via exposure to specific pain-related activities that are feared or avoided (i.e., *in vivo* exposure; Bailey et al., 2010) have been shown in numerous studies to be effective in reducing pain severity and improving function. This may occur through physical reconditioning as well as amelioration of fear of pain and/or anxiety sensitivity. Consequently, increased physical activity is an attractive treatment consideration for people with co-occurring PTSD and chronic pain.

Liedl and colleagues (2011) have provided the only study to systematically evaluate whether the addition of physical activity to other treatment efforts is effective in people with both PTSD and chronic pain; specifically, they added physical activity to a 10-session CBT program for pain management (comprising psychoeducation, relaxation training alone and with imaginal exposure of painful situations, and cognitive restructuring; also see Muller et al., 2009) and assessed whether this would improve outcomes in 30 refugees with probable PTSD and chronic pain. Manualized exercises comprised 20 minutes of stretching, endurance training, and muscular strength training, introduced with psychoeducation regarding the effects of avoidance and inactivity on maintenance of pain (i.e., in the context of a fear-avoidance model of chronic pain). Participants receiving each of the CBT pain management program and the CBT program plus physical activity had improvements on all pain-related and anxiety outcome measures relative to a wait-list group, but effect sizes were larger in the participants also receiving physical activity. In short, those receiving the CBT program plus physical activity had the largest pre- to posttreatment improvements in PTSD symptom severity, pain severity, and pain-related coping. Moreover, a greater number of participants in the CBT plus physical activity group showed clinically significant improvement in pain-related coping than did those in the CBT-alone group. These findings, although preliminary, suggest that physical activity is a valuable addition to pain management offered to people with co-occurring PTSD and chronic pain. Given the manner in which the physical activity was introduced—using psychoeducation in line with the fear-avoidance model of chronic pain—the findings also suggest that *in vivo* exposure to specific activities that are avoided due to association with trauma and pain may prove effective in these cases. In Jamie's case, we worked together to gradually increase his participation in regular physical activity as part of his posttreatment plan for extending treatment gains.

Attention Modification

Altering attentional biases (i.e., the stimuli to which a person directs his or her attention) is associated with treatment gains for people with various anxiety disorders (Amir, Elias, Klumpp, & Przeworski, 2003; Hope, Heimberg, & Klein, 1990). Recent evidence suggests attentional biases can be modified using variations of the paradigms used to identify those biases (Koster, Fox, & MacLeod, 2009). For example, an adapted version of the dot-probe paradigm allows training that aids people in learning to shift attention from threatening to neutral stimuli. In essence, the standard dot-probe task requires people to respond as quickly as possible by hitting a computer key upon seeing a probe, typically a dot, which follows in the position of either the threat or neutral word of word-pair presentations. Selective attention is indicated when responses to probes that follow threat words are speeded relative to responses that follow neutral words. In the adapted version of the paradigm, the computer is programmed such that probes only follow in the position of neutral words of the threat and neutral word pairings, effectively training a person over repeated sessions (e.g., 20-minute sessions twice weekly for 4 weeks) to direct attention away from threat words. Recent evaluations of the adapted paradigm in people with various anxiety disorders have shown that attention modification significantly reduces anxiety symptom severity (Amir, Beard, Burns, & Bomyea, 2009; Koster et al., 2009; Najmi & Amir, 2010; Schmidt, Richey, Buckner, & Timpano, 2009), although this effect is not observed when threat and neutral words are replaced with graphics of emotional and neutral faces (Boettcher, Berger, & Renneberg, 2012). Carleton, Richter, and Asmundson (2011) recently reported that the modified paradigm, but not a standard dot-probe (i.e., control) paradigm, resulted in significant reductions in pain severity and on measures of various individual difference factors (e.g., fear of pain, anxiety sensitivity, injury/illness sensitivity) in people with fibromyalgia. It remains to be determined whether attention modification would be beneficial in treating people with co-occurring PTSD and chronic pain; however, when considered in the context of the role attentional biases may play in each condition and their co-occurrence, this approach appears to hold promise. Attention modification training was not used in Jamie's treatment.

SUMMARY AND CLINICAL RECOMMENDATIONS

It is now well established that PTSD and chronic pain frequently co-occur. Several models have proposed a number of maintenance and shared vulnerability (i.e., risk) factors through which these conditions are associated and, as the research community continues to evaluate these factors, empirical support has been mounting. This research, combined with pain- and PTSD-specific treatment outcome research, has stimulated development of treatments specific to people, like Jamie, who present with both PTSD and chronic pain.

Jamie was referred to our clinic for assessment and potential treatment of PTSD. Pain was not mentioned in the initial referral, but details of his leg injuries and physical rehabilitation were documented in a summary medical report that was provided. In addition to PTSD symptoms, Jamie also mentioned continuing daily pain of moderate-to-high severity in his knees and surrounding muscles. We conducted a comprehensive assessment with Jamie that, among other important information, yielded pretreatment severity ratings of pain, pain-related functional limitations, fear of pain, anxiety sensitivity, and PTSD symptom severity. Serial measures were taken at the outset of each subsequent treatment session. Based on the assessment, it was collaboratively agreed upon that PTSD would be the primary focus of treatment; as such, we implemented a CBT-based treatment comprising psychoeducation, emotion regulation strategies (e.g., grounding, progressive relaxation), cognitive restructuring, trauma-related exposure, and relapse prevention programming. After the first few sessions it was apparent that Jamie was becoming increasingly anxious about his condition. He was specifically worrying that his continued leg pain meant he would never "get back to normal," that there was something else physically wrong, and that his lack of focus in treatment and elsewhere (e.g., drifting off to thoughts of the IED blast and all that followed) meant he was losing his mind. It was at this point that we discussed the option of IE. The rationale of IE appealed to Jamie; as such, we worked to identify some exercises that provoked sensations similar to those concerning him (e.g., jogging on spot increased overall arousal as well as muscle tension and feelings of fatigue; spinning in a chair to induce deprsonalization; lightly tensing leg muscles increased muscle tension as well as muscle trembling and shakiness), practiced how to properly conduct IE exercises, and then sent him home to practice and monitor progress. After 3 weeks of in-session practice and homework (daily for approximately 20 minutes), Jamie was reporting significantly reduced anxious arousal and pain in response to the IE exercises, and scores on presession measures of anxiety sensitivity, fear of pain, and pain severity diminished significantly. While he continued to experience generally persistent moderate pain, it was no longer a source of distress or concern. Jamie also reported that his general concentration had improved somewhat and that he and his wife were both pleased that he indicated interest for, and participated in, a game of tennis with her. In the weeks that followed Jamie was able to resume and successfully complete the CBT-based PTSD treatment.

Based on the information presented above we have formulated several early intervention recommendations when dealing with a person in the days shortly after experiencing an event that is potentially traumatic and painful, and for treating those presenting with co-occurring PTSD and chronic pain. These are as follows:

1. In the period prior to transition from acute distress and pain to PTSD and chronic pain, we recommend an intervention comprising:
   a. Graded physical activity that encourages confrontation of pain and activities associated with pain.
   b. If responsible administration is possible, the addition of one or both of an opioid analgesic prescription and interoceptive exposure.
2. For those people who present for treatment at a later stage (i.e., with co-occurring PTSD and chronic pain), and where specialized integrated treatment programs are not available:
   a. Begin with treatment as usual for PTSD, with initial assessment of pain and monitoring of its impact on treatment progress.
   b. If progress is hampered by pain, add one or both of interceptive exposure and increased physical activity within the context of the PTSD treatment protocol.
   c. Consider attention modification only if the requisite specialized computer software makes it feasible.

While evidence from case observation and emerging systematic evaluation support the promise of the various early intervention and treatment strategies described above, there is much work that remains. It is our hope that the ideas presented in this chapter not only identify actionable clinical strategies for clinicians who treat people with co-occurring PTSD and chronic pain but also that the ideas stimulate further clinical practice and research developments that systematically move forward the agenda of improving the lives of these people.

REFERENCES

American Psychiatric Association. (2013). *Diagnostic and statistical manual of mental disorders* (5th ed.). Arlington, VA: Author.

Amir, N., Beard, C., Burns, M., & Bomyea, J. (2009). Attention modification program in individuals with generalized anxiety disorder. *Journal of Abnormal Psychology, 118,* 28–33.

Amir, N., Elias, J., Klumpp, H., & Przeworski, A. (2003). Attentional bias to threat in social phobia: Facilitated processing of threat or difficulty disengaging attention from threat? *Behaviour Research and Therapy, 41,* 1325–1335.

Asmundson, G. J. G., Coons, M. J., Taylor, S., & Katz, J. (2002). PTSD and the experience of pain: Research and clinical implication of shared vulnerability and mutual maintenance models. *Canadian Journal of Psychiatry, 47*, 930–937.

Asmundson, G. J. G., & Katz, J. (2009). Understanding the co-occurrence of anxiety disorders and chronic pain: State-of-the-art. *Depression and Anxiety, 26*, 888–901.

Asmundson, G. J. G., McMillan, K. A., & Carleton, R. N. (2011). Understanding and managing clinically significant pain in patients with an anxiety disorder. *Focus: The Journal of Lifelong Learning in Psychiatry, 9*, 264–272.

Asmundson, G. J. G., Norton, P. J., & Norton, G. R. (1999). Beyond pain: The role of fear and avoidance in chronicity. *Clinical Psychology Review, 19*, 97–119.

Asmundson, G. J. G., & Taylor, S. (2006). PTSD and chronic pain: Cognitive-behavioral perspective and practical implications. In G. Young, A. W. Kane, & K. Nicholson (Eds.), *Causality: Psychological knowledge and evidence in court* (pp. 225–241). New York: Springer.

Asmundson, G. J. G., Wright, K. D., & Hadjistavropoulos, H.D. (2000). Anxiety sensitivity and disabling chronic health conditions: State of the art and future directions. *Scandinavian Journal of Behaviour Therapy, 29*, 100–117.

Bahrke, M. S., & Morgan, W. P. (1978). Anxiety reduction following exercise and meditation. *Cognitive Therapy and Research, 2*, 323–333.

Bailey, K. M., Carleton, R. N., Vlaeyen, J. W., & Asmundson, G. J. G. (2010). Treatments addressing pain-related fear and anxiety in patients with chronic musculoskeletal pain: A preliminary review. *Cognitive Behaviour Therapy, 39*, 46–63.

Bar-Haim, Y., Lamy, D., Pergamin, L., Bakermans-Kranenburg, M. J., & van IJzendoorn, M. H. (2007). Threat-related attentional bias in anxious and non-anxious individuals: A meta-analytic study. *Psychological Bulletin, 133*, 1–24.

Beck, J. G., & Clapp, J. D. (2011). A different kind of comorbidity: Understanding posttraumatic stress disorder and chronic pain. *Psychological Trauma: Theory, Research, Practice, and Policy, 3*, 101–108.

Beck, J. G., Coffey, S. F., Foy, D. W., Keane, T. M., & Blanchard, E. B. (2009). Group cognitive behaviour therapy for chronic posttraumatic stress disorder: An initial randomized pilot study. *Behavior Therapy, 40*, 82–92.

Beck, J. G., DeMond, G., Clapp, J., & Palyo, S. (2009). Understanding the interpersonal impact of trauma: Contributions of PTSD and depression. *Journal of Anxiety Disorders, 23*, 443–450.

Beck, J. G., Freeman, J. B., Shipherd, J. C., Hamblen, J. L., & Lackner, J. M. (2001). Specificity of Stroop interference in patients with pain and PTSD. *Journal of Abnormal Psychology, 110*, 536–543.

Beckham, J. C., Crawford, A. L., Feldman, M. E., Kirby, A. C., Hertzberg, M. A., Davidson, R. J. T., et al. (1997). Chronic posttraumatic stress disorder and chronic pain in Vietnam combat veterans. *Journal of Psychosomatic Research, 43*, 379–389.

Breivik, H., Collett, B., Ventafridda, V., Cohen, R., & Gallacher, D. (2006). Survey of chronic pain in Europe: Prevalence, impact on daily life, and treatment. *European Journal of Pain, 10*, 287–333.

Bryant, R. A., Creamer, M., O'Donnell, M., Silove, D., & McFarlane, A. C. (2010). Sleep disturbance immediately prior to trauma predicts subsequent psychiatric disorder. *Sleep, 33*, 69–74.

Boettcher, J., Berger, T., & Renneberg, B. (2012). Internet-based attention training for social anxiety: A randomized controlled trial. *Cognitive Therapy and Research, 36,* 522–536..

Broman-Fulks, J. J., Berman, M. E., Rabian, B.A., & Webster, M. J. (2004). Effects of aerobic exercise on anxiety sensitivity. *Behaviour Research and Therapy, 42,* 125–136.

Carleton, R. N., Richter, A. A., & Asmundson, G. J. G. (2011). Attention modification in persons with fibromyalgia: A double blind, randomized clinical trial. *Cognitive Behaviour Therapy, 40*(4), 279–290.

Chaouloff, F. (1997). Effects of acute physical exercise on central serotonergic systems. *Medical Science Sports Exercise, 29,* 58–62.

Clark, M. E., Bair, M. J., Buckenmaier, C. C. III, Gironda, R.J., & Walker, R.L. (2007). Pain and OIF/OEF combat injuries: Implications for research and practice. *Journal of Rehabilitation Research and Development, 44,* 179–194.

Craft, L. L. (2005). Exercise and clinical depression: Examining two psychological mechanisms. *Psychology of Sport and Exercise, 6,* 151–171.

Deahl, M., Srinivasan, M., Jones, N., Thomas, J., Neblett, C., & Jolly, A. (2000). Preventing psychological trauma in soldiers: The role of operational stress training and psychological debriefing. *British Journal of Medical Psychology, 73,* 77–85.

Dworkin, R. H., Turk, D. C., Farrar, J. T., Haythomthwait, J. A., Jensen, M. P., Katze, N. P., et al. (2005). IMMPACT: Core outcome measures for chronic pain in clinical trials: IMMPACT recommendations. *Pain, 113,* 9–19.

Ehlers, A., & Clark, D. M. (2000). A cognitive model of posttraumatic stress disorder. *Behaviour Research and Therapy, 38,* 319–345.

Farmer Teh, C., Zaslavsky, A. M., Reynolds, C. F., & Cleary, P. D. (2010). Effect of depression treatment on chronic pain outcomes. *Psychosomatic Medicine, 72,* 61–67.

Fedoroff, I. C., Taylor, S., Asmundson, G. J. G., & Koch, W. J. (2000). Cognitive factors in traumatic stress reaction: Predicting PTSD symptoms from AS and beliefs about harmful events. *Behavioural and Cognitive Psychotherapy, 28,* 5–15.

Flink, I. K., Nicholas, M. K., Boersma, K., & Linton, S. J. (2009). Reducing the threat value of chronic pain. A preliminary replicated single-case study of interoceptive exposure versus distraction in six individuals with chronic back pain. *Behaviour Research and Therapy, 47,* 721–728.

Foa, E. B., Steketee, G., & Rothbaum, B. O. (1989). Behavioral/cognitive conceptualisation of post-traumatic stress disorder. *Behavior Therapy, 20,* 155–176.

Gabert-Quillen, C. A., Fallon, W., & Delahanty, D. L. (2011). PTSD after traumatic injury: An investigation of the impact of injury severity and peritraumatic moderators. *Journal of Health Psychology, 16,* 678–687.

Gatchel, R. J., Polatin, P. B., Noe, C., Gardea, M., Pulliam, C., & Thompson, J. (2003). Treatment- and cost-effectiveness of early intervention for acute low-back pain patients: A one-year prospective study. *Journal of Occupational Rehabilitation, 13,* 1–9.

Goodwin, R. D. (2003). Association between physical activity and mental disorders among adults in the United States. *Preventive Medicine, 36,* 698–703.

Gureje, O., Von Korff, M., Simon, G. E., & Gater, R. (1998). Persistent pain and well-being: A World Health Organization study in primary care. *Journal of the American Medical Association, 280,* 147–151.

Guzman, J., Esmail, R., Karjalainen, K., Malmivaara, A., Irvin, E., & Bombardier, C. (2001). Multidisciplinary rehabilitation for chronic low back pain: Systematic review. *British Medical Journal, 322,* 1511–1516.

Hofmann, S. G. (2008). Cognitive processes during fear acquisition and extinction in animals and humans: Implications for exposure therapy of anxiety disorders. *Clinical Psychology Review, 28,* 199–210.

Holmes, A., Williamson, O., Hogg, M., Arnold, C., Prosser, A., Clements, J., et al. (2010). Predictors of pain 12 months after serious injury. *Pain Medicine, 11,* 1599–1611.

Holbrook, T. L., Galarneau, M. R., Dye, J. L., Quinn, K., & Dougherty, A. L. (2010). Morphine use after combat injury in Iraq and post-traumatic stress disorder. *New England Journal of Medicine, 362,* 110–117.

Hope, D. A., Heimberg, R. G., & Klein, J. F. (1990). Social anxiety and the recall of interpersonal information. *Journal of Cognitive Psychotherapy: An International Quarterly, 4,* 185–195.

Hopko, D. R., Lejuez, C. W., Ruggiero, K. J., & Eifert, G. H. (2003). Contemporary behavioural activation treatments for depression: Procedures, principles, and progress. *Clinical Psychology Review, 23,* 699–717.

International Association for the Study of Pain. (1986). Classsification of chronic pain. Descriptions of chronic pain syndromes and definitions of terms. *Pain,* (Suppl. 3), 51–226.

Jakupcak, M., Osborne, T., Michael, S., Cook, J., Albrizio, P., & McFall, M. (2006). Anxiety sensitivity and depression: Mechanisms for understanding somatic complaints in veterans with posttraumatic stress disorder. *Journal of Traumatic Stress, 19,* 471–479.

Katz, J., McCartney, C. J. L., & Rashiq, S. (2008). Why does pain become chronic? In S. Rashiq, D. Schopflocher, P. Taenzer, & E. Jonsson (Eds.), *Chronic pain: A health policy perspective* (pp. 69–84). Hoboken, NJ: Wiley-Blackwell.

Koch, W. J., & Taylor, S. (1995). Assessment and treatment of victims of motor vehicle accidents. *Cognitive and Behavioral Practice, 2,* 327–342.

Koster, E. H., Fox, E., & MacLeod, C. (2009). Introduction to the special section on cognitive bias modification in emotional disorders. *Journal of Abnormal Psychology, 118,* 1–4.

Kroenke, K., Krebs, E. E., & Bair, M. J. (2009). Pharmacotherapy of chronic pain: A synthesis of recommendations from systematic reviews. *General Hospital Psychiatry, 31,* 206–219.

Lang, A. J., Sorrell, J. T., Rodgers, C. S., & Lebeck, M. M. (2006). Anxiety sensitivity as a predictor of labor pain. *European Journal of Pain, 10,* 263–270.

Liedl, A., & Knaevelsrud, C. (2008). Chronic pain and PTSD: The perpetual avoidance model and its treatment implications. *Torture, 18,* 69–76.

Liedl, A., Muller, J., Morina, N., Karl, A., Denke, C., & Knaevelsrud, C. (2011). Physical activity within a CBT intervention improves coping with pain in traumatized refuges: Results of a randomized controlled design. *Pain Medicine, 12,* 234–245.

Litz, B. T., Gray, M. J., Bryant, R. A., & Adler, A. B. (2002). Early interventions for trauma: Current status and future directions. *Clinical Psychology: Science and Practice, 9*, 112–134.

Manger, T. A., & Motta, R. W. (2005). The impact of an exercise program on posttraumatic stress disorder, anxiety, and depression. *International Journal of Emergency Mental Health, 7*, 49–57.

Marshall, G. N., Miles, J.N. V., & Stewart, S. H. (2010). Anxiety sensitivity and PTSD symptom severity are reciprocally related over time: Evidence from a longitudinal study of physical injury survivors. *Journal of Abnormal Psychology, 119*, 143–150.

Martin, A. L., McGrath, P. A., Brown, S. C., & Katz, J. (2007). Anxiety sensitivity, fear of pain and pain-related disability in children and adolescents with chronic pain. *Pain Research and Management, 12*, 267–272.

Mathews, A., & MacLeod, C. (2002). Induced processing biases have causal effects on anxiety. *Cognition and Emotion, 16*, 331–354.

Mayou, R., Ehlers, A., & Hobbs, M. (2000). Psychological debriefing for road traffic accident victims: Three-year follow-up of a randomised controlled trail. *British Journal of Psychiatry, 176*, 589–593.

McGeary, D., Moore, M., Vriend, C. A., Peterson, A. L., & Gatchel, R. J. (2011). The evaluation and treatment of comorbid pain and PTSD in a military setting: An overview. *Journal of Clinical Psychology in Medical Settings, 18*, 155–163

Mogg, K., & Bradley, B. P. (1998). A cognitive-motivational analysis of anxiety. *Behaviour Research and Therapy, 36*, 809–848.

Morgan, C. A., Krystal, J. H., & Southwest, S. M. (2003). Toward early pharmacological post- traumatic stress intervention. *Biological Psychiatry, 53*, 834–843.

Morley, S., Williams, A., & Hussain, S. (2008). Estimating the clinical effectiveness of cognitive behavioural therapy in the clinic: Evaluation of a CBT informed pain management programme. *Pain, 137*, 670–480.

Muller, J., Karl, A., Denke, C., Mathier, F., Dittmann, J., Rohleder, N., et al. (2009). Biofeedback for pain management in traumatized refuges. *Cognitive Behaviour Therapy, 38*, 184–190.

Muse, M. (1986). Stress-related, posttraumatic chronic pain syndrome: Behavioral treatment approach. *Pain, 25*, 389–394.

Najmi, S., & Amir, N. (2010). The effect of attention training on a behavioral test of contamination fears in individuals with subclinical obsessive–compulsive symptoms. *Journal of Abnormal Psychology, 119*, 136–142.

Newman, C. L., & Motta, R. W. (2007). The effects of aerobic exercise on childhood PTSD, anxiety, and depression. *International Journal of Emergency Mental Health, 9*, 133–158.

O'Donnell, M. L., Bryant, R. A., Creamer, M., & Carty, J. (2008). Mental health following traumatic injury: Toward a health system model of early psychological intervention. *Clinical Psychology Review, 28*, 387–406.

Otis, J. D., Keane, T. M., & Kerns, R. D. (2003). An examination of the relationship between chronic pain and post-traumatic stress disorder. *Journal of Rehabilitation Research and Development, 40*, 397–406.

Otis, J. D., Keane, T. M., Kerns, R. D., Monson, C., & Scioli, E. (2009). The development of an integrated treatment for veterans with comorbid chronic pain and posttraumatic stress disorder. *Pain Medicine, 10,* 1300–1311.

Poundja, J., Fikretoglu, D., & Brunet, A. (2006). The co-occurrence of posttraumatic stress disorder symptoms and pain: Is depression a mediator? *Journal of Traumatic Stress, 19,* 747–751.

Resick, P. A., Monson, C. M., & Rizvi, S. L. (2008). Posttraumatic stress disorder. In D. H. Barlow (Ed.), *Clinical handbook of psychological disorders: A step-by-step treatment manual* (4th ed., pp 65–122). New York: Guilford Press.

Rose, S., Brewin, C. R., Andrews, B., & Kirk, M. (1999). A randomized controlled trial of individual psychological debriefing for victims of violent crime. *Psychological Medicine, 29,* 793–799.

Rosenfeld, M., Gunnarsson, R., & Borenstein, P. (2000). Early intervention in whiplash-associated disorders: A comparison of two treatment protocols. *Spine, 25,* 1782–1787.

Roth, R. S. Geisser, M. E., & Bates, R. (2008). The relation of post-traumatic stress symptoms to depression and pain in patients with accident-related chronic pain. *Journal of Pain, 9,* 588–596.

Rothbaum, B. O., Hodges, L. F., Ready, D., Graap, K., & Alacron, R. D. (2001). Virtual reality exposure therapy for Vietnam veterans with posttraumatic stress disorder. *Journal of Clinical Psychiatry, 62,* 617–622.

Rothbaum, B. O., & Schwartz, O. (2002). Exposure therapy for posttraumatic stress disorder. *American Journal of Psychotherapy, 56,* 59–75.

Sareen, J., Cox, B. J., Clara, I., & Asmundson, G. J. G. (2005). The relationship between anxiety disorders and physical disorders in the U.S. National Comorbidity Survey. *Depression and Anxiety, 21,* 192–202.

Schmidt, N. B., Richey, J. A., Buckner, J. D., & Timpano, K. R. (2009). Attention training for generalized social anxiety disorder. *Journal of Abnormal Psychology, 118,* 5–14.

Seedat, S., & Stein, M B. (2001). Post-traumatic stress disorder: A review of recent findings. *Current Psychiatry Reports, 3,* 288–294.

Sharp, T. J., & Harvey, A. G. (2001). Chronic pain and posttraumatic stress disorder: Mutual maintenance? *Clinical Psychology Review, 21,* 857–877.

Shiperd, J. C., Beck, J. G., Hamblen, J. L., Lackner, J. M., & Freeman, J. B. (2003). A preliminary examination of treatment for posttraumatic stress disorder in chronic pain patients: A case study. *Journal of Traumatic Stress, 16,* 451–457.

Shiperd, J. C., Keyes, M., Jovanovic, T., Ready, D. J., Baltzell, D., Worley, V., et al. (2007). Veterans seeking treatment for posttraumatic stress disorder: What about comorbid chronic pain? *Journal of Rehabilitation Research and Development, 44,* 153–166.

Smeeding, S. J. W., Bradshaw, D.H., Kumpfer, K. L., Trevithick, S., & Stoddard, G. J. (2011). Outcome evaluation of the Veterans Affairs Salt Lake City Integrative Health Clinic for chronic non-malignant pain. *Clinical Journal of Pain, 27,* 146–155.

Smits, J. A. J., Berry, A. C., Rosenfield, D., Powers, M. B., Behar, E., & Otto, M. (2008). Reducing anxiety sensitivity with exercise. *Depression and Anxiety, 25,* 689–699.

Stathopoulou, G., Powers, M. B., Berry, A. C., Smits, J. A. J., & Otto, M. W.

(2006). Exercise interventions for mental health: A quantitative and qualitative review. *Clinical Psychology: Science and Practice, 13*, 179–193.

Taylor, S. (2006). *Clinician's guide to PTSD: A cognitive-behavioral approach.* New York: Guilford Press.

Taylor, S., Fedoroff, I. C., Koch, W. J., Thordarson, D. S., Fecteau, G., & Nicki, R. M. (2001). Posttraumatic stress disorder arising after road traffic collisions: Patterns of response to cognitive-behavior therapy. *Journal of Consulting and Clinical Psychology, 69*, 541–551.

Taylor, S., Koch, W. J., & McNally, R. J. (1992). How does anxiety sensitivity vary across the anxiety disorders? *Journal of Anxiety Disorders, 6*, 249–259.

Thorn, B. E. (2004). *Cognitive therapy for chronic pain: A step-by-step guide.* New York: Guilford Press.

Turk, D. C. (2002). A diathesis–stress model of chronic pain and disability following traumatic injury. *Pain Research and Management, 7*, 9–19.

Turk, D. C., & Rudy, T. E. (1988). Towards an empirically derived taxonomy of chronic pain patients: Integration of psychological assessment data. *Journal of Consulting and Clinical Psychology, 56*, 233–238.

van Etten, M. L., & Taylor, S. (1998). Comparative efficacy of treatments for posttraumatic stress disorder: A meta-analysis. *Clinical Psychology and Psychotherapy, 5*, 126–144.

Vlaeyen, J. W., & Linton, S. J. (2000). Fear-avoidance and its consequences in chronic musculoskeletal pain: A state of the art. *Pain, 85*, 317–332.

Wald, J., & Taylor, S. (2005). Interoceptive exposure therapy combined with trauma-related exposure therapy for post-traumatic stress disorder: A case report. *Cognitive Behaviour Therapy, 34*, 34–40.

Wald, J., & Taylor, S. (2007). Efficacy of interoceptive exposure therapy combined with trauma-related exposure therapy for posttraumatic stress disorder: A pilot study. *Journal of Anxiety Disorders, 21*(8), 1050–1060.

Wald, J., & Taylor, S. (2008). Responses to introspective exposure in people with posttraumatic stress disorder (PTSD): A preliminary analysis of induced anxiety reactions and trauma memories and their relationship to anxiety sensitivity and PTSD symptom severity. *Cognitive Behaviour Therapy, 37*, 90–100.

Wald, J., Taylor, S., Chiri, L. R., & Sica, C. (2010). Posttraumatic stress disorder and chronic pain arising from motor vehicle accidents: Efficacy of introspective exposure plus trauma-related exposure therapy. *Cognitive Behaviour Therapy, 39*, 104–113.

Wald, J., Taylor, S., & Fedoroff, I. C. (2004). The challenge of treating PTSD in the context of chronic pain. In S. Taylor (Ed.), *Advances in the treatment of posttraumatic stress disorder* (pp. 197–222). New York: Springer.

Wall, P. W. (1978). On the relation of injury to pain. *Pain, 6*, 253–264.

Watt, M. C., Stewart, S. H., Lefaivre, M.-J., & Uman, L. (2006). A brief cognitive-behavioural approach to reducing anxiety sensitivity decreases pain-related anxiety. *Cognitive Behaviour Therapy, 35*, 248–256.

Williams, J. M. G., Mathews, A., & MacLeod, C. (1996). The emotional Stroop task and psychopathology. *Psychological Bulletin, 120*, 3–24.

Wright, A., & Sluka, K. A. (2001). Nonpharmacological treatments for musculoskeletal pain. *Clinical Journal of Pain, 17*, 33–46.

Young Casey, C., Greenberg, M. A., Nacassio, P. M., Harpin, R. E., & Hubbard, D. (2008). Transition from acute to chronic pain and disability: A model including cognitive, affective and trauma factors. *Pain, 134,* 69–79.

Zatzick, D. F., Kang, S. M., Muller, H. G., Russo, J. E., Frederick, R., Wayne, K., et al. (2002). Predicting posttraumatic distress in hospitalized trauma survivors with acute injuries. *American Journal of Psychiatry, 159,* 941–946.

Chapter 13

The Crucial Role of Social Support

Norah C. Feeny, Nina K. Rytwinski,
and Lori A. Zoellner

Ann had always wanted to be in the military and joined the Army as soon as she turned 18. Her mom, dad, and boyfriend were supportive of her choice and threw her a big good-bye party before she left for basic training. She was handling being away from home and the grueling schedule well until, 2 weeks before the end of training, one of her superiors raped her. He threatened that if she told anyone, her career would be ruined, and said that no one would believe her anyway. Ann believed him and told no one in her squad what happened. She withdrew from her squad mates, kept to herself as much as possible, and began to call home whenever there was a chance. After about a week, Ann told her mom in vague terms that she had been sexually attacked. Her mom was horrified and started to cry; she wanted Ann to come home. A couple days later, Ann called her boyfriend to tell him what had happened. He fell silent. He was shocked and didn't know what to say. Eventually he sputtered, "What were you doing alone with him anyway?" The rest of the conversation was awkward and filled with periods of silence. After his reaction, Ann vowed not to tell anyone else. Following basic training, Ann went home for several weeks before deploying. When she got home, it was very difficult for her to talk to her mother or father about what had happened, and she ended up staying in her room most of the time. Ann's mother was extremely sad and angry about the assault but did not know what to say to her daughter to help. At one point she put her arm around Ann and told her things might be better if she could just put this behind her; when Ann looked back at her with a hurt expression, her mom decided not to say anything else. Ann's father was overwhelmed by what had happened to her, and in the weeks following her return home couldn't look at her without feeling like he might start to cry. Ann felt very lonely and distant from everyone, and knew her boyfriend thought she was to blame. She could not stop thinking about the attack and how it had changed her forever. No one understood what she was going through and no one was there to help her.[1]

When we think about factors associated with facilitating and impairing recovery, probably one of the most important postevent factors is social support, or one's connectedness to and help from loved ones, friends, and community. In recent summaries of research exploring recovery following trauma exposure (Brewin, Andrews, & Valentine, 2000; Ozer, Best, Lipsey, & Weiss, 2003), *lack of social support* emerged as one of the strongest predictors of posttraumatic stress disorder (PTSD). In fact, lack of support predicted PTSD better than other factors such as prior trauma history or prior mental illness and even severity of the event itself. Indeed, the absence of social support, or the presence of negative support (e.g., blame), including the unhelpful reactions of friends and relatives, may be an especially important factor in impeding recovery (Zoellner, Foa, & Brigidi, 1999).

How does social support impact responses to traumatic events? Ann's boyfriend and parents care about her, but their reactions are most likely not helpful. What should people who want help do and say? What do we know about how important positive, helpful responses are to trauma survivors' ability to recover following these experiences? What about the impact of negative reactions? What happens to social support over time following trauma? In this chapter, we address these questions by defining social support, addressing the impact of negative and positive social support, and discussing the clinical implications for trauma survivors. Broadly, we argue that reducing the presence and impact of negative social support is crucial in helping trauma survivors to recover successfully. However, eliminating negative social support is not sufficient; it is important to also bolster positive social support and protect against the erosion of existing social support.

---

[1]This case represents a mixture of various clients whom we have seen in our clinical work who have experienced trauma. Any resemblance to a specific individual is purely coincidental.

WHAT IS SOCIAL SUPPORT?

Although most of us believe we know what social support is, the construct itself is multifaceted. Thus, it is important to begin this chapter with a definition that encompasses all aspects of social support. One definition of social support that may be helpful for our purposes was put forth by Hobfoll and Stephens (1990, p. 455), suggesting that social support is "those social interactions or relationships that provide actual assistance or a feeling of attachment to a person or group that is perceived as caring or loving." This definition highlights key aspects important to understanding the nature of social support. One important idea here is that the benefits of social support can lie in the belief that one has support available or in the actual receipt of such support (e.g., Stewart, 1989). The definition also highlights that support is provided not only by individuals but also by groups. Consistent with this, the concept of a "social network" raises questions of whether more avenues for social connectedness are better than a few avenues of strong connectedness. Finally, this definition highlights the importance of a sense of attachment and having the perception that one is loved and cared for. Thus, social support can be positive (i.e., support that makes us feel loved and cared for) or negative (i.e., support that has the opposite effect and makes us feel unloved and isolated). Along these lines, after we discuss the detrimental impact of negative social support and the buffering effect of positive social support, we then focus on five facets of social support and their relative import to recovery following trauma: quality versus quantity of support, perceived versus actual/objective received support, emotional versus practical support, informal versus formal support, and sustained versus acute support.

NEGATIVE SOCIAL SUPPORT

When you think of social support, thoughts of positive, helpful relationships might come to mind. Unfortunately, in the wake of trauma, there is also the distinct possibility that trauma survivors will experience negative social reactions from friends, family, and/or individuals in a position of authority (e.g., police officers, physicians, therapists). Negative social interactions may take the form of reactions that are intended or perceived to be critical, blaming, or grossly insensitive. For example, following a rape, a trauma survivor may experience negative reactions in response to the assault itself (e.g., "At least he didn't use a weapon—you're lucky"), a person's response to it (e.g., " It's over, try to put it behind you"), or to the situation in which it occurred (e.g., "Why were you alone with him in his room? You should have been more careful . . . "). In contrast to overtly hostile or blaming reactions, negative social support may also take the form of indifference (e.g., changing the topic or failing to acknowledge the impact of the trauma) or encouraging avoidance (e.g., "Just stop thinking about it"). These negative reactions can have a profound impact on an individual's ability to cope following a stressor (e.g., Ullman & Filipas, 2001; Zoellner et al., 1999). In fact, a growing body of evidence suggests that negative social reactions may be more directly related to worse long-term psychological functioning than the presence of positive social support is in terms of facilitating resilience (e.g., Andrews, Brewin, & Rose, 2003; Brewin et al., 2000; Davis, Brickman, & Baker, 1991; Dunmore, Clark, & Ehlers, 2001; Guay, Billette, & Marchand, 2006; Ozer et al., 2003; Ullman, 1996; Ullman & Filipas, 2001; Zoellner et al., 1999). Thus, let's examine the effects of these two forms of negative social support in turn.

Overtly Negative Support

Overtly negative social reactions may be powerful determinants of lack of recovery following trauma. Indeed, a mounting body of evidence suggests that when both positive social support and negative social reactions are examined, overtly negative social reactions are stronger predictors of PTSD (e.g., Andrews et al., 2003; Davis et al., 1991; Dunmore et al., 2001; Ullman, 1996; Ullman & Filipas, 2001; Zoellner et al., 1999). Moreover, these sorts of reactions are not uncommon; many trauma survivors report negative social reactions from at least one person they consider part of their support network (Campbell, Ahrens, Sefl, Wasco, & Barnes, 2001).

So, what are these negative reactions? Three common types of negative reactions are blame, doubt, and criticism (e.g., Holeva, Tarrier, & Wells, 2001; Ullman, 1996). Blame implies that the survivor is culpable or responsible for the traumatic event itself or his or her reaction to it to a certain degree. Blame can be overt—"You shouldn't have been out that late; had you come straight home, none of this would have happened"—or more indirect—"Were you being careful?" Doubtful reactions often take the form of questioning the accuracy of a victim's description of events, or, if they were as "traumatic" as described. Take the case of a rape survivor, for example, being asked by a police officer if what she described was "really" rape. Think about a child who confides sexual abuse to parents or teachers and is asked if this is "really" what happened. Criticism, like blame and doubt, may be quite explicit, "Stop talking about it—it's over!," or more subtle, "You might want to just put this behind you . . . ".

There is good evidence at this point that reactions of blame, doubt, and criticism are associated with worse psychological health and persistent maladaptive reactions to trauma (e.g., Frazier, Davis-Ali, & Dahl, 1995; Frazier & Schauben, 1994; Ullman, Townsend, Filipas, & Starzynski, 2007). In three studies of women who had been assaulted, negative reactions to disclosing the assault to others (e.g., perceived blame for assault; Ullman, 1996; Ullman & Filipas, 2001) and interpersonal friction (Zoellner et al.,

1999), but not positive support, were associated with worse psychological adjustment. Similarly, among recent motor vehicle accident survivors, those who perceived high levels of negative support (i.e., criticism) were more vulnerable to the development of acute stress (Holeva et al., 2001). It is important to note that this work maps on to a broader literature examining the impact of impaired family functioning, criticism, and intrusive, overinvolved family relationships on psychopathology in general. Indeed, there is significant evidence (see Hooley & Gotlib, 2000) that these types of responses are powerful predictors of worse outcomes and relapse for serious psychiatric illnesses such as schizophrenia, bipolar disorder, and depression (e.g., Butzlaff & Hooley, 1998; Hooley, Orley, & Teasdale, 1986; Keitner et al., 1995; Marom, Munitz, Jones, Weizman, & Hermesh, 2005; Miklowitz, Goldstein, Nuechterlein, Snyder, & Mintz, 1988).

Indifference/Invalidation of the Trauma

Another type of negative social support to consider is indifference to, or invalidation of, a person's experience of trauma or his or her reactions to it. Although less well understood than the impact of overtly hostile reactions, there is growing evidence that such forms of negative social support may be particularly harmful to recovery (e.g., Maercker & Müller, 2004; Mueller, Moergeli, & Maercker, 2008; Pruitt & Zoellner, 2008). In one interesting analogue study, Pruitt and Zoellner (2008) directly manipulated the nature of social support received following a distressing video; they compared positive, negative, and neutral reactions to automobile accidents. Those who received neutral reactions (e.g., brief acknowledgment of event, discussion of unrelated events, not addressing emotions) rather than negative support (e.g., victim blaming, discouraging disclosure), had more upsetting intrusive thoughts and rated the event itself as more severe. This suggests that neutral reactions do not appear to be neutral in their impact. Instead, they may indirectly challenge the legitimacy of one's experience. When a person's experience and his or her subsequent emotion or behavior are not acknowledged, this invalidation may shut down future emotion expression. This, in turn, may lead to an increase in overall emotional arousal, further contributing to the development and maintenance of trauma-related psychopathology (Fruzzetti & Iverson, 2004; Sayrs & Fruzzetti, 2003). Overtly negative reactions may actually sometimes be easier to dismiss as wrong or misguided. Thus, such invalidating reactions may be as, or even more, damaging than overtly negative social reactions.

The Impact of Negative Social Support

Why is negative social support potentially so harmful? One of the ways that overtly negative, critical reactions may impede recovery among trauma survivors is via the suppression of natural coping responses like talking about what happened with others or thinking about and trying to make sense of it (e.g., Ehlers & Clark, 2000; Ullman, 1996). It may be that such negative environments divert attention from actively processing the trauma by inhibiting discussion of fears and worries and preventing corrective feedback (e.g., normalizing) about the meaning of the event and one's reactions to it (Holeva et al., 2001). More simply, as Ahrens (2006) suggests, these sorts of negative reactions can silence survivors; it may be that when a negative reaction occurs, it not only impedes the relationship where it occurs but it also makes it less likely that the survivor will disclose information in any other similar relationships.

Similarly, in the case of indifferent reactions, it is likely that victims get the message that they should not talk about what happened. If one's experience is not acknowledged, perhaps it really wasn't that bad and they "should" be over it. So, attempts to talk about what happened and potentially garner emotional support are totally shut down. In our example, we see Ann told by her mom to "Put this behind you." While well intentioned, this remark clearly gives Ann the message that she *should* be able to move on and that her mother does not want to hear more. Thus, Ann stops actively reaching out. She stops talking about what happened, and despite her distress, she abandons healthy attempts to cope.

More broadly, negative reactions may initiate or reinforce negative thinking. Indeed, as our chapter on cognitions highlights, many models of PTSD emphasize the role of individuals' negative beliefs about self, others, and the world in the development of such chronic reactions (e.g., Ehlers & Clark, 2000; Epstein, 1991; Foa & Rothbaum, 1998; Foa, Steketee, & Rothbaum, 1989; Janoff-Bulman, 1985, 1992; McCann & Pearlman, 1990; Resick & Schnicke, 1992). For example, imagine how Ann felt when her boyfriend said, "What were you doing alone with him?" after she'd been raped? If she hadn't already questioned her role in the assault, it would be hard not to in the face of such a comment from someone she trusted.

Negative social reactions may also be reflective of interpersonal processes that are thought to contribute to the development and maintenance of depression and other psychopathology (e.g., Sacco & Vaughn, 2006). In their model of depression, for example, Sacco and Vaughn (2006) propose that negative reactions such as blame, criticism, and argumentativeness lead to negative appraisals and lack of support, and that this, in turn, negatively influences self-esteem, mood, and behavior. Indeed, perceptions of negative reactions and accompanying reductions in social support are thought to be the most proximal causes of depression (Gotlib & Hammen, 2002). Similar interpersonal processes may well account for the impact of negative social reactions among trauma survivors.

Finally, it is important to note that negative features of relationships are typically considered more powerful in terms of their psychological impact than positive social interactions (Coyne & Bolger, 1990; Lakey, Tardiff, &

Drew, 1994; Turner, 1994). A common adage in marital therapy or parental coaching, for example, is that 10 positive interactions are needed to
compensate for the impact of one negative interaction (e.g., Barkley, 2000).
Thus, even if a trauma survivor has adequate positive support, the addition
of negative social support may negate the beneficial effects of the positive
support he or she has received.

Summary and Clinical Recommendations

To summarize what we know about negative social support, let's consider
how Ann, in our opening vignette, was affected by negative reactions from
her boyfriend. Ann tells her boyfriend, someone she loves and trusts, that
she has been raped. His response is blaming: "What were you doing alone
with him any way?" While this may seem like an innocuous question,
simply clarifying the situation, his response was harmful, as it either was
overtly blaming or interpreted as blaming. Further attempts to talk about
what happened were awkward, and Ann's sense that maybe she did something wrong was reinforced. This is exactly what is meant by natural coping being shut down. Ann's response is to tell no one else. If her boyfriend
had avoided statements that could be interpreted in a negative light, Ann
may have been able to continue to talk about her trauma and over time
her symptoms may have subsided and their relationship may have been
strengthened.

Clinically, the implications of such negative interactions are clear. Even
one negative response such as indifference, blame, doubt, or criticism of
trauma survivors for their traumatic experiences or their reactions to them,
can impede recovery by reducing a survivor's willingness to discuss his or
her experiences and by contributing to negative self-appraisals. Furthermore, negative responses can negate the helpful effects of positive social
support (which will be discussed shortly). Thus, it is crucial for anyone who
learns about a trauma (e.g., friends, family, and professionals) to listen in a
supportive manner and avoid comments that could be perceived to be negative or invalidating. At a very basic level, what happened needs to be taken
at face value; accept the event as traumatic and listen to the story. Similarly,
normalize reactions and encourage active coping.

Of course, avoiding statements that could be interpreted negatively
and normalizing the trauma survivor's feelings are somewhat obvious sug-
gestions. More often, negative reactions that are harmful are not intended
to be. Ann's boyfriend presumably cares about her, but he says something
that is harmful, perhaps without even realizing its effect on Ann. It can
be quite difficult in emotionally charged situations to regulate one's own
emotions, let alone do so and be appropriately supportive at the same time.
Likely, Ann's boyfriend was overwhelmed by his own reaction to her attack
and said something negative without considering how his words would

affect Ann. Similarly, because it is scary to recognize that bad things can happen randomly (e.g., any one of us could be raped, attacked, or in a serious accident today), we may have a tendency to "blame the victim" when we hear about a trauma. By finding some fault in the victim's actions, it renews our sense of justice (Lerner, 1980) and makes us feel like we (and the victim) can avoid similar misfortunes by acting differently in the future (Dalbert, 2001). Of course, although this style of thinking is natural and helps us regulate our own emotions, it is flawed. Bad things happen to innocent people on a regular basis. Even if the victim's behavior may have put him or her at greater risk of experiencing a trauma (e.g., walking home alone at night in a dangerous area; drinking to the point of intoxication), the trauma is not his or her fault and pointing out what he or she could have done differently is unhelpful. In fact, rather than helping to keep the victim safe in the future, it may have the opposite effect. Blaming reactions may actually increase the risk of revictimization (Mason, Ullman, Long, Long, & Starzynski, 2008), possibly by increasing the likelihood that the victim will resort to risk behaviors (e.g., excessive drinking and substance use) to cope with the distress associated with the trauma (Ullman, Starzynski, Long, Mason, & Long, 2008). Thus, in such a situation, try to stay calm, and focus on the survivor him- or herself, rather than on one's own reactions. It may be helpful to take time later to think about or talk with others about your own feelings and how to deal with them.

It is also easy in such a situation to make assumptions that may or may not be helpful. For example, to say "You did the right thing by *not* pressing charges" is well intentioned but may leave a crime survivor feeling like everything she does is being judged or boxed in if she wants to later change her mind. Alternatively, to say "You did the right thing by pressing charges" is also well intentioned but may also dismiss how difficult the experience of pressing charges was and how much she now regrets it. While there is not a straightforward formula for sensitively responding to people who have been through traumatic experiences, probably the best place to start is by attempting to take the perspective of the survivor. In these situations, whether a friend or a professional, slowing down and thinking about what to say that will likely be perceived as nonjudgmental and caring is critical. One of the simplest things to do is ask survivors "What can I do that would be helpful?" Another simple response is to have a conversation with the trauma survivor about how even the most well-intentioned folks don't know how to respond when someone goes through a horrific event and, in fact, may unintentionally say things that are hurtful. That is, in some respects, normalizing how difficult it is for others to respond well in these situations is helpful to the victim.

Similarly, trauma survivors themselves can help shape their own support as well by giving feedback to people about what is helpful. That is, when they recognize something that feels appropriate or supportive, to simply say things like "Thanks" or "I really appreciate you saying that" can help shape future supportive responses. This type of response lets the giver know that he or she was on the right track. In contrast, for the trauma survivor to directly say that something is not helpful or negative may further shut down the person attempting to support him or her by convincing him or her that he or she just can't do it. While there are most likely some scenarios where direct negative feedback is appropriate, ultimately reinforcing the positive and attempting to ignore the negative may help to better shape future supportive behaviors.

POSITIVE SOCIAL SUPPORT

Given the harmful impact of negative social support, one might logically hypothesize that removing negative social support would be adequate to improve outcomes in the wake of a trauma. Although removing negative social support is helpful, it is *not* adequate. Indeed, as we highlighted earlier, both meta-analyses of PTSD risk (Brewin et al., 2000; Ozer et al., 2003) found that the *lack* of social support was related to increased risk for PTSD. Perceived or actual lack of support may lead to, or be intertwined with, a general sense of social alienation and disconnection. Some of the earliest work in this area was focused on war veterans and what was protective or harmful when they came home. Consistent with the later meta-analyses, among Vietnam veterans (Fontana & Rosenheck, 1994) and Operations Enduring Freedom and Iraqi Freedom (OEF/OIF) veterans (Pietrzak, Johnson, Goldstein, Malley, & Southwick, 2009), lack of support from family and friends emerged as a powerful predictor of PTSD. Similarly, among Lebanese War veterans, those who were poorly socially integrated and perceived little social appreciation when they returned home were most vulnerable to severe posttrauma difficulties (Solomon, Mikulincer, & Flum, 1989). Lack of appreciation may lead soldiers to question their actions in war in ways similar to those we described following overtly negative reactions. Upon returning home, soldiers may already be unsure about how they will fit back into society and perhaps about their behavior during war. Lacking social support means that potentially there is little opportunity for corrective feedback in these areas. Thus, in addition to minimizing negative social support, it is imperative to also ensure that trauma survivors have positive social support.

What are the beneficial effects of positive social support? In line with theoretical models, and perhaps our own intuitive models, in the broader health literature, social support is often associated with better health outcomes (e.g., Berkman & Syme, 1979; Cohen & Wills, 1985; House, Landis, & Umberson, 1988). In the aftermath of trauma exposure, higher levels of social support are often associated with less severe PTSD (e.g., Galea et al.,

2008; Kaniasty & Norris, 1993; King, King, Fairbank, Keane, & Adams, 1998; Martz, Bodner, & Livneh, 2010; Thompson et al., 2000). Similarly, following mass trauma (e.g., terrorism; Galea et al., 2002; Hobfoll, Canetti-Nisim, & Johnson, 2006), disasters (e.g., hurricanes; Norris & Kaniasty, 1996), interpersonal violence (e.g., child abuse and rape; Schumm, Briggs-Phillips, & Hobfoll, 2006) and combat (e.g., Vietnam; Barrett & Mizes, 1988), positive social support is also often associated with better functioning. In the months following September 11, 2001, over 1,000 New Yorkers were asked about their experiences of emotional support (such as "someone to love you and make you feel wanted"), instrumental support (such as "someone to help you if you were confined to bed"), and appraisal support (such as "someone to give you good advice in a crisis"). Perhaps not surprisingly, those who reported that they felt highly supported in these ways were less likely to develop both PTSD (4.4%) and depression (5.6%) than those who said they had little support (PTSD: 10.2%; depression: 15.5%; Galea et al., 2002). Simply said, social ties following September 11, 2001, appeared broadly protective. More anecdotally, many New Yorkers reflecting on the events of September 11, 2001, often comment on the importance of spending time with friends and family: people with whom they have meaningful connections. Stories similar to this were common: a man who lost several friends in the attack said that he'd never have gotten through the days and weeks following September 11, 2001, without his wife; "She kept me sane," he said, "She'd let me cry, hold my hand, and then make me get out of bed. She reminded me just by being there that there was still some good in the world when I really wasn't sure." Similarly, others reported things like saving family messages on answering machines and listening to them when lonely or scared. These sorts of interactions are very meaningful and kept many survivors from feeling very disconnected and alienated from the rest of the world. Overall, social support is associated with better psychological and physical functioning.

The Impact of Positive Social Support

How does positive social support help? Positive social support provides a buffer that blocks, or helps mitigate, the experience of whatever stress someone is undergoing (e.g., Cohen & Wills, 1985; Gottlieb, 1987; Lazarus & Folkman, 1984; Norris, Friedman, & Watson, 2002; Sarason, Sarason, & Pierce, 1994; Vaux, 1988). In their classic book on stress and coping, Lazarus and Folkman (1984, p. 243) write, "The social environment . . . provides vital resources which the individual can and must draw upon to survive and flourish. That people gain sustenance and support from social relationships has been known intuitively for a long time, and should be, in a sense, obvious. What is less obvious is how this works." Relationships, or social support, likely "buffer," or help minimize the impact of stress in multiple ways. Theorists propose that social support aids coping in the aftermath of stress (e.g., Lazarus & Folkman, 1984; Thoits, 1986), and protects other resources helpful to coping (e.g., self-esteem; Hobfoll, 1988). Thus, one of the major roles of social support is, in essence, to reduce the impact of the stressor. In Ann's case, for example, had her mother said something like, "I'm so very sorry about what happened honey, I love you, what can I do to help? Let's talk about what you're going through . . . ", Ann may have been less likely to stay isolated in her room, more likely to talk about her feelings with her mom, and perhaps able to begin to develop a plan for how to cope with her difficulties resulting from the rape and her upcoming deployment. Her mother's words, and Ann's perception that she is available, could potentially help buffer or mitigate some of the negative impact of the assault on Ann.

Additionally, positive social support may aid in recovery by helping individuals to develop a more adaptive view of their trauma. For example, Prati and Pietrantoni (2009) demonstrated that social support is related to traumatic growth, possibly because social support encourages a more favorable appraisal of the event (Schaefer & Moos, 1998) and/or offers new perspectives on the trauma (Tedeschi & Calhoun, 2004). Thus, if Ann's mother or boyfriend had encouraged her to talk about the trauma and provided positive feedback (e.g., "Wow, you were brave," or "I know it's hard, but I am impressed by how you have dealt with the situation"), Ann may have developed a more adaptive view of the assault (e.g., that she was not to blame for the assault) and possibly gained something positive from the experience (e.g., that she is stronger than she thought she was).

Taken together, positive social support has a buffering role, protecting trauma survivors to a certain degree from trauma-related difficulties such as PTSD. Yet, this research tells us very little about what is actually supportive or not and really lacks a fine-grained analysis of the nature of positive social support. That is, what does a positive socially supportive response after trauma exposure actually look like? In the following sections, we discuss five aspects of social support: quality versus quantity of support, perceived versus received support, emotional versus practical support, informal versus formal support, and sustained versus acute support.

Quantity versus Quality of Social Connections

One way to start breaking down positive social support is to examine the *amount (i.e., structural support)* and *type (i.e., functional support)* of social connections a person has (e.g., Cohen & Syme, 1985; Stokes, 1983). Social networks models examining structural support attempt to capture how connected a person is socially: how many connections someone has (such as with friends, neighbors, and family members), and how many interactions he or she has (such as seeing or talking on the phone with them). This is an attempt to *quantify* an individual's social ties and the diversity of such ties. Implicit in the social network model is that larger networks are better and that by having a relationship you, in essence, automatically garner support from it. In other words, having the connection ensures that support will be received. For example, in a very simplified network model, Ann has three significant relationships (mother, father, and boyfriend) and multiple contacts with each should be better off than someone with only one such relationship. By having more access to social resources, that is, a larger network, Ann theoretically should be able to gather more information, more resources, and more emotional support. Although this approach is intuitively appealing, as should be obvious when thinking of Ann, with more social connections there are also more opportunities for negative consequences. Although Ann has multiple significant relationships, her boyfriend had a profoundly negative impact that indirectly affected other areas of her social network. Moreover, this sort of network model basically only provides a rough index of potentially available support (e.g., Cohen & Wills, 1985). Even though it makes sense that "how many" relationships one has should relate to "how much" actual support is received, the association between the two is generally weak (e.g., Barrera, 1981; Sarason, Levine, Basham, & Sarason, 1983). In other words, more connections and interactions do not necessarily translate into more support. Quantity in and of itself does not equate with quality.

Quality of support (i.e., functional support), on the other hand, is likely quite important. Loosely, *quality* is the connection and acceptance that make relationships meaningful. Quality is about relatedness, as opposed to contact. The quality of social support is really about one's perceived closeness to others and the perceptions of social interactions as helpful or unhelpful. As you can imagine, this aspect of social support appears to be particularly important. Think about a really important relationship with a close friend who is empathetic and understanding but with whom you speak only rarely. This is the kind of person you might turn to or call to mind when you need help. Evidence for the importance of quality of support comes from findings that measures of network size or frequency of interactions tend to be less predictive than measures that take the quality of interactions into account (Kessler, Price, & Wortman, 1985; Sarason, Shearin, Pierce, & Sarason, 1987; Shinn, Lehmann, & Wong, 1984). Indeed, a close relationship with the supporter seems to be central to the positive impact of support (Sarason, Sarason, & Gurung, 1997). Building on this, we may learn most about the protective effects of social ties by examining specific relationships, rather than focusing on global notions of social support or networks of connections (e.g., Pierce, Sarason, Sarason, 1991; Sarason, Sarason, & Pierce, 1995). Specific, meaningful relationships (e.g., spouses [Fredman et al., 2010], parents [Vigna, Hernandez, Paasch, Gordon, &

Kelley, 2009], and peers [Wilcox, 2010]) appear to be those with the most power to protect or buffer.

Despite the clear importance of close social relationships, the role of a large network may be more important following a communitywide disaster than an individually experienced event. For example, perceived community support was associated with reduced PTSD symptoms among individuals who were rendered homeless following Hurricane Katrina (Kloos, Flory, Hankin, Cheely, & Segal, 2009) and among survivors of the 2004 Indian Ocean tsunami (Bisson et al., 2011). In a communitywide disaster, such as a hurricane, earthquake, or cyclone, having a broad support network may be essential (Hobfoll et al., 2007). Knowing and talking with other survivors may provide useful survival information (e.g., where to go that is safe), actual help (e.g., food, transportation), and later, empathy and connectedness around a shared survival experience. In a refugee camp or a war-torn community, the number and quality of relationships may be important to survival and well-being. Such connections afford protection and perhaps help to return a sense of normalcy. Yet, in the aftermath of such situations, social networks are often damaged or even eliminated (e.g., Norris, Baker, Murphy, & Kaniasty, 2005). Consequently, in the immediate aftermath, reestablishing social connections might be very important. Social connections can foster information gathering, tangible help (e.g., sharing food), and coping. A related notion is that of community resilience (Hall, Norwood, Ursano, & Fullerton, 2003). This refers to a community's ability to bounce back as a collective and overcome traumatic experiences through cohesion (Landau & Saul, 2004). Obviously, such resilience is challenged in the face of trauma because of the disruptions of individual connections (Landau & Saul, 2004). This further argues for the importance of networks of connection in the immediate aftermath of community disasters. After safety and normalcy has been re-established, it is likely that good close relationships (i.e., quality) play an equally important role in fostering resilience for those who have experienced communal events as for those who have experienced other sorts of trauma.

Perceived versus Received Social Support

Another way to start understanding the nature of social support is to examine whether or not this support is perceived to be available or is actually received (e.g., Dolbier & Steinhardt, 2000; Yap & Devilly, 2004). Perceived support is support that is interpreted to be available in the environment. Specifically, perceived support focuses on how people cognitively view or appraise their available support, regardless of the accuracy of this appraisal. For example, a person who has perceived support would answer yes to the following questions: "Do I feel valued by others?" "Do I have people I trust?" "Do I feel the moral support I need?" This is the sense that one is cared about by others and that help is available if needed. Received support, on the other hand, captures actual assistance provided (such as financial, informational, or relational help). This quantifies how much actual assistance a person receives. It is easy to imagine that one could feel very supported without receiving actual support (such as "I know that a lot of people care about me and are there for me if I need them"). Furthermore, the reverse could also be true; that despite actual assistance, the perception could be that one is alone and has no one to rely on (such as "I know that someone has given me clothing, food, and a place to stay, but I still feel as though no one is really there to listen to me or help me"). Many argue that it is the perception of available support that is more important than actual support (e.g., Dolbier & Steinhardt, 2000; Stewart, 1989; Yap & Devilly, 2004). Research findings also underscore the impact of perceptions of support on recovery, both in reaction to generally stressful events (e.g., Wethington & Kessler, 1986) and among trauma survivors (e.g., Holeva et al., 2001; Joseph, Yule, Williams, & Andrews, 1993; Ozer et al., 2003; Thompson et al., 2000). Women who experience domestic violence, for example, when compared to those who have not experienced such violence, perceive little available social support in their environments. Most importantly, perhaps, their low appraisals of available support explain their higher levels of psychological distress (Thompson et al., 2000). How we interpret what supports are available to us, whether we are right or wrong, appear to substantially impact resilience following both stressful and traumatic events.

It may be that this appraisal process, "People care about me and will help me if and when I need it," impacts the *appraisal of the stressor* and one's ability to manage it as well. Indeed, it is the case that models of stress typically include interpretation of the stressor and one's ability (or not) to successfully cope with it as determinants of how stressful an event is (e.g., Lazarus, 1966; Lazarus & Folkman, 1984). Thus, perceiving that people will help and support you can influence both how threatening the event seems and how possible successful coping is. It is also the case that those who develop PTSD often have distorted appraisals of themselves and their abilities to cope (Valentiner, Foa, Riggs, & Gershuny, 1996) that may extend to or be impacted by negative perceptions of the availability of support.

However, despite our emphasis on perceptions of support, that does not mean that actual support is unimportant. It is quite likely the case that receiving support has a role in shaping appraisals of available support (e.g., Norris & Kaniasty, 1996; Wethington & Kessler, 1986). That is, when one gets actual help, this can be indirectly helpful to mental health in that it improves, or prevents worsening of, perceptions of support. For example, over time following Hurricanes Hugo and Andrew in Florida, providing help (e.g., food, shelter) to victims was related to their views of the availability of support, and this contributed to less distress overall (Norris & Kaniasty, 1996). So, providing concrete help to trauma survivors is likely helpful in the long run, perhaps indirectly through shifting perceptions of support.

Emotional versus Instrumental Social Support

A third way to look at social support is to divide it into *emotional* support, or support aimed at meeting emotional needs, and *instrumental* support, or support aimed at meeting practical needs (e.g., Sarason, Pierce, & Sarason, 1994). Emotional support taps into how well an individual's emotional needs are being met. Examples of this are reassurance from friends and loved ones and the availability to talk with someone trusted about problems. Instrumental support, on the other hand, is not aimed at emotional sustenance or interpersonal connectedness, but is instead related to available practical help. Examples of this are having someone who would be willing to drive you to an appointment or lend you money. In many ways, these concepts overlap with perceived and received support; however, the critical difference here is the *functional* purpose of the support. Both emotional support and instrumental support can be either perceived or actually received.

Is it emotional support or practical help that trauma survivors need? While the answer is likely not black and white, when emotional connectedness is examined separately from other aspects of social support, emotional support typically looks most helpful to recovery (e.g., Dikel, Engdahl, & Eberly, 2005; King, King, Foy, Keane, & Fairbank, 1999; Schnurr, Lunney, & Sengupta, 2004). Among World War II prisoners of war (POWs), for example, when social support after the war was looked at as a global construct, it was not associated with PTSD (Dikel et al., 2005); however, when support was divided into two dimensions, emotional and instrumental, the results looked very different. Lack of emotional support was among the best predictors of PTSD. The only more influential contributor to PTSD was the actual severity of their POW camp experiences. Several other studies with veterans have shown a similar pattern of results (King et al., 1999; Schnurr et al., 2004). When looking at multiple aspects of social support and risk for PTSD in over 500 Vietnam veterans, emotional sustenance appeared most important (Schnurr et al., 2004). Men who returned home after experiencing a range of traumatic combat experiences, and perceived that people did not welcome them home and did not support them, were the most vulnerable to develop trauma-related difficulties (Schnurr et al., 2004). Similarly, in terms of the persistence of PTSD, again only poor *emotional sustenance* predicted failure to recover (Schnurr et al., 2004). This means many years after trauma exposure, men's current appraisals that they are not understood or loved are important contributors to persistent, impairing symptoms. This is good evidence of the import of emotional closeness and connectedness in recovery.

Clearly, emotional support seems to be central to resilience and recovery. But what does emotional support really look like? At its core is the message that one is "loved, valued, and unconditionally accepted" (Sarason et al., 1994, p. 110). Emotional support is rooted in genuine caring. In order to foster resilience, existing sources of support such as family, friends, colleagues, social groups, and clergy ought to be mobilized. However, it is *feeling* understood, valued, and listened to by such people that are of the utmost value. Making a casserole is a kind gesture, and may well be appreciated. Sitting down with a survivor (or calling him or her or writing a letter), letting him or her know you care about how he or she is doing, and are open to talking about what happened, is critical. Part of this is also being able to listen to and tolerate what a survivor has endured; try not to change the subject because the conversation is difficult. Many times survivors of trauma get the message that no one really wants to hear what they've been through and feel alone and misunderstood as a result. To the extent that they are willing and emotionally able, let survivors of trauma talk about their experiences and feelings. Help them to feel understood by normalizing their reactions. Caring, listening, and understanding—these sorts of emotional elements of social support, as opposed to the practical, appear to be more important to emotional recovery.

Formal versus Informal Support

Still another way to begin to understand positive social support in a more refined way is to look at the type of relationship with the support provider as either formal or informal. Informal support is that support that is offered via existing informal relationships, like those with spouses, family, or friends (e.g., Gottlieb, 1997; Ullman & Filipas, 2001). Formal support, on the other hand, is that offered or sought through professional support networks such as health care, mental health counselors, or police officers (e.g., Gottlieb, 1996; Ullman & Filipas, 2001). Generally, in line with the idea that connectedness is quite important, informal, as opposed to formal, support seems to be sought often and may be most helpful in the aftermath of trauma (Golding, Siege, Sorenson, Burnam, & Stein, 1989; Ullman & Filipas, 2001).

In terms of formal support, probably one of the most common forms is that of mental health crisis providers or, depending on the event, grief counselors on scene in the immediate aftermath of a traumatic event. Often we as mental health care professionals feel the moral imperative to do something to help. This is admirable and understandable. Yet, given what is known about formal support in general, does this extend to mental health providers in the immediate aftermath as well? As discussed in

Chapter 1, most people who experience trauma are resilient in the long run, do not have persistent trauma-related mental health problems, and do not need formal professional intervention. Indeed, somewhat counter-intuitively, what we know about the helpfulness of early formal efforts to provide brief, one-time mental health intervention efforts to all survivors is not encouraging (Rose, Bisson, & Wessely, 2003). Moreover, unhelpful responses may sometimes be more common when seeking formal support; among rape survivors, for example, negative responses to disclosing (e.g., blame and criticism) the assault were reported more often from formal (police and physicians) than informal support providers (Ullman, 1996). Similarly, formal support in the form of four to five sessions of support-ive counseling in the aftermath of trauma, seems to be minimally helpful in preventing PTSD (Bryant, Harvey, Dang, Sackville, & Basten, 1998; Bryant, Sackville, Dang, Moulds, & Guthrie, 1999). Why would this be? Perhaps, most simply, support is more easily or naturally obtained by peo-ple with whom a trauma survivor has established relationships. Knowing someone well, and trusting him or her, likely makes it easier to disclose the details of a trauma and emotions about it. It is also probably the case that formal networks are more likely to provide practical aid (e.g., food, shelter, legal advice) and that informal support providers are more likely to provide emotional support, which we have argued is often more helpful to enhancing resilience.

This leads to several concrete recommendations. Friends and family need to reach out to trauma survivors, provide reassurance that things will get better, and normalize their reactions by encouraging the gradual return to normal routines (e.g., work, school, sleep, meal preparation). If formal support providers (e.g., counselors, mental health professionals, crisis workers) are to be helpful in the immediate aftermath of trauma, several things they can do are to encourage survivors to seek support from loved ones (i.e., existing social support networks) and normalize their stress reactions. Similarly, if survivors need shelter or need to be relocated, these forms of assistance should be made with the priority of maintaining natu-ral social groups (e.g., families, church groups, neighborhoods). Survivors who are very distressed and clearly not functioning well may benefit from more direct mental health intervention. The best evidence we have thus far in terms of what helps to prevent PTSD, in terms of formalized interven-tions, is for multiple-session, cognitive-behavioral interventions for those with significant trauma-related symptoms (Bryant et al., 1998, 1999; Foa, Hearst-Ikeda, & Perry, 1995; Foa, Zoellner, & Feeny, 2006). Interest-ingly, among treatment-seeking individuals with PTSD, informal support was associated with a stronger therapeutic alliance early in therapy, which was positively associated with treatment completion and adherence (Keller, Zoellner, & Feeny, 2010). Thus, even among those who require formal sup-port from mental health care providers, informal support may improve the victim's ability to engage in treatment (Thrasher, Power, Morant, Marks, & Dalgleish, 2010).

Sustained versus Acute Support

In addition to the quality and type of social support, it is important to consider the fact that social support is most likely not a static entity, but rather dynamic and changing over time (e.g., Hobfoll, 1988; Kaniasty & Norris, 1993). In fact, social support may actually deteriorate over time (Kaniasty, Norris, & Murrell, 1990; Lepore, Evans, & Schneider, 1991; Norris & Kaniasty, 1996). This deterioration of perceived support over time is one way that traumatic events can adversely influence mental health outcomes (e.g., Barrera, 1986; Kaniasty & Norris, 1993). Hobfoll (1998) calls this a "loss spiral," a pattern in which a loss of resources like social support, which are needed to replenish other resources depleted by a trauma, contributes to additional loss. Poor social support, for example, may contribute to the development of PTSD, and PTSD symptoms themselves (e.g., detachment) may further erode the social support needed to foster resilience.

Generally, in trauma survivors, social support levels are often low (e.g., Schumm et al., 2006; Thompson et al., 2000) and further decline in the months following stress or trauma exposure (e.g., Kaniasty et al., 1990; Lepore et al., 1991; Norris et al., 2005). Among victims of interpersonal violence, social support is lowest among those most severely or multiply traumatized (Schumm et al., 2006; Thompson et al., 2000). Likewise, Croatian war veterans with PTSD have lower perceived support from family and friends than veterans without PTSD (Jelusić et al., 2010). Among women who have experienced partner violence, those who report the worst violence also perceive the least support (Thompson et al., 2000). Similarly, among sexual assault survivors, those who experience both childhood and adulthood assault are about 4.5 times more likely to report low social support than women who had never been abused (Schumm et al., 2006). So, trauma may have an erosive impact on the perception that support is available.

Actual social support may also deteriorate over time among those who are most vulnerable. In line with this idea, data from Vietnam veterans suggests that among those who develop PTSD, support after they are discharged and beyond is lower than before they were deployed; however, for those who do not develop PTSD, support levels stay the same or increase (Keane, Scott, Chavoya, Lamparski, & Fairbank, 1985). Notably, across studies, individuals reporting less support showed higher rates of PTSD, especially when more time elapsed between the traumatic event and the assessment of PTSD. Specifically, in their meta-analysis, Ozer and colleagues (2003) reported that the association between low levels of social support and higher levels of trauma-related symptoms was strongest in studies in which more than 3 years had elapsed since the traumatic event, and weakest in studies in which 1 to 6 months had elapsed. Thus, it may be that social support becomes more important over time with regard to its impact on recovery.

Why might support lessen over time among those who need it most? In the immediate aftermath of traumatic events, often support is abundant; but with time, it naturally diminishes. Perhaps those who are very symptomatic require so much support early on that the resources become depleted (such as a friend who feels like it is too much for him or her to handle) and no longer available as they continue to still need it. Alternatively, it could be that among those with PTSD symptoms, interpersonal skills are also impacted (such as PTSD symptoms of feeling detached and not interested in people or activities) and that, with time, leads to further social distancing and interpersonal conflicts that in turn exacerbates PTSD symptoms. There is good evidence that those with PTSD do experience interpersonal difficulties (e.g., Beckham, Lytle, & Feldman, 1996; Soloman & Mikulincer, 1987). Moreover, when King, Taft, King, Hammond, and Stone (2006) examined the directionality of the relationship between PTSD and social support among a sample of Gulf War I veterans, they found that PTSD symptoms more strongly predicted subsequent social support than social support predicted subsequent PTSD symptoms. Kaniasty and Norris (2008) added to this research by demonstrating that among flood victims in Mexico, less social support predicted more PTSD symptoms 6 to 12 months following the flood. However, 18–24 months posttrauma, more PTSD predicted less social support. These findings are consistent with the idea that interpersonal problems associated with PTSD negatively influence one's support resources. Social support, in essence, may burn out over time. It is also possible that social support may function as a kind of secondary prevention. Most people recover naturally over time following traumatic events (Rothbaum, Foa, Riggs, Murdock, & Walsh, 1992), but for those with persistent reactions, ongoing social support likely functions to foster help-seeking behavior. People who care about the survivor, for example, and who notice that he or she is continuing to suffer may be the catalyst to encourage the survivor to seek outside help. If Ann's symptoms persist with time, maybe her mother or father will encourage her to seek professional help. Perhaps for those with enduring difficulties who have little or diminished support, no one gives them the feedback that they are not doing well, and no one encourages them to get additional help. Thus, continued social support may be particularly important in helping individuals cope with trauma.

Summary and Clinical Implications

In the previous sections we summarized five different aspects of social support that can be helpful for trauma survivors. Let's now review what we know about positive social support and consider the practical implications of this research by imagining what aspects of the social world might really help to buffer Ann and facilitate resilience following her assault. Generally, the presence of support is important, but let's be more specific.

First, *meaningful relationships*: We hope that Ann has people, or at least one person, in her life who cares about her and to whom she feels connected. Those relationships could be with family, close friends, clergy, or coworkers: people who she knows, who she can talk to, who will sit with her, and who will listen. Concretely, of course this connection can take a variety of forms—phone calls, visits, e-mails, letters. Coffee with her favorite aunt, weekly phone calls with her sister, regular time to talk with a friend about how things are going—these are the kinds of interactions that should be fostered.

If Ann's relationships had been damaged or were nonexistent, an important point of intervention might be to help her develop or cultivate new supportive relationships. This might include helping Ann to contact and/or schedule visits with family or friends she has not been in touch with. Alternatively, if she had few healthy relationships, beginning to develop relationships with existing community institutions may be a good option, for example, starting to attend church or a community center regularly. For those with less existing support, a warm, therapeutic relationship may be important. Similarly, social support groups whose focus is to coalesce around a shared trauma experience may provide support for those without strong preexisting support. Yet, even here, these relationships should be used to build a bridge toward facilitating more long-term self-sustaining social support outside of the therapeutic relationship or the traumatic experience itself. The goal ultimately is for Ann to have the sense that she is cared about and help is available, if needed. Furthermore, established and meaningful relationships, even just one such relationship, are probably more important following trauma than having a large network of friends and acquaintances, or than acquiring "out-of-network" help.

Second, regardless of what concrete help is offered, we hope Ann *perceives* that there is support for her in her social network. That is, that she appraises people as being approachable and willing to help. Unfortunately, the cognitive distortions associated with PTSD (e.g., "People are malevolent," "I am damaged/not loveable," "The world is unsafe") and symptoms of PTSD (e.g., social withdrawal, feeling disconnected from others) may make it difficult for Ann to see the support that is available to her. However, corrective feedback from individuals in her support network (e.g., "I am here for you if you need me and will be no matter what") or perhaps indirectly via the provision of help (e.g., "Can I make you dinner? I know that things are difficult for you right now") may help Ann to have a more accurate perception of the help that is available to her.

Third, ideally, when support is offered, the focus should be on how she is doing *emotionally*: helping to calm and soothe her, normalizing her reactions, and if necessary, helping her return to her regular routine. Being supportive emotionally is likely more powerful than concrete help, though both ought to be offered.

Fourth, if possible, Ann's *informal*, already established support networks are utilized, and if need be mobilized. For many trauma survivors, being with and talking with friends and family will most likely be more important in increasing resilience than talking with a counselor or other professionals. If Ann was a member of a sports team, book club, or meditation group, going to the regular activities and connecting with friends afterward for dinner would be good way to remind her of the support available to her and help her feel less alone. Informal support can facilitate return to normal routines. These facets of positive social support singly and collectively appear to be important to fostering resilience in the aftermath of trauma.

Finally, it is imperative that this support continues, ideally forever, but at least until her symptoms subside. Friends and family need to recognize that single acts of kindness (e.g., sending a letter, giving Ann flowers, making her dinner) are helpful but not enough. It is more helpful to provide continued support. Furthermore, it is important to recognize that caring for someone with PTSD can be an emotionally difficult experience. Thus, caregivers may need to reach out to others for support in order to maintain the psychological resources required to care for both themselves and Ann.

CHAPTER SUMMARY AND CLINICAL IMPLICATIONS

In this chapter, we have tried to convey in different ways that good relationships and a supportive environment are likely important resources to draw upon in the aftermath of trauma. Meaningful relationships with people who are perceived to be emotionally available and supportive are broadly protective. However, as opposed to the power of social support in its capacity to buffer the effects of stress, it appears that social support is most powerful in its absence, that is, when social supports are perceived to be lacking or when they are negative in nature. So, while we would certainly suggest that in order to foster resilience following trauma individuals should attempt to draw on existing sources of support in their lives (e.g., family, friends, colleagues, social groups, and clergy), we would emphasize even more strongly the long-term import of having people available who are nonjudgmental, open to talking about what happened, and emotionally supportive. The emotional aspects of social support, as opposed to the practical aspects, appear to be most important in their role in recovery. In the context of therapeutic recovery, social support can be just as important—not as an intervention, but as part of the glue that helps people complete known helpful treatments (e.g., prolonged exposure, cognitive therapy).

With all this in mind, let's end this chapter with the basic elements of a concrete plan for optimizing social support in the aftermath of trauma. This plan could be the building blocks for responding to an individual or group following a traumatic event and is based on the principles we have tried to illuminate in this chapter: *validate, connect, contain, encourage,* and *sustain.*

Validate

First, remember that overtly negative reactions (e.g., blaming or criticizing the victim for the trauma or his or her reaction to the trauma) and invalidating responses (e.g., not allowing the victim to talk about the trauma) in response to a trauma victim can have a long-lasting, negative impact. In fact, these negative responses may be able to override the benefits of positive social support. Thus, if you learn of a trauma, avoid saying or doing things that are or could be perceived to be negative. Instead, validate the victim's feelings and reactions. Although this advice may sound simple, it can be difficult to respond appropriately when you are emotionally upset or caught off-guard by learning about a trauma. So, if you realize that your emotions are making it too difficult for you to respond in a validating, helpful manner, it may be beneficial to take time to sort out your feelings surrounding the victim's disclosure before providing support to the victim. Similarly, if your emotions do get the best of you and you say something that could be perceived in a negative light, don't beat yourself up. Instead, talk it out with the trauma survivor. Much emotional damage can likely be undone by apologizing to the trauma survivor and explaining what happened.

Connect

Next, connect survivors with family and friends. For example, in the case of a large disaster, make phones available to survivors and/or make calls to loved ones updating them of the status of the situation. Similarly, keep natural affinity groups together. For example, at a college, try to keep students from the same dorms together, and if this is not practical, make sure there are ways, like bulletin boards, meeting spaces, blogs, or chat groups where people can easily connect with people who are familiar to them. At the individual level, this same principle applies. In a hospital setting, for example, encourage the assault, robbery, or motor vehicle accident survivor to be picked up by and go home with someone he or she knows, regardless of the level of his or her injuries. Help a survivor to make phone calls, encourage him or her to talk about what happened to his or her loved ones, and help him or her to schedule times to be with others, if necessary.

Contain

Encourage survivors to talk about what happened if they'd like to. If they do not feel ready, let them know you're available to talk when they are ready. While not shutting down emotions, help survivors calm down when very upset and stay calm enough yourself that you convey you can hear about their experiences and tolerate them. Slow down and think about what might be helpful and, if unsure about what to say, quietly offer a hand to hold or an ear to just listen. Keep in mind that there is no one right way to react to trauma.

Encourage

Encourage recovery by normalizing what they are going through. Reassure survivors that they are coping the best they can and encourage them to stick with or reestablish normal routines. More specifically, encourage them to get out of the house, to get to school or work, and to spend time with people they are close to. Encourage them to talk about their experiences to the extent they are able. Encourage reaching out by asking "What would be helpful?" Finally, when reactions are severe and persistent (not sleeping, not leaving house) encourage survivors to seek outside help.

Sustain

As suggested above, support routinely declines with time, and support is often least available for those who need it most. If a friend or family member, plan for regular, ongoing contact with loved ones who are recovering following trauma. Schedule a weekly lunch date or talk on the phone weekly. Ask about how to be helpful. If a mental health counselor or in a similar role, plan routine check-ins with trauma survivors. If trauma survivors withdraw, seek them out. Finally, remember that caring for a trauma survivor can be emotionally draining. So, don't forget to take time to care for yourself in order to have the resources to continue to support others.

ACKNOWLEDGMENTS

We would like to thank Stephanie Keller for her careful reading of and comments on this chapter.

REFERENCES

Ahrens, C. E. (2006). Being silenced: The impact of negative social reactions on the disclosure of rape. *American Journal of Community Psychology, 38,* 263–274.

Andrews, B., Brewin, C. R., & Rose, S. (2003). Gender, social support, and PTSD in victims of violent crime. *Journal of Traumatic Stress, 16,* 421–427.

Barkley, R. A. (2000). *Taking charge of ADHD: The complete, authoritative guide for parents* (rev. ed.). New York: Guilford Press.

Barrett, T. W., & Mizes, J. S. (1988). Combat level and social support in the development of posttraumatic stress disorder in Vietnam veterans. *Behavior Modification, 12,* 100–115.

Barrera, M. Jr. (1981). Social support in the adjustment of pregnant adolescents: Assessment issues. In B. Gottlieb (Ed.), *Social networks and social support* (pp. 69–95). Beverly Hills, CA: Sage.

Barrera, M. Jr. (1986). Distinctions between social support concepts, measures, and models. *American Journal of Community Psychology, 14,* 413–445.

Beckham, J. C., Lytle, B. L., & Feldman, M. E. (1996). Caregiver burden in partners of Vietnam veterans with posttraumatic stress disorder. *Journal of Consulting and Clinical Psychology, 64,* 1068–1072.

Berkman, L. F., & Syme, S. L. (1979). Social networks, host resistance and mortality: A nine-year follow-up study of Alameda County residents. *American Journal of Epidemiology, 109,* 186–204.

Bisson, J. I., Lewis, C., Howlett, M., Corallo, D., Davies, E., & Norris, V. (2011). Perceived support and psychological outcome following the 2004 tsunami: A mixed-methods study. *The Psychiatrist, 35,* 283–288.

Brewin, C. R., Andrews, B., & Valentine, J. D. (2000). Meta-analysis of risk factors for posttraumatic stress disorder in trauma exposed adults. *Journal of Consulting and Clinical Psychology, 68,* 748–766.

Bryant, R. A., Harvey, A. G., Dang, S. T., Sackville, T., & Basten, C. (1998). Treatment of acute stress disorder: A comparison of cognitive-behavioral therapy and supportive counseling. *Journal of Consulting and Clinical Psychology, 66,* 862–866.

Bryant, R. A., Sackville, T., Dang, S. T., Moulds, M., & Guthrie, R. (1999). Treating acute stress disorder: An evaluation of cognitive behavior therapy and supportive counseling techniques. *American Journal of Psychiatry, 156,* 1780–1786.

Butzlaff, R. L., & Hooley, J. M. (1998). Expressed emotion and psychiatric relapse: A meta-analysis. *Achieves of General Psychiatry, 55,* 547–552.

Campbell, R., Ahrens, C. E., Sefl, T., Wasco, S. M., & Barnes, H. E. (2001). Social reactions to rape victims: Healing and hurtful effects on psychological and physical health outcomes. *Violence and Victims, 16,* 287–302.

Cohen, S., & Syme, S. L. (1985). *Social support and health.* New York: Academic Press.

Cohen, S., & Wills, T. A. (1985). Stress, social support, and the buffering hypothesis. *Psychological Bulletin, 98,* 310–357.

Coyne, J. C., & Bolger, N. (1990). Doing without social support as an explanatory concept. *Journal of Social and Clinical Psychology, 9,* 148–158.

Dalbert, C. (2001). *The justice motive as a personal resource: Dealing with challenges and critical life events.* New York: Kluwer Academic/Plenum Press.

Davis, R. C., Brickman, E., & Baker, T. (1991). Supportive and unsupportive responses of others to rape victims: Effects on concurrent victim adjustment. *American Journal of Community Psychology, 19,* 443–451.

Dikel, T. N., Engdahl, B., & Eberly, R. (2005). PTSD in former prisoners of war: Prewar, wartime, and postwar factors. *Journal of Traumatic Stress, 18,* 69–77.

Dolbier, C. L., & Steinhardt, M. A. (2000). The development and validation of the Sense of Support Scale. *Behavioral Medicine, 25*(4), 169–179.

Dunmore, E., Clark, D. M., & Ehlers, A. (2001). A prospective investigation of the role of cognitive factors in persistent posttraumatic stress disorder after physical or sexual assault. *Behaviour Research and Therapy, 39,* 1063–1084.

Ehlers, A., & Clark, D. M. (2000). A cognitive model of posttraumatic stress disorder. *Behaviour Research and Therapy, 38,* 319–345.

Epstein, S. (1991). The self-concept, the traumatic neurosis, and the structure of personality. In D. Ozer, J. M. Healy Jr., & J. Stewart (Eds.), *Perspectives in personality* (Vol. 3, pp. 63–98). London, UK: Jessica Kingsley.

Foa, E. B., Hearst-Ikeda, D., & Perry, K. J. (1995). Evaluation of a brief cognitive-behavioral program for prevention of chronic PTSD in recent assault victims. *Journal of Consulting and Clinical Psychology, 63,* 948–955.

Foa, E. B., & Rothbaum, B. O. (1998). *Treating the trauma of rape: Cognitive-behavioral therapy for PTSD.* New York: Guilford Press.

Foa, E. B., Steketee, G., & Rothbaum, B. O. (1989). Behavioral/cognitive conceptualizations of post-traumatic stress disorder. *Behavior Therapy, 20,* 155–176.

Foa, E. B., Zoellner, L. A., & Feeny, N. C. (2006). An evaluation of three brief programs for facilitating recovery after assault. *Journal of Traumatic Stress, 19,* 29–43.

Fontana, A., & Rosenheck, R. (1994). Posttraumatic stress disorder among Vietnam theater veterans: A causal model of etiology in a community sample. *Journal of Nervous and Mental Disease, 182,* 677–684.

Frazier, P. A., Davis-Ali, S. H., & Dahl, K. E. (1995). Stressors, social support, and adjustment in renal transplant patients and their spouses. *Social Work in Health Care, 21,* 89–104.

Frazier, P. A., & Schauben L. J. (1994). Stressful life events and psychological adjustment among female college students. *Measurement and Evaluation in Counseling and Development, 27,* 280–292.

Fredman, S. J., Monson, C. M., Schumm, J. A., Adair, K. C., Taft, C. T., & Resick, P. A. (2010). Associations among disaster exposure, intimate relationship adjustment, and PTSD symptoms: Can disaster exposure enhance a relationship? *Journal of Traumatic Stress, 23,* 446–451.

Fruzzetti, A. E., & Iverson, K. M. (2004). Mindfulness, acceptance, validation, and "individual" psychopathology in couples. In S. C. Hayes, V. M. Follette, & M. M. Linehan (Eds.), *Mindfulness and acceptance: Expanding the cognitive-behavioral tradition* (pp. 168–191). New York: Guilford Press.

Galea, S., Ahern, J., Resnick, H., Kilpatrick, D., Bucuvalas, M., Gold, J., et al. (2002). Psychological sequelae of the September 11 terrorist attacks in New York City. *New England Journal of Medicine, 346,* 982–987.

Galea, S., Ahern, J., Tracy, M., Hubbard, A., Cerda, M., Goldmann, E., et al.

(2008). Longitudinal determinants of posttraumatic stress in a population-based cohort study. *Epidemiology, 19,* 47–54.

Golding, J. M., Siege, J. M., Sorenson, S. B., Burnam, M. A., & Stein, J. A. (1989). Social support sources following sexual assault. *Journal of Community Psychology, 17,* 92–107.

Gotlib, I. H., & Hammen, C. L. (Eds.). (2002). *Handbook of depression.* New York: Guilford Press.

Gottlieb, B. H. (1987). Using social support to protect and promote health. *Journal of Primary Prevention, 8,* 49–70.

Gottlieb, B. H. (1997). *Coping with chronic stress.* New York: Plenum Press.

Guay, S., Billette, V., & Marchand, A. (2006). Exploring the links between posttraumatic stress disorder and social support: Processes and potential research avenues. *Journal of Traumatic Stress, 19,* 327–338.

Hall, M. J., Norwood, A. E., Ursano, R. J., & Fullerton, C. S. (2003). The psychological impacts of bioterrorism. *Biosecurity and Bioterrorism: Biodefense Strategy, Practice, and Science, 1,* 139–144.

Hobfoll, S. E. (1988). *The ecology of stress.* New York: Hemisphere.

Hobfoll, S. E. (1998). *Stress, culture and community: The psychology and philosophy of stress.* New York: Plenum Press.

Hobfoll, S. E., Canetti-Nisim, D., & Johnson, R. J. (2006). Exposure to terrorism, stress-related mental health symptoms, and defensive coping among Jews and Arabs in Israel. *Journal of Consulting and Clinical Psychology, 74,* 207–218.

Hobfoll, S. E., & Stephens, M. P. (1990). Social support during extreme stress: Consequences and intervention. In B. R. Sarason (Ed.), *Social support: An interactional view* (pp. 454–481). New York: Wiley.

Hobfoll, S. E., Watson, P., Bell, C. C., Bryant, R. A., Brymer, M. J., Friedman, M. J., et al. (2007). Five essential elements of immediate and mid-term mass trauma intervention: Empirical evidence. *Psychiatry, 70,* 283–315.

Holeva, V., Tarrier, N., & Wells, A. (2001). Prevalence and predictors of acute stress disorder and PTSD following road traffic accidents: Thought control strategies and social support. *Behavior Therapy, 32,* 65–83.

Hooley, J. M., & Gotlib, I. H. (2000). A diathesis–stress conceptualization of expressed emotion and clinical outcome. *Applied and Preventive Psychology, 9*(3), 135–151.

Hooley, J. M., Orley, J., & Teasdale, J. D. (1986). Levels of expressed emotion and relapse in depressed patients. *British Journal of Psychiatry, 148,* 642–647.

House, J. S., Landis, K. R., & Umberson, D. (1988). Social relationships and health. *Science, 241,* 540–545.

Janoff-Bulman, R. (1985). The aftermath of victimization: Rebuilding shattered assumptions. In C.R. Figley (Ed.), *Trauma and its wake: The study and treatment of post-traumatic stress disorder* (pp. 15–35). New York: Brunner/Mazel.

Janoff-Bulman, R. (1992). *Shattered assumptions: Toward a new psychology of trauma.* New York: Free Press.

Jelusić, I., Stevanović, A., Frandiaković, T., Grković, J., Suković, Z., & Knezović, Z. (2010). Social support and posttraumatic stress disorder in combat veterans in Croatia. *Collegium Antropologicum, 34,* 853–858.

Joseph, S., Yule, W., Williams, R., & Andrews, B. (1993). Crisis support in the aftermath of disaster: A longitudinal perspective. *British Journal of Clinical Psychology, 32,* 177–185.

Kaniasty, K., & Norris, F. H. (1993). A test of the social support deterioration model in the context of natural disaster. *Journal of Personality and Social Psychology, 64,* 395–408.

Kaniasty, K., & Norris, F. H. (2008). Longitudinal linkages between perceived social support and posttraumatic stress symptoms: Sequential roles of social causation and social selection. *Journal of Traumatic Stress, 21,* 274–281.

Kaniasty, K., Norris, F., & Murrell, S. A. (1990). Received and perceived social support following natural disaster. *Journal of Applied Social Psychology, 20,* 85–114.

Keane, T. M., Scott, W. O., Chavoya, G. A., Lamparski, D. M., & Fairbank, J. A. (1985). Social support in Vietnam veterans with posttraumatic stress disorder: A comparative analysis. *Journal of Consulting and Clinical Psychology, 53,* 95–102.

Keitner, G. I., Ryan, C. E., Miller, I. W., Kohn, R., Bishop, D. S., & Epstein, N. B. (1995). Role of family in recovery and major depression. *American Journal of Psychiatry, 152,* 1002–1008.

Keller, S. M., Zoellner, L. A., & Feeny, N. C. (2010). Understanding factors associated with early therapeutic alliance in PTSD treatment: Adherence, childhood sexual abuse history, and social support. *Journal of Consulting and Clinical Psychology, 78,* 974–979.

Kessler, R. C., Price, R. H., & Wortman, C. B. (1985). Social factors in psychopathology: Stress, social support, and coping processes. *Annual Review of Psychology, 36,* 531–572.

King, D. W., King, L. A., Fairbank, J. A., Keane, T. A., & Adams, G. A. (1998). Resilience–recovery factors in post-traumatic stress disorder among female and male Vietnam veterans: Hardiness, postwar social support, and additional stressful life events. *Journal of Personality and Social Psychology, 74,* 420–434.

King, D. W., King, L. A., Foy, D. W., Keane, T. M., & Fairbank, J. A. (1999). Posttraumatic stress disorder in a national sample of female and male Vietnam veterans: Risk factors, war zone stressors, and resilience–recovery variables. *Journal of Abnormal Psychology, 108,* 164–170.

King, D. W., Taft, C. T., King, L. A., Hammond C., & Stone E. R. (2006). Directionality of the association between social support and posttraumatic stress disorder: A longitudinal investigation. *Journal of Applied Social Psychology, 36,* 2980–2992.

Kloos, B., Flory, K., Hankin, B. L., Cheely, C. A., & Segal, M. (2009). Investigating the roles of neighborhood environments and housing-based social support in the relocation of persons made homeless by Hurricane Katrina. *Journal of Prevention, 37,* 143–154.

Lakey, B., Tardiff, T. A., & Drew, J. B. (1994). Negative social interactions: Assessment and relations to social support, cognitions, and psychological distress. *Journal of Social and Clinical Psychology, 13,* 42–62.

Landau, J., & Saul, J. (2004). Facilitating family and community resilience in response to major disaster. In F. Walsh & M. McGoldrick (Eds.), *Living beyond loss* (2nd ed., pp. 285–309). New York: Norton.

Lazarus, R. S. (1966). *Psychological stress and the coping process*. New York: McGraw-Hill.

Lazarus, R. S., & Folkman, S. (1984). *Stress, appraisal, and coping*. New York: Springer.

Lepore, S. J., Evans, G. W., & Schneider, M. L (1991). Dynamic role of social support in the link between chronic stressors and psychological distress. *Journal of Personality and Social Psychology, 61,* 899–909.

Lerner, M. J. (1980). *The belief in a just world: A fundamental delusion*. New York: Plenum Press.

Maercker, A., & Müller, J. (2004). Social acknowledgment as a victim or survivor: A scale to measure a recovery factor of PTSD. *Journal of Traumatic Stress, 17,* 345–351.

Marom, S., Munitz, H., Jones, P. B., Weizman, A., & Hermesh, H. (2005). Expressed emotions: Relevance to rehospitalization in schizophrenia over 7 years. *Schizophrenia Bulletin, 31,* 751–758.

Martz, E., Bodner, T., & Livneh, H. (2010). Social support and coping as moderators of perceived disability and posttraumatic stress levels among Vietnam theater veterans. *Health, 2,* 332–341.

Mason, G. E., Ullman, S., Long, S. E., Long, L., & Starzynski, L. (2008). Exploring the relationships of women's sexual assault disclosure, social reactions, and problem drinking. *Journal of Community Psychology, 37,* 58–72.

McCann, I. L., & Pearlman, L. A. (1990). Vicarious traumatization: A framework for understanding the psychological effects of working with victims. *Journal of Traumatic Stress, 3,* 131–149.

Miklowitz, D. J., Goldstein, M. J., Nuechterlein, K. H., Snyder, K. S., & Mintz, J. (1988). Family factors and the course of bipolar affective disorder. *Archives of General Psychiatry, 45,* 225–231.

Mueller, J., Moergeli, H., & Maercker, A. (2008). Disclosure and social acknowledgement as predictors of recovery from posttraumatic stress: A longitudinal study in crime victims. *Canadian Journal of Psychiatry, 53*(3), 160–168.

Norris, F. H., Baker, C. K., Murphy, A. D., & Kaniasty, K. (2005). Social support mobilization and deterioration after Mexico's 1999 flood: Effects of context, gender, and time. *American Journal of Community Psychology, 36,* 15–28.

Norris, F. H., Friedman, M. J., & Watson, P. J. (2002). 60,000 disaster victims speak: Part II. Summary and implications of the disaster mental health research. *Psychiatry—Interpersonal and Biological Processes, 65*(3), 240–260.

Norris, F. H., & Kaniasty, K. (1996). Received and perceived social support in times of stress: A test of the social support deterioration deterrence model. *Journal of Personality and Social Psychology, 71,* 498–511.

Ozer, E. J., Best, S. R., Lipsey, T. L., & Weiss, D. S. (2003). Predictors of posttraumatic stress disorder and symptoms in adults: A meta-analysis. *Psychological Bulletin, 129,* 52–73.

Pierce, G. R., Sarason, I. G., & Sarason, B. R. (1991). General and relationship-based perceptions of social support: Are two constructs better than one? *Journal of Personality and Social Psychology, 61,* 1028–1039.

Pietrzak, R. H., Johnson, D. C., Goldstein, M. B., Malley, J. C., & Southwick, S. M. (2009). Psychological resilience and postdeployment social support

protect against traumatic stress and depressive symptoms in soldiers returning from Operations Enduring Freedom and Iraqi Freedom. *Depression and
Anxiety, 26,* 745–751.

Prati, G., & Pietrantoni, L. (2009). Optimism, social support, and coping strategies as factors contributing to posttraumatic growth: A meta-analysis. *Journal of Loss and Trauma, 14,* 364–388.

Pruitt, L. D., & Zoellner, L. A. (2008). The impact of social support: An analogue
investigation of the aftermath of trauma exposure. *Journal of Anxiety Disorders, 22,* 253–262.

Resick, P. A., & Schnicke, M. K. (1992). Cognitive processing therapy for sexual
assault victims. *Journal of Consulting and Clinical Psychology, 60,* 748–
756.

Rose, S., Bisson, J., & Wessely, S. (2003). A systematic review of single-session
psychological interventions ("debriefing") following trauma. *Psychotherapy
and Psychosomatics, 72,* 176–184.

Rothbaum, B. O., Foa, E. B., Riggs, D. S., Murdock, T., & Walsh, W. (1992).
A prospective examination of post-traumatic stress disorder in rape victims.
Journal of Traumatic Stress, 5, 455–475.

Sacco, W. P., & Vaughan, C. A. (2006). Depression and the response of others: A
social–cognitive interpersonal process model. In T. E. Joiner, J. S. Brown, &
J. Kistner (Eds.), *The interpersonal, cognitive, and social nature of depression*
(pp. 101–132). Mahwah, NJ: Erlbaum.

Sarason, I. G., Levine, H. M., Basham, R. B., & Sarason, B. R. (1983). Assessing
social support: The Social Support Questionnaire. *Journal of Personality and
Social Psychology, 44,* 127–139.

Sarason, I. G., Pierce, G. R., & Sarason, B. R. (1994). General and specific perceptions of social support. In W. R. Avison & I. H. Gotlib, *Stress and mental
health* (pp. 153–178). New York: Plenum Press.

Sarason, B. R., Sarason, I. G., & Gurung, R. A. R. (1997). Close personal relation-
ships and health outcomes: A key to the role of social support. In S. Duck
(Ed.), *Handbook of personal relationships* (2nd ed., pp. 547–573). New York:
Wiley.

Sarason, I. G., Sarason, B. R., & Pierce, G. R. (1994). Social support: Global and
relationship-based levels of analysis. *Journal of Social and Personal Relationships, 11,* 295–312.

Sarason, I. G., Sarason, B. R., & Pierce, G. R. (1995). Social and personal relationships: Current issues, future directions. *Journal of Social and Personal
Relationships 24,* 613–619.

Sarason, B. R., Shearin, E. N., Pierce, G. R., & Sarason, I. G. (1987). Interrelations
of social support measures: Theoretical and practical implications. *Journal of
Personality and Social Psychology, 52,* 813–832.

Sayrs, J. H. R., & Fruzzetti, A. E. (2003). *Couple intimacy as a predictor of less
aversive and less aggressive parenting behaviors.* Unpublished manuscript,
Reno, NV.

Schaefer, J., & Moos, R. (1998). The context for posttraumatic growth: Life crises,
individual and social resources, and coping. In R. Tedeschi, C. Park, & L.
Calhoun (Eds.), *Posttraumatic growth: Positive changes in the aftermath of
crisis* (pp. 99–126). Mahwah, NJ: Erlbaum.

Schnurr, P. P., Lunney, C. A., & Sengupta, A. (2004). Risk factors for the development versus maintenance of posttraumatic stress disorder. *Journal of Traumatic Stress, 17,* 85–95.

Schumm, J. A., Briggs-Phillips, M., & Hobfoll, S. (2006). Cumulative interpersonal traumas and social support as risk and resiliency factors in predicting PTSD and depression among inner city women. *Journal of Traumatic Stress, 19,* 825–836.

Shinn, M., Lehmann, S., & Wong, N. W. (1984). Social interaction and social support. *Journal of Social Issues, 40*(4), 55–76.

Solomon, Z., & Mikulincer, M. (1987). Combat stress reactions, post traumatic stress disorder and social adjustment: A study of Israeli veterans. *Journal of Nervous and Mental Disease, 175,* 277–285.

Solomon, Z., Mikulincer, M., & Flum, H. (1989). The implications of life events and social integration in the course of combat-related post-traumatic stress disorder. *Social Psychiatry and Psychiatric Epidemiology, 24,* 41–48.

Stewart, M. J. (1989). Social support: Diverse theoretical perspectives. *Social Science and Medicine, 28,* 1275–1282.

Stokes, J. (1983). Predicting satisfaction with social support from social network structure. *American Journal of Community Psychology, 11,* 141–152.

Tedeschi, R. G., & Calhoun, L. G. (2004). Posttraumatic growth: Conceptual foundations and empirical evidence. *Psychological Inquiry, 15,* 1–18.

Thoits, P. A. (1986). Social support as coping assistance. *Journal of Consulting and Clinical Psychology, 54,* 416–423.

Thompson, M. P., Kaslow, N. J., Kingree, J. B., Rashid, A., Puett, R., Jacobs, D., et al. (2000). Partner violence, social support, and distress among inner-city African American women. *American Journal of Community Psychology, 28,* 127–143.

Thrasher, S., Power, M., Morant, N., Marks, I., & Dalgleish, T. (2010). Social support moderates outcome in a randomized controlled trial of exposure therapy and (or) cognitive restructuring for chronic posttraumatic stress disorder. *Canadian Journal of Psychiatry, 55*(3), 187–190.

Turner, H. (1994). Gender and social support: Taking the bad with the good. *Sex Roles, 30,* 521–541.

Ullman, S. E. (1996). Social reactions, coping strategies, and self-blame attributions in adjustment to sexual assault. *Psychology of Women Quarterly, 20,* 505–526.

Ullman, S. E., & Filipas, H. H. (2001). Predictors of PTSD symptom severity and social reactions in sexual assault victims. *Journal of Traumatic Stress, 14,* 369–389.

Ullman, S. E., Starzynski, L. L., Long, S., Mason, G., & Long, L. M. (2008). Exploring the relationships of women's sexual assault disclosure, social reactions, and problem drinking. *Journal of Interpersonal Violence, 23,* 1235–1257.

Ullman, S. E., Townsend, S. M., Filipas, H. H., & Starzynski, L. L. (2007). Structural models of the relations of assault severity, social support, avoidance coping, self blame and PTSD among sexual assault survivors. *Psychology of Women Quarterly, 31,* 23–37.

Valentiner, D. P., Foa, E. B., Riggs, D. S., & Gershuny, B. S. (1996). Coping strategies and posttraumatic stress disorder in female victims of sexual and nonsexual assault. *Journal of Abnormal Psychology, 105,* 455–458.

Vaux, A. (1988). *Social support: Theory, research and intervention.* New York: Praeger.

Vigna, J. F., Hernandez, B. C., Paasch, V., Gordon, A. T., & Kelley, M. L. (2009). Positive adjustment in youth post-Katrina: The impact of child and maternal social support and coping. In K. E. Cherry (Ed.), *Lifespan perspectives on natural disasters: Coping with Katrina, Rita, and other storms* (pp. 45–64). New York: Springer.

Wethington, E., & Kessler, R. C. (1986). Perceived support, received support, and adjustment to stressful life events. *Journal of Health and Social Behavior, 27,* 78–89.

Wilcox, S. (2010). Social relationships and PTSD symptomatology in combat veterans. *Psychological Trauma: Theory, Research, Practice, and Policy, 2,* 175–182.

Yap, M. B. H., & Devilly, G. J. (2004). The role of perceived social support in crime victimization. *Clinical Psychology Review, 24,* 1–14.

Zoellner, L. A., Foa, E. B., & Brigidi, B. (1999). Interpersonal friction and PTSD in female victims of sexual and non-sexual assault. *Journal of Traumatic Stress, 12,* 689–700.

Part IV

INTEGRATION AND FUTURE DIRECTIONS

Chapter 14

Conclusion

Risk and Resilience Following Trauma Exposure

Norah C. Feeny *and* Lori A. Zoellner

As soon as she was able, Mora (see Chapter 1) started going to church, reaching out to her friends, and began physical rehabilitation. Although she thought about the crash on occasion, she started to drive as soon as she was medically cleared. As she continued to do these things, Mora's earlier depression also dissipated, and she threw out the bottle of pills she earlier thought about using to end her life. Similarly, over the next few months, her fears around having another car accident also started to disappear.

As we have conveyed throughout this volume, resilience is the norm following trauma exposure. This is one of the remarkable findings emerging from the study of psychological reactions to traumatic events. With this point, we have also tried to convey realistic hope, both for those who have experienced trauma and for those who witness its impact up close (e.g., clinicians, family, friends). Experiencing a trauma simply is not synonymous with psychopathology and long-term disability. As cases such as Mora's throughout this book illustrate, many men and women bounce back following even the most devastating events. As we think of it, being resilient does not necessarily mean a lack of a reaction to a traumatic event. Instead, resilience allows for an initial and appropriate marked reaction to a traumatic stressor, but also includes a pattern of recovery to prior functioning.

As described in the Introduction, resilience is an ability to spring back or recover.

Why are some resilient and not others? How do we harness the forces that underlie such resilience? Or even more broadly, how do we reduce the psychological impact of trauma?

REDUCING THE IMPACT OF TRAUMA: PREVENTING TRAUMA EXPOSURE

One clear solution to reducing the psychological impact of trauma is to reduce trauma. This book emerges against a backdrop of public debate and concern about trauma and violence in the United States and around the world. Unfortunately, exposure to trauma is not rare. In epidemiological studies, 50–70% of adults report they have experienced at least one traumatic event (e.g., Kessler, Sonnega, Bromet, Hughes, & Nelson, 1995). Close to one in three American women report being raped or sexually assaulted at some time in their lives (Resnick, Kilpatrick, Dansky, Saunders, & Best, 1993). With two recent U.S. wars and close to two million soldiers deployed since 2001, many have experienced trauma during active duty (e.g., being shot at, injured, handling dead bodies, death of friends, rape). Natural disasters like Hurricane Katrina, which devastated New Orleans, and the 2004 South Asian tsunami leave many people in their wakes who have been exposed to death, injury, unsafe conditions, and destruction of their homes and communities. Besides these large-scale disasters, trauma also takes the form of more everyday events such as fires, motor vehicle accidents, and sudden deaths of loved ones. Trauma is common.

Those of us psychologists, social workers, and psychiatrists who study reactions after trauma and work with trauma survivors don't often see preventing traumatic events as under our purview. Perhaps we should. Reducing exposure to violence and trauma is the most straightforward way to reduce the psychological impact of trauma. Despite our best intentions, though, we will never eliminate traumatic events. So we still must carefully consider how and when to intervene in their aftermath.

HOW TO HARNESS FORCES OF NATURAL RECOVERY

Attending to Basic Human Needs

Following trauma, be it at the individual or community level, basic human needs should be met. Maslow (1954) proposed that human needs were organized hierarchically and that those at the bottom of the hierarchy, those required for human survival, must be met before needs of a more psychological nature can be addressed. We should not underestimate the psychological healing power of food, water, sleep, clothing, shelter, and ways to contact family and friends. In the aftermath of natural disasters and in war-torn locations, these basic needs may be vast and difficult to meet consistently. In such situations, food, clean water, safe toilets, and temporary shelters are necessary for life. They allow for calming, for a sense of safety, and for predictability to begin to be restored. Years ago, both authors worked on a prevention project, screening for mental health difficulties soon after trauma. In one setting, people were seeking help after their houses had been damaged or destroyed by fire. We were there to figure out who was in psychological distress and offer them intervention. Despite this, people kept asking us for housing vouchers, where to pick up pajamas and shoes for their children, what the phone number was for food assistance, and so on. Neither of us forgot that experience. In the immediate aftermath of trauma, no matter our training, often the best psychological help we can give is delivered in boxes and bottles.

Beyond meeting essential basic needs, there are certainly other things that can be done in the immediate aftermath of trauma to foster resilience. Here we will highlight some basic ways to harness natural resilience: reinforcing social ties, getting back to life, and dealing with thoughts and memories.

Social Ties

As described in Chapter 13, meaningful, supportive social ties are some of the most critical factors that may help enhance recovery. To foster resilience, professionals should encourage trauma survivors to spend time with friends and family to whom they are connected and trust. The flip side to this recommendation is that friends and family should be encouraged to reach out as well. It can be tempting to stay away from a person who has just been through something tragic. As one of our young daughters recently said about going to her friend's mom's funeral, "I don't know what to say," "I might make her cry," "It's too sad," "There will be lots of people there." Adults often feel the same way. Friends and family can be told something like this: "It's all right if you don't know what to say. Go anyway. Hold hands. Listen. Be present."

This support needs to be sustained to some degree over time (e.g., Hobfoll, 1998). Sometimes being available and supportive is relatively easy to do in the short run but more difficult in the long run. Accordingly, for trauma survivors, social support tends to fade over time (e.g., Kaniasty, Norris, & Murrell, 1990; Lepore, Evans, & Schneider, 1991; Norris & Kaniasty, 1996). One of us has an uncle in the hospital right now following a serious car accident. People visit him daily. They ask how he's doing and remind him he's loved. There is a blog updating his status, and food for the family is delivered by neighbors and friends daily. What will happen when he goes home? Much of this support will fade away. Surely this is natural, as he will be getting better physically. Psychologically, however, the social ties that got him through his hospital stay will remain important to his resilience over time.

Social support and connectedness are important not just at the individual level. At the community level, support may look different but is equally, if not more, important (e.g., Bisson et al., 2011; Hobfoll et al., 2007; Kloos, Flory, Hankin, Cheely, & Segal, 2009). After disasters, for example, important community institutions (schools, churches) may be damaged and natural social rhythms and routines disrupted. Facilitating the connection of established social groups—neighborhoods, church groups, classrooms, parent–teacher associations, soccer teams—can be reassuring, can begin to restore a sense of belongingness, and can facilitate organization (e.g., cleaning up, organizing fund raising, coordinating meals). Similarly, in refugee shelters, there should be structural acknowledgment of the import of social and familial bonds. Families should be housed together and eat together. Ideally, families that lived in the same neighborhood should be placed in proximity to one another. News of family whereabouts should be shared quickly and consistently, and a communal meeting place should be established. No matter the setting or trauma, social ties are important facilitators of recovery (Norris, Stevens, Pfefferbaum, Wyche, & Pfefferbaum, 2008). Any plan aimed at fostering resilience in the aftermath of trauma should attend to supporting these meaningful connections as vital.

Getting Back to Life

After a person experiences a life-threatening event, once he or she is safe, reestablishing a sense of normalcy as much as is feasibly possible and as quickly as can be managed is important. There are lots of benefits to reconnecting with familiar surroundings, people, and routines, and it's probably one of the most powerful ways to harness natural recovery. Avoidance of trauma-related reminders is a common coping mechanism; it makes sense, but it is also a trap. As discussed in Chapter 11, learning to be afraid is easy (Bolles, 1972). Once you are afraid, learning not to be afraid is much harder (e.g., Bouton, 2004; Foa & Kozak, 1986). From the start, clear advice should be provided to those who have experienced trauma to get back as soon as possible to their normal routines, including aspects of life that are trauma-related. For example, if you have been in a car accident, look at the car, sit in the car, and drive in the car. Getting back to life should also include seeking out positive experiences. Instead of shutting down feelings, we can recommend doing things that are enjoyable. For each person, this will be different, of course. Begin to paint again, play basketball, walk the dogs, swim, listen to music, and so on. Each of the authors routinely gets calls seeking advice from recent trauma survivors or their family members. Most often these are recent rape survivors. It is rare that we make an appointment for them. Instead, we encourage them to spend time with those they love and trust, to make sure they try get enough sleep, not to drink or use drugs to cover up feelings, to talk about what happened when they are ready, and perhaps most important, get back to school/work/ parenting/living as soon as they can. We encourage them to recognize the strong urge to avoid trauma-related thoughts, feelings, and places, but to move forward and reclaim their lives regardless.

Dealing with Thoughts and Memories: Actively Making Meaning

As is described in Chapter 7, to help buffer against the impact of trauma, we should encourage trauma survivors to allow themselves to remember the trauma memory and their thoughts about it. This includes thinking about it when it comes to mind, journaling about it, talking about it with supportive family and friends when ready, and appropriately disclosing what has happened to others when ready. Avoiding the memory can be just as problematic as avoiding getting back to life. We say this with the caveat that if the memory is not problematic (e.g., no nightmares, no distressing and frequent thoughts and images), this is not necessary. Trauma memories are to some degree malleable, just like other memories. Active recalling of the trauma memory can shape how it is remembered in the future. The meaning of the event can be shaped, in part, by incorporating new elements of the event. The useful pieces to focus on may be those that highlight one's actions or inactions (e.g., "I did try to stop him—I kept saying NO," or, conversely, "If I would have fought back, he would have killed me"), challenge unhelpful thoughts (e.g., "It was not all my fault—I slammed on the brakes and swerved"), or help link to a bigger meaning system (e.g., "Sometimes bad things happen to good people for no reason"). This active meaning making can help shift the memory in a more adaptive direction.

Working with their thoughts can be quite counterintuitive to trauma survivors, who understandably want to shut their trauma memories down. It can also feel counterintuitive to those who want to help the trauma survivor, who may say things like "Don't think about it. It'll just upset you," "What's over is over," or "Put it behind you." By framing the memory as something to work with, something to actively call up and to some degree "sculpt," we give trauma survivors a tool to combat the powerfulness of the initial memory. We can encourage trauma survivors to allow themselves to purposely think or talk about what happened, rather than avoid it, and to purposely focus on the adaptive parts of the memory.

From a community perspective, this kind of active meaning making may be facilitated by open acknowledgment of the events that happened, accurate media portrayal of the events, and opportunity for discussion and reflection. Of course, it may not happen at all, to the detriment of the community and its members. For example, one of us (Feeny) was invited to Kosovo recently to talk about the psychological impact of the 1998 Kosovo War. The informal invitation said in essence that the tragedies that occurred during the war between Serbians and ethnic Albanians were "festering." Instead of looking back and making sense as a community, there was silence. People were still suffering. In contrast, on the first anniversary of the 2012 Chardon school shooting, the entire high school was invited (but not obligated) to take part in a day of remembrance. The students were engaged in shaping this event and were asked how they would like to remember the tragedy, but also (critically) how they wanted to acknowledge the strength of their community. They responded that they wanted to help others because so many had reached out to help them. On their remembrance day, they made blankets for hospitalized children. They made dog leashes and cookies for the first responders. They also made meaning: We won't forget what happened, but there are still good people in the world and we want to give back even though we've suffered.

It is worth nothing that although these sorts of community events can be very powerful for some, they are not necessarily helpful for everyone. People should be free to choose if they would like to be involved; there is no "right way" for a survivor to respond in the wake of a trauma. Both adaptive individual and community remembering can dramatically shape how a trauma is remembered in future and help to facilitate resilience.

HOW TO INTERVENE LATER

Most people don't seek treatment for trauma-related difficulties for many years, if at all (e.g., Wang et al., 2005). There are likely many reasons for this, one being stigma both about *being traumatized* and about *needing treatment*. Many women and men who are raped are reluctant to tell anyone. Reporting rates to the police are notoriously low (Langton, Berzofsky, Krebs, & Smiley-McDonald, 2012). Sexual assault victims often describe themselves as "marked," "damaged," or "broken." The very fact of being a survivor of a trauma can be stigmatizing. Seeking treatment can be similarly stigmatizing. In the military, soldiers are supposed to be tough, to act if necessary without feeling, and to defend their nation no matter what. Seeking treatment can be perceived as weak or may be perceived as hurting career advancement. Although there are active efforts underway to shift this culture and encourage active treatment seeking, the reluctance remains. We need to work to reduce stigma and other barriers to effective interventions. A delay of receiving an effective treatment translates directly into prolonged suffering.

We have good treatments for trauma-related psychopathology, which work on average both in the short- and long-term (i.e., gains are maintained for years after treatment; Institute of Medicine, 2007; Resick, Williams, Suvak, Monson & Gradus, 2012). Treatments have been tested in randomized controlled trials on real people with real, complex trauma-related problems (see Powers, Halpern, Ferenschak, Gillihan, & Foa, 2010). There is a concern among some in the trauma community that these treatments have been tested in rarified conditions and won't work in the trenches, where men and women don't come for posttraumatic stress disorder (PTSD) treatment in a nice DSM or ICD diagnostic box but present with multiple problems (e.g., Bradley, Greene, Russ, Dutra, & Westen, 2005; Zayfert et al., 2005). However, the idea that short-term, trauma-focused treatments don't work for those with "complex" PTSD is not well supported. The markers that we typically think of as characterizing complex PTSD (or clinical complexity more broadly) such as child sexual abuse, multiple traumas, dissociation, and emotional dysregulation are not good predictors for who will or will not benefit from empirically supported, short-term interventions (e.g., Clarke, Rizvi, & Resick, 2008; Cloitre, Koenen, Cohen, & Han, 2002; Feeny, Zoellner, & Foa, 2002; Resick, Nishith, & Griffin, 2003). Similarly, the idea that empirically supported interventions have only been tested on those with "pure" PTSD is not accurate. In our PTSD treatment research, for example, most men and women are multiply traumatized, with chronic symptoms, other disorders, severely impaired interpersonal relationships, and significant ongoing life stressors. Even under these conditions, on average, established treatments work (e.g., Feeny et al., 2002; Foa et al., 2005). More people should have access to them. The false notion that PTSD cannot be treated stands in contrast to the bulk of the data accumulated over the past 20-plus years. There is still work to be done, for sure. New treatments need to meet the same standards and be as good, or better, than existing treatments. Accordingly, we should be wary of new "quick fixes." The next generation of trauma-related interventions should grow out of our accumulated knowledge to date.

How do we know who will do well in treatment? How do we optimize therapy outcomes? We don't yet have clear, consistent predictors of therapy outcome or of how to match people to particular treatments. From an intuitive, clinical perspective, we do have a sense of those who may do well and how to help those who are struggling. Well-validated therapies for PTSD typically include addressing unhelpful trauma-related beliefs (e.g., "PTSD symptoms mean I'm going crazy") and addressing avoidance of the trauma memory, trauma-related feelings, and trauma-related situations. Early in treatment, the rationale for these therapy targets is carefully explained. There are people who "get it" and take the proverbial ball and run with it—doing homework, thinking about situations they've been avoiding and need to approach, tackling their thoughts actively. It's the "getting it" that we think is important. When working with someone who is not under-standing or buying-in to the treatment rationale, it's essential to address this early on. Another piece that we think is important is being willing to tolerate short-term distress for long-term benefit. More specifically, asking those with PTSD to revisit and engage with their trauma memories and things that remind them of them is asking them to do something that is dif-ficult. Those who realize that while it is painful to think about their trauma and look at how it has shifted their beliefs about themselves and the world, but are willing to tolerate this distress in order to get better, are the ones who succeed. This is not suggesting that people need to be taught this abil-ity before treatment. The idea is that during treatment we talk about that fact that facing painful memories is hard, but that at the same time, as one sits with the distress, one learns that one can sit with it. It is the willingness to "sit with it" that we think is important. Most people with PTSD benefit substantially from treatment; a firm grasp of the treatment rationale and being willing to endure short-term distress for long-term benefit are two important pieces that we think facilitate improvement.

CLOSING THOUGHTS

In the last 20-plus years, we have learned a great deal about how people respond to traumatic events and what shapes that response. Resilience, as we have conceptualized it, is the norm following traumatic stressors. Fur-thermore, we can foster resilience by better understanding the principles that underlie natural recovery. Here we have focused on several such core principles including meeting basic human needs following trauma, facilitat-ing short- and longer-term social support, combating the powerful urge to avoid by getting back to life, and actively recalling and working with the trauma memory to make it more adaptive. We think these are some of the most powerful processes that undergird people's natural ability to recover following even the most devastating traumatic events. Our treatments for PTSD, a disorder often conceptualized as a failure of natural recovery, also attempt to harness these processes, albeit in more structured ways. In our careers, we have been surprised, moved, and honestly staggered by peoples' ability to rebound and even grow from great suffering. But, what if people could suffer less? That's why we developed this book.

ACKNOWLEDGMENTS

Preparation of this chapter was supported in part by Grant Nos. R01MH066348 (Norah C. Feeny, Principal Investigator) and R01MH066347 (Lori A. Zoellner, Principal Investigator).

REFERENCES

Bisson, J. I., Lewis, C., Howlett, M., Corallo, D., Davies, E., & Norris, V. (2011). Perceived support and psychological outcome following the 2004 tsunami: A mixed-methods study. *The Psychiatrist, 35,* 283–288.

Bolles, R. C. (1972). Reinforcement, expectancy, and learning. *Psychological Review, 79,* 394–409.

Bouton, M. E. (2004). Context and behavioral processes in extinction. *Learning and Memory, 11,* 485–494.

Bradley, R., Greene, J., Russ, E., Dutra, L., & Westen, D. (2005). A multidimensional meta-analysis of psychotherapy for PTSD. *American Journal of Psychiatry, 162,* 214–227.

Clarke, S. B., Rizvi, S. L., & Resick, P. A. (2008). Borderline personality characteristics and treatment outcomes in cognitive-behavioral treatments for PTSD in female rape victims. *Behavior Therapy, 39,* 72–78.

Cloitre, M., Koenen, K. C., Cohen, L. R., & Han, H. (2002). Skills training in affective and interpersonal regulation followed by exposure: A phase-based treatment for PTSD related to childhood abuse. *Journal of Consulting and Clinical Psychology, 70,* 1067–1074.

Feeny, N. C., Zoellner, L. A., & Foa, E. B. (2002). Treatment outcomes for chronic PTSD among female assault victims with borderline personality characteristics: A preliminary examination. *Journal of Personality Disorders, 16,* 30–40.

Foa, E. B., Hembree, E. A., Cahill, S. P., Rauch, S. A. M., Riggs, D. S., Feeny, N. C., et al. (2005). Randomized trial of prolonged exposure for posttraumatic stress disorder with and without cognitive restructuring: Outcome at academic and community clinics. *Journal of Consulting and Clinical Psychology, 73,* 953–964.

Foa, E. B., & Kozak, M. J. (1986). Emotional processing of fear: Exposure to corrective information. *Psychological Bulletin, 99,* 20–35.

Hobfoll, S. E. (1998). *Stress, culture and community: The psychology and philosophy of stress.* New York: Plenum Press.

Hobfoll, S. E., Watson, P., Bell, C. C., Bryant, R. A., Brymer, M. J., Friedman, M. J., et al. (2007). Five essential elements of immediate and mid-term mass trauma intervention: Empirical evidence. *Psychiatry, 70,* 283–315.

Institute of Medicine. (2007). *Treatment of PTSD: An assessment of the evidence.* Washington, DC: National Academies Press.

Kaniasty, K., Norris, F. H., & Murrell, S. A. (1990). Received and perceived social support following natural disaster. *Journal of Applied Social Psychology, 20,* 85–114.

Kessler R. C., Sonnega, A., Bromet, E., Hughes, M., & Nelson, C. B. (1995). Posttraumatic stress disorder in the national comorbidity survey. *Archives of General Psychiatry, 52,* 1048–1060.

Kloos, B., Flory, K., Hankin, B. L., Cheely, C. A., & Segal, M. (2009). Investigating the roles of neighborhood environments and housing-based social support in the relocation of persons made homeless by Hurricane Katrina. *Journal of Prevention and Intervention in the Community, 37,* 143–154.

Langton, L., Berzofsky, M., Krebs, C., & Smiley-McDonald, H. (2012). Victimizations not reported to the police, 2006–2010. *Bureau of Justice Statistics*

National Crime Victimization Survey, 2006–2010. Washington, DC: U.S. Department of Justice, Bureau of Justice Statistics.

Lepore, S. J., Evans, G. W., & Schneider, M. L (1991). Dynamic role of social support in the link between chronic stressors and psychological distress. *Journal of Personality and Social Psychology, 61,* 899–909.

Maslow, A. H. (1954). *Motivation and personality.* New York: Harper & Row.

Norris, F. H., & Kaniasty, K. (1996). Received and perceived social support in times of stress: A test of the social support deterioration deterrence model. *Journal of Personality and Social Psychology, 71,* 498–511.

Norris, F. H., Stevens, S. P., Pfefferbaum, B., Wyche, K. F., & Pfefferbaum, R. L. (2008). Community resilience as a metaphor, theory, set of capacities, and strategy for disaster readiness. *American Journal of Community Psychology, 41,* 127–150.

Powers, M. B., Halpern, J. M., Ferenschak, M. P., Gillihan, S. J., & Foa, E. B. (2010). A meta-analytic review of prolonged exposure for posttraumatic stress disorder. *Clinical Psychology Review, 30,* 635–641.

Resick, P. A., Nishith, P., & Griffin, M. G. (2003). How well does cognitive-behavioral therapy treat symptoms of complex PTSD?: An examination of child sexual abuse survivors within a clinical trial. *CNS Spectrums, 8,* 340–355.

Resick, P. A., Williams, L. F., Suvak, M. K., Monson, C. M., & Gradus, J. L. (2012). Long-term outcomes of cognitive-behavioral treatments for posttraumatic stress disorder among female rape survivors. *Journal of Consulting and Clinical Psychology, 80,* 201–210.

Resnick, H. S., Kilpatrick, D. G., Dansky, B. S., Saunders, B. E., & Best, C. L. (1993). Prevalence of civilian trauma and posttraumatic stress disorder in a representative national sample of women. *Journal of Consulting and Clinical Psychology, 61,* 984–991.

Wang, P. S., Berglund, P., Olfson, M., Pincus, H. A., Wells, K. B., & Kessler, R. C. (2005). Failure and delay in initial treatment contact after first onset of mental disorder in the National Comorbidity Survey Replication. *Archives of General Psychology, 62,* 603–613.

Zayfert, C., DeViva, J. C., Becker, C. B., Pike, J. L., Gillock, K. L., & Hayes, S. A. (2005). Exposure utilization and completion of cognitive behavioral therapy for PTSD in a "real world" clinical practice. *Journal of Traumatic Stress, 18,* 637–645.

Index

Page numbers followed by *f* indicate figure, *t* indicate table.